Patient Recruitment in Clinical Trials

OTHER BOOKS BY THE AUTHORS

EDITED BY JOYCE A. CRAMER AND BERT SPILKER:
Patient Compliance in Medical Practice and Clinical Trials
    Raven Press, 1991

BY BERT SPILKER:
*Guide to Clinical Studies and Developing Protocols**
    Raven Press, 1984
*Guide to Clinical Interpretation of Data**
    Raven Press, 1986
*Guide to Planning and Managing Multiple Clinical Studies**
    Raven Press, 1987
Multinational Drug Companies: Issues in Drug Discovery and Development
    Raven Press, 1989
Inside the Drug Industry
    (Bert Spilker and Pedro Cuatrecasas) Prous Science Publishers, 1990
Quality of Life Assessments in Clinical Trials
    (Edited by Bert Spilker) Raven Press, 1990
Presentation of Clinical Data
    (Bert Spilker and John Schoenfelder) Raven Press, 1990
Guide to Clinical Trials
    Raven Press, 1991
Data Collection Forms in Clinical Trials
    (Bert Spilker and John Schoenfelder) Raven Press, 1991

BY JOYCE A. CRAMER:
Alcohol and Seizures
    (Edited by RJ Porter, RH Mattson, JA Cramer, and I Diamond) F. A. Davis & Co.,
    1990

* Out of Print

Patient Recruitment in Clinical Trials

Bert Spilker, Ph.D, M.D.

Director
Project Coordination
Burroughs Wellcome Co.
Research Triangle Park, North Carolina
Adjunct Professor of Pharmacology
and Adjunct Professor of Medicine
University of North Carolina School of Medicine
Clinical Professor of Pharmacy
University of North Carolina School of Pharmacy
Chapel Hill, North Carolina

Joyce A. Cramer, B.S.

Project Director
Health Services Research
Department of Veterans Affairs Medical Center
Department of Neurology
Yale University School of Medicine
New Haven, Connecticut

Raven Press ⬦ New York

Raven Press, Ltd., 1185 Avenue of the Americas, New York, New York 10036

Made in the United States of America

Library of Congress Cataloging-in-Publication Data

Spilker, Bert.
    Patient recruitment in clinical trials / Bert Spilker, Joyce A.
Cramer.
      p.   cm.
    Includes bibliographical references and index.
    ISBN 0-88167-931-3
    1. Clinical trials.   I. Cramer, Joyce A. II. Title.
    [DNLM: 1. Clinical trials. 2. Patients.   QV 771 S756p]
  RA853.C55S66 1992
  615.5′028′7—dc20
  DNLM/DLC
  for Library of Congress   92-12023
                                              CIP

9 8 7 6 5 4 3 2 1

To all patients and volunteers who enroll in clinical trials
to help advance the art and science of medicine.

Contents

LIST OF TABLES

Part I

LIST OF FIGURES

Part I

Part II

Part III

Preface

Recruitment problems are undoubtedly the single most important reason for the failure of clinical trials. There are editorials stating that poor recruitment is hampering clinical research (Macintyre, 1991), but there are no comprehensive overviews of this critically important topic. Each of the other links in the clinical trials chain has been described in standard monographs, including planning, design, conduct, analysis, interpretation, and publication. In a sense, this book represents the missing link in the descriptive literature on the clinical trial process.

This book is written for experienced clinical trialists and trial coordinators, as well as for those who are new to clinical research in multicenter or single-site studies. It describes practical approaches to preventing recruitment problems from occurring and to solving those that do occur. This book focuses on the concept of developing a strategy for successful patient recruitment in clinical trials. Each element of recruitment strategy is described along with the approach to creating and using it.

Part I presents the framework for reviewing recruitment and defines the numerous terms used during the creation of a successful strategy. Using an overall frame of reference and clear definitions of numerous terms, investigators and others will be better able to plan their approaches to this topic. Perspectives of various groups that deal with patient recruitment are also discussed.

Part I also includes a chapter on each of the major elements of recruitment: sources of patients, methods to use, ethical issues, economic issues, as well as other specific or general issues that arise in selected situations. These chapters provide a descriptive catalogue of available approaches to recruitment.

Part II shows how the elements of recruitment are brought together to create a strategy. Insofar as possible, a standardized approach is described. The other chapters in Part II discuss related aspects and problems of a strategy, such as establishing quotas and goals, enhancing poor recruitment rates, and publishing data on the recruitment process.

Part III explores some of the consequences of the recruitment process. The consequences include various problems that arise (as well as succinct approaches to help solve each) and the extrapolatability of data. The book concludes with a synopsis of the golden rules of patient recruitment, a series of principles to help guide investigators and others involved in clinical trials.

In addition, the book contains numerous pages of actual newspaper advertisements and brochures used to recruit patients, letters sent to physicians to request referral of patients, newspaper stories published about clinical trials in response to press releases, and similar types of documents. These can serve as models for those who wish to use tested approaches.

The authors hope that the frame of reference and practical approach provided throughout this book will help investigators improve the recruitment of patients into their clinical trials and resolve problems that arise.

Acknowledgments

The authors appreciate the time and effort given by many colleagues to review and offer suggestions that enhanced this book: Marvin B. Cramer, Beverly De Vries, Daniel Deykin, M.D., Mary Foulkes, Ph.D., Jacqueline French, M.D., Barbara Hawkins, M.S., William Henderson, Ph.D., Robert Kerns, Ph.D., Susan Mayne, Ph.D., Jeffrey Probstfield, M.D., Nancy Santilli, RN, PNP, MN, Dennis Smith, M.D., and William Williford, Ph.D. Many thanks for technical assistance to Lynne Spencer and Anne Dwane, and to Laura Mansberg for reviewing the manuscript.

Patient Recruitment in Clinical Trials

PART I

Overview and Elements of Recruitment

Complacency should be avoided, because the first hurdle of any clinical trial, and often the most difficult to overcome, is the problem of recruitment.
—Schoenberger (1987)

Although one can learn from others, each trial has its own set of problems.
—Borhani et al. (1989)

In any investigation involving human subjects the most difficult part is getting hold of them. It is expensive and takes a long time.
—Hamilton (1985)

Population samples have a habit of dwindling when one is seeking them.
—Zifferblat (1975)

Excessively strict entry criteria hamper enrollment, lead to lower control event rates than anticipated, and limit generalizability. As trials get larger and larger, simple entry criteria become essential.
—Deykin (1991)

1

A Frame of Reference for Patient Recruitment Issues

The subject of recruitment is a broad one with numerous definitions, perspectives, and topics that overlap with other subjects (e.g., informed consent, randomization, use of placebos, blinding of a trial, and many other clinical trial design topics). This chapter describes the approaches taken in subsequent chapters and provides an overall framework for reading this book and thinking about recruitment. For the purposes of this framework, the periods, stages, and durations of recruitment are described and an overview of published reports on patient recruitment issues is provided.

WHY STUDY RECRUITMENT?

It is important to study patient recruitment because flaws in recruitment are the major cause of a clinical trial's failure. Many investigators would respond to the preceeding statement with ''Maybe so, but not in my trial because I know how to be successful.'' While this statement could be true, and the investigator may never

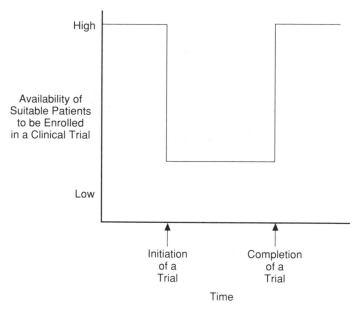

FIG. 1.1. Lasagna's Law or Muench's Third Law.

have a problem with recruitment, it is also likely that the investigator is incorrect. So many investigators (and others) have been wrong about the likelihood of conducting recruitment successfully that it has given rise to "Lasagna's Law," popularized after comments by Dr. Louis Lasagna, Dean of Tufts University Medical School and by Bearman et al.(1974) who list a "third law" as part of "Muench's Postulates, Laws, and Corollaries." Both point to the same principle, that investigators overestimate many-fold the pool of available patients who meet the inclusion criteria and would be willing to enroll in a particular trial (Fig. 1.1). Williford et al.(1987) reported that in eight of nine multicenter trials conducted within the Department of Veterans Affairs (VA) Cooperative Studies Program, the original recruitment projections were grossly overrated.

Lasagna's Law and Muench's Third Law hold true because inclusion criteria restrict the availability of many patients considered eligible by the investigator. Furthermore, investigators may overestimate patient recruitment because they (1) are naive, (2) do not adequately consider the patients' willingness to adhere to the protocol's requirements, and (3) do not understand the patients' true interest in the treatments being tested. Even experienced investigators have recruitment problems. Thus it is important that both currently active and future investigators become more knowledgeable about recruitment.

The importance of recruitment is becoming increasingly recognized. There has been an enormous increase in the number of articles and editorials published on this subject over the last decade (Macintyre, 1991).

DEFINITIONS

Before describing the frame of reference and stages of patient recruitment, the terms recruitment and screening are defined.

Recruitment

In this book, the term recruitment refers to the process of enrolling volunteers or patients in a clinical trial. This process includes up to ten stages that are described below. Other types of recruitment also exist for clinical trials. Three types of recruitment that are not discussed at length in this book are (1) recruitment of investigators to conduct a clinical trial, (2) enlisting the assistance of health professionals to operate specific equipment or to conduct specific tests as part of a clinical trial, and (3) enrollment of an organization to sponsor a clinical trial. Nonetheless, many of the principles and approaches described in this book for patient recruitment also may be used for these other types of recruitment. O'Hara et al. (1991) describe recruitment strategies for enrolling school districts in a health promotion study and their approaches were almost identical to those for clinical trials.

Screening

Screening may be conducted to (1) identify patients who are potentially eligible to enter a clinical trial (e.g., by reviewing medical records), or (2) to identify patients who either have a disease (e.g., tuberculosis, hypertension, hypercholesterolemia, breast cancer) or are at high risk of getting that disease (by utilizing a specific test such as chest x-ray, blood pressure, cholesterol level, or mammogram). This screening laboratory test may be conducted as part of a broad population screen to identify patients at risk who are then encouraged to seek medical care, or to identify patients for possible entrance into clinical trials. Screening is also conducted to ensure that volunteers do not have certain diseases or other medical abnormalities.

Five specific types of screening are listed. Actual use of the first three is uncommon. Almost all clinical trials use method number 4, but most trials using one of the first three methods would not use number 4 also. Method 5 is used in most prospective trials.

1. *Chart reviews*: evaluation of medical records to screen patients for possible invitation to enter a trial.
2. *Community-based screening*: to identify patients at risk or with a medical problem so that they may seek (or be offered) medical information and follow-up care.
3. *Community-based screening*: to identify patients for possible entry into a specific clinical trial.
4. *Primary screening*: Interview over the telephone or in person to assess whether potential patients meet inclusion criteria and are also suitable for a trial (e.g., availability, interest). A specific list of questions may be posed to patients by letter to identify (i.e., screen) those who are eligible for a clinical trial.
5. *Secondary screening*: Testing of all parameters in the screening's time and events section (i.e., summary of activities to be done at each clinic visit is usually presented in one table) of the protocol to ensure that patients meet the inclusion criteria. This may be done on one or over several days. The battery of tests and examinations (e.g., ophthalmology, electrocardiogram) may even be repeated on two or more occasions as part of the secondary screen. Additional interviews and discussions to assess the patient, and during which the patient may consider entering the trial, are also part of secondary screening.

Conclusion of the Recruitment Period

There are at least five possible models for indicating the conclusion of the patient recruitment period (Fig. 1.2). In Model A, the model used throughout this book, enrollment in the trial is said to occur upon signing the informed consent and this time marks the end of recruitment activities relating to that patient. However, the recruitment period does not necessarily end in all people's view when the informed consent is signed (as in Model A). Models B and C illustrate randomization to a treatment arm occurring before screening and actual initiation of the treatment in

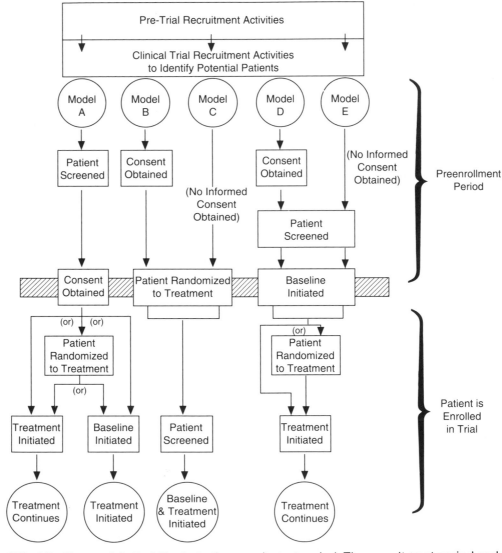

FIG. 1.2. Five models that illustrate the recruitment period. The recruitment period ends at the time that the hatched bar is reached. Model A is used throughout this book, although the other models may be used. A common definition (i.e., model) must be used by all sites participating in a multicenter trial.

the trial. Models D and E illustrate screening leading to baseline, followed by treatment within the trial.

It is important to define the point at which the recruitment period is complete for individual patients because that marks the official point of enrollment into the clinical trial. Thus, the total number of patients passing through the recruitment period into the trial may be calculated. The models are important for record keeping, particularly in multicenter trials where all sites must concur on definitions and the categories used must be identical. If randomization preceeds the baseline period, then any adverse reactions are deemed as treatment-related using an intention-to-treat analysis. If baseline occurs prior to randomization it prevents this possibility from occurring which is usually viewed in a positive way. Whichever model is selected, the definitions should be established during protocol planning, making it clear when the patient recruitment period ends and enrollment occurs.

PERIODS OF RECRUITMENT

The total period of recruitment is the period of time from initiation of the plan to enroll patients until all patients have provided their informed consent. At the point when each patient signs or verbally provides informed consent they are considered to be enrolled in a trial and the period of recruitment is completed. The recruitment period for a clinical trial may be approximately equivalent to that for a single patient, if all patients begin the trial simultaneously. At the other extreme, the duration of recruitment for a clinical trial may be nearly as long as the entire duration of the clinical trial. The periods of recruitment may be considered as a pipeline with four parts or periods (Fig. 1.3). These are described below.

Period One: Planning the Recruitment Strategy

This is the first of four principal recruitment periods (i.e., planning, initiation, conduct, and review of recruitment). All four recruitment periods may be conducted at the same time after the trial is underway. Obviously, advance planning is optimum, but it is possible to consider and reconsider a strategy during a trial. Later chapters describe this aspect in greater detail. One of the initial decisions is whether to enroll the entire group at one time or sequentially (Figs. 1.4 and 1.5), as well as whether to replace patients who drop out.

Period Two: Initiating Recruitment

During this period the investigator may appoint one or more clinical or research staff to assist with recruitment. The specific role of recruitment coordinator does not exist in most clinical trials, but it could involve the hiring of a different recruitment coordinator at each participating site in a multicenter trial. Another important series of recruitment activities conducted during this period is to contact each of the sources identified during the planning phase that will be part of the recruitment strategy.

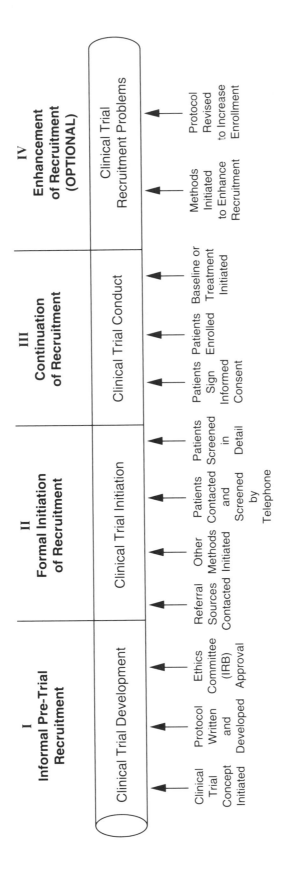

FIG. 1.3. Recruitment pipeline. This illustrates the four periods of recruitment during a clinical trial and several of the types of recruitment-related activities that occur.

A. Entire Group Starts the Clinical Trial Simultaneously

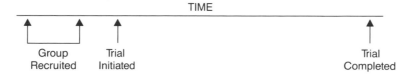

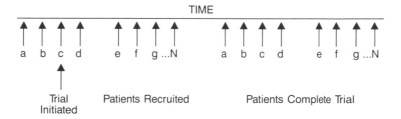

B. Patients Enter the Clinical Trial Sequentially

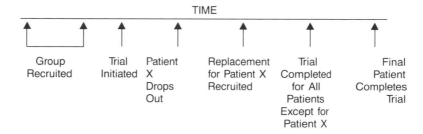

C. Variation of Model A to Replace Patient Dropouts

TIME

| Group Recruited | Trial Initiated | Patient X Drops Out | Replacement for Patient X Recruited | Trial Completed for All Patients Except for Patient X | Final Patient Completes Trial |

This last model may be avoided by enrolling a few patients above the minimal number desired to complete the trial.

FIG. 1.4. Models of patient enrollment. Simultaneous (A) and sequential (B) enrollment models are illustrated, plus a model (C) where patient dropouts are replaced. Each letter in model B represents a separate patient. One way to avoid model C is to enroll a few patients above the minimum number desired to complete the trial using model A.

Period Three: Conducting Recruitment

Recruitment of patients often begins as soon as the protocol is approved and informed consent forms are available. Screening record forms are also often created for each trial (Fig. 1.6). Flow diagrams may be created to simplify the process used to implement each method of recruitment used. A flow diagram describing use of a chart review is shown in Fig. 1.7. Later chapters describe sources and methods used to conduct recruitment. Some patients may have been waiting for the trial to start and others are found in the initial survey of the investigator's clinic population. There is usually a substantial time lag between the initial telephone or mail contact with the patient and the actual meeting with potential enrollees. In the Coronary Primary

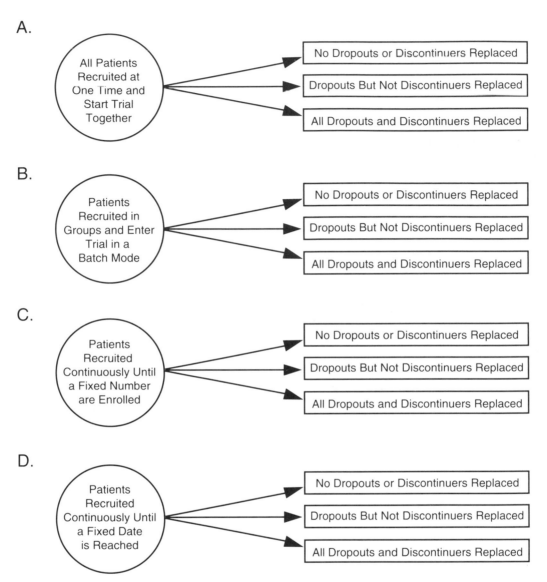

FIG. 1.5. Common patterns of patient recruitment and enrollment.

Prevention Trial, this period averaged 10 weeks at many sites (Lipid Research Clinics Program, 1983), but the specific length of time is likely to differ for each trial.

Period Four: Reviewing Recruitment Progress

Every trial should include a plan to periodically review the progress of patient recruitment to assess whether too few, too many, or an adequate number of patients are being enrolled. Use of goals and quotas as aids in the review process are described in Chapter 9.

VA COOPERATIVE STUDY #264 — CARBAMAZEPINE RX VS VALPROIC AC RX
FORM 7 — SCREENING RECORD

Medical Center Name _____ Medical Center No. ____ ____ ____

Patient Name _____ Patient No. ____ ____ ____ ____

Form Completed By _____ Date ___ ___ — ___ ___ — ___ ___
 (Mo) (Day) (Yr)

(Data Collected By) .... _____

 Card 1:
 1. Age (in years) .... ____ ____ (30-31)

 2. Sex (1 = Male, 2 = Female) .... _____ (32)

 3. Race .... _____ (33)

   1 = American Indian or Alaskan Native
   2 = Asian or Pacific Islander
   3 = Black, not of Hispanic origin
   4 = Hispanic
   5 = White, not of Hispanic origin

 4. Code predominant seizure type .... _____ (34)
   (1 = Tonic-clonic, 2 = Complex partial, 3 = Other, 4 = Unknown)

REASONS FOR REJECTION (Code: 1 = Yes, 2 = No, 3 = Not Evaluated)

 5. Diagnosis of epilepsy not confirmed .... _____ (35)

 6. Classification of specific seizure type not possible .... _____ (36)

 7. Patient has generalized seizures but not tonic-clonic .... _____ (37)

 8. Patient has only simple partial seizures .... _____ (38)

 9. Patient now receiving more than one antiepileptic drug ..... _____ (39)

10. Patient now receiving one antiepileptic drug with levels in or just below
   therapeutic range .... _____ (40)

11. Patient is abuser of alcohol or has alcohol withdrawal seizures .... _____ (41)

12. Patient is abuser of other drugs .... _____ (42)

13. Patient has progressive medical or neurological disorder (e.g., brain lesion,
   tumor, cancer, liver or kidney failure) .... _____ (43)

14. Patient has unstable neurological or medical disorder (e.g., diabetes, TIAs) .. _____ (44)

FIG. 1.6. Screening record form used in VA Cooperative Study # 264 to study two-medicines in patients with epilepsy. The numbers in parentheses refer to coding for data entry.

STUDY #264 — FORM 7 (Page 2 of 2)   Medical Center No. ____ ____ ____

                                           Patient No.   ____ ____ ____ ____

REASONS FOR REJECTION (Continued) (Code: 1 = Yes, 2 = No, 3 = Not Evaluated)

15. Patient has recurrent major affective disorder, schizophrenia, personality
    disorder or borderline state that requires use of long-term psychoactive
    drugs or hospitalization .... _____ (45)

16. Patient using other drugs which would interfere with antiepileptic drugs .... _____ (46)

17. Patient has below normal intelligence (IQ < 85) .... _____ (47)

18. Patient's age < 18 or > 65 .... _____ (48)

19. Patient is a known noncomplier (≥ 50% fluctuation in serum levels in
    previous 3 months .... _____ (49)

20. Seizure etiology is neoplastic, degenerative, metabolic, demyelinating, or
    active infection .... _____ (50)

21. Patient allergic to study drugs .... _____ (51)

22. Patient unwilling to participate in randomized study .... _____ (52)

23. Other, specify _____ .... _____ (53-54)

24. If accepted, date study medication began: Mo __ __ Day __ __ Yr __ __   (55-60)

PATIENT IS EXCLUDED IF **ANY** "YES" RESPONSE IS GIVEN IN QUESTIONS 5-23.

FIG. 1.6. *Continued.*

The four periods of patient recruitment has been divided into ten stages (Table
1.1) and each of these stages is described. The order in which these stages occur
may vary from trial to trial. Moreover, not all stages will be conducted within any
one trial.

TABLE 1.1. *Stages of patient recruitment[a]*

Prescreen
I Develop a plan to contact or reach patients
II Contact referral groups (optional)
III Utilize media advertising to attract patients (optional)
IV Contact patients directly

Screening
V Discussion of the clinical trial
VI Assess initial interest
VII Conduct initial screening questions
VIII Conduct initial physical and laboratory screen
IX Rescreen or conduct a more detailed secondary screen
X Obtain the patient's informed consent

[a] The patient is usually considered enrolled when the informed consent is given. See text for a discussion of this
point.

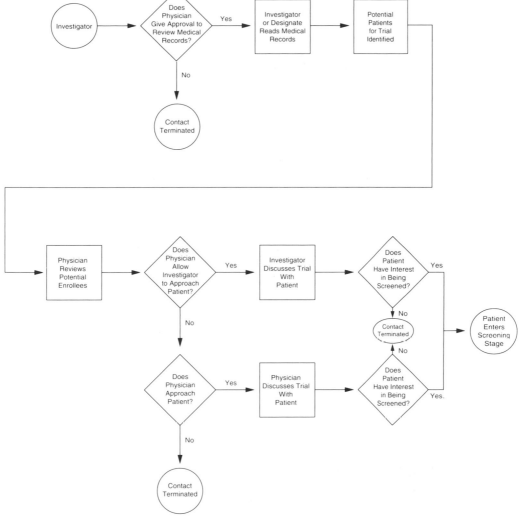

FIG. 1.7. Flow diagram to illustrate use of a recruitment method (i.e., chart review). See Chapter 3 for additional details.

STAGES OF RECRUITMENT

Stage I: Develop a Plan to Contact Patients

It is usually desirable to initiate discussions on patient recruitment while the protocol is being conceptualized. This allows the protocol design and requirements to reflect the types of patients who are desired, and those who are believed to be available for enrollment in the trial (Fig 1.8). For example, either inpatients or outpatients could be enrolled. The choice is often based on their expected availability. If inpatient trials are to last for four weeks it must be ascertained whether patients would be willing to spend that much time in the hospital, and also, how their stay

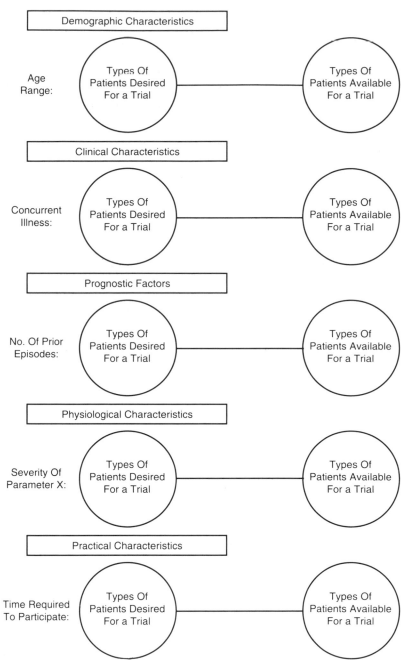

FIG. 1.8. Representative spectra to consider in establishing inclusion criteria. If the difference between the two poles is great it may jeopardize the trial.

would be financed. These considerations may affect the decision of whether to enroll in- or outpatients.

Initial discussions on patient recruitment should include factors such as:

1. Actual or estimated size of the pool of patients.
2. Requirements of the clinical trial that would affect recruitment and whether any criteria could be relaxed without affecting the clinical trial's integrity.
3. Whether to seek true volunteers, true patients, or patient volunteers (Fig 1.9).
4. Estimating the likelihood that the desired type of patients would be willing to enroll in the clinical trial. This likelihood is largely based on the consideration of potential risks and benefits to the patient.
5. Developing a plan (e.g., a pilot screening) to test the likelihood that a sufficient number of patients will enroll.
6. Determination of where the desired patients would be most likely to be found (e.g., specialty clinics, emergency room, inpatients).
7. A determination of the necessity to seek referrals, and if so from which sources and with which methods.
8. A determination of the necessity to advertise for patients.
9. Evaluating the likelihood that these approaches will be successful.
10. Determination of the desired rate of enrollment (e.g., two patients per month or all at once).

If the recruitment plans are developed after the clinical protocol is complete, it may be more difficult to create a plan that will recruit all patients within the scheduled time period. Nonetheless, this is the situation that often occurs when a different person or group prepares the protocol from the one that conducts the trial. Those who conduct multicenter trials can only hope that the organizers have clearly and

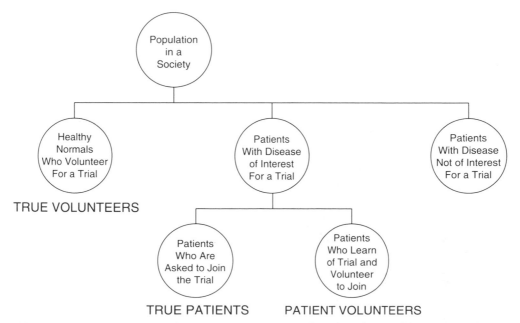

FIG. 1.9. Illustrating the distinction among true patients, patient volunteers, and true volunteers.

completely evaluated and appropriately dealt with the issues of recruitment in the protocol and have sufficient resources to apply to recruiting patients.

Recruitment plans (i.e., strategies) do not always have to be elaborate. However, the most successful large scale clinical trials [e.g., those conducted by the National Heart, Lung, and Blood Institute (NHLBI)] were meticulously planned in advance and rigidly adhered to their schedules. A variety of plans are described in Chapter 7. Plans can be as elaborate as those devised for the Lipid Research Clinics (1983) or as simple as one of the plans listed below.

Plan 1. Ask all appropriate patients (i.e., based on the protocol's inclusion criteria and protocol requirements) in the Wednesday morning clinic if they would like to join the clinical trial.

Plan 2. Put notices about the clinical trial on bulletin boards in the Emergency Room so that physicians there will call the medical resident when appropriate patients are seen.

Plan 3. Call Drs. X, Y, and Z about the clinical trial and ask them to refer patients to the investigator's clinic for evaluation.

The principal point is that a clear plan tied to a recruitment calendar or timetable should be developed for all clinical trials. A plan consists of any number of individual approaches such as the three mentioned. These approaches may all be initiated at the same time, staged to occur at different time points, or staged to occur when triggered by different degrees of need. The timing of these approaches is discussed in Chapter 8 (developing a strategy to enhance recruitment).

Stage II: Contact Referral Groups (Optional)

The stage of contacting referral groups is optional because many clinical trials do not require patient referrals. For those trials where referrals are an important issue, a plan to obtain referrals must be developed. This plan would include consideration of:

1. Type of organizations, centers, groups, or individuals to be contacted for referrals.
2. Number of organizations, centers, groups, or individuals to be contacted.
3. Times when each group will be contacted relative to the initiation of the clinical trial or relative to various milestones (or recruitment problems) that may arise.
4. Identification of concerns that each center or group may have about referring patients (e.g., the patient will not return for future treatment) and means of addressing each of these.
5. Inducements that will be used to encourage each group to refer patients.

Stage III: Utilize Media Advertising to Attract Patients (Optional)

The stage of utilizing the media to advertise for patients is also optional. A plan must be developed if this approach is to be used. Essential factors to consider include:

1. Types of media to consider for advertising (e.g., radio, television, newspaper).
2. Anticipated yield from each type of advertisement.

3. Budget for this activity.
4. Steps to ensure appropriate patient appointments and recruitment for those who contact the site.

Stage IV: Contact Volunteers/Patients Directly

This step may be conducted via a telephone or written interview, or by a face-to-face discussion. The purpose of the initial contact is to attract patients to consider joining the trial and to initiate the screening process. This step is often a brief contact conducted during the prescreen stage and preceding a face-to-face interview. Telephone contact is particularly well-suited for screening patients who are recruited by advertisements. Telephone contact may be used for almost all methods of recruitment. In some cases it is more likely that patients will contact the investigator(s) (e.g., in response to advertisements) and in others (e.g., seeking referrals) investigators may contact potential patients. Written interviews (e.g., questionnaires) may be used when a large pool of patients is being screened. Face-to-face methods are usual in most clinical trials, even though these verbal interviews are often preceded by a telephone screen.

Steps described as stages five through ten may either be combined into a smaller number or subdivided into a larger number of relatively independent steps.

Stage V: Discuss the Clinical Trial

Once a patient is contacted, or the patient contacts the staff person who is to conduct the initial discussion, recruitment passes from the prescreen stage to the screening stage (Fig. 1.3). This first step of the screening stage provides the prospective enrollee with information about the planned or ongoing clinical trial so that the patient may begin to assess both advantages and disadvantages of joining the trial.

Stage VI: Assess the Patient's Initial Interest

Assessing the patient's initial interest is an important step and usually is conducted after presenting information about the trial and prior to posing various screening questions. In order to assess patient interest, the amount of effort, inconvenience, and risk involved in the trial must be described. In addition, the appropriateness of the patient for the trial should be considered.

Stage VII: Conduct Initial Screening Questions

The process of screening usually is conducted in two or more separate steps. The exact number and nature of these steps depends on the protocol as well as practical considerations, but should be planned logically to make efficient use of staff time. If the number of patients interested in joining a trial is relatively large, it is preferable to screen patients initially with a few key questions. These questions could be chosen based on the most common or easiest means of eliminating patients (e.g., Are you over 21? Have you had your disease for more than two years? Do you have more than two episodes per month?).

The questions in the initial screen may be written on checklist forms for review with individuals to ensure that the patients or volunteers meet all relevant inclusion criteria, and that they understand and have an interest in participating in the trial.

Stage VIII: Conduct Initial Physical and Laboratory Screen

Physical, laboratory, and other tests may be conducted at the same time as or separately from the asking of initial screening questions. It is usually important to eliminate unsuitable patients in Stage VII and to conduct the tests of Stage VIII only on those who have passed the hurdle of Stage VII. This saves time, money, and effort.

Stage IX: Rescreen or Conduct a More Detailed Secondary Screen (Optional)

The conduct of a more detailed secondary screen is not required in many clinical trials. Reasons for including this step would be (1) to confirm that patient values (e.g., cholesterol levels) were constant on a repeated test or remained within a certain range; (2) to probe into more details of one or more aspects of inclusion criteria (e.g., compliance with medication or a diet); (3) to schedule more time-consuming or expensive tests that would be inconvenient or too expensive to conduct on all patients who entered Stage VIII; and (4) to schedule tests (e.g., fundoscopy) with other medical departments (e.g., ophthalmological) that are necessary to meet the inclusion criteria, but which could not be conveniently or appropriately scheduled for all patients who entered Stage VIII.

Stage X: Obtain the Patient's Informed Consent

This stage is the last part of patient recruitment because in most clinical trials, only patients who sign or otherwise provide an informed consent may be said to be enrolled. However, many people do not consider an informed consent to be part of recruitment. In many respects, this stage differs from the first nine stages; in particular, numerous ethical issues are involved. Because of the unique nature of the stage, and the many articles and books written on this subject (Levine, 1986; Spilker, 1991), it is not discussed in detail in this book.

One variation of the stages described occurs in clinical trials where the informed consent is obtained from patients prior to their formal screening. For example, if it is believed that patients may have apprehension about enrolling in a trial and the screening process is either time intensive or expensive (e.g., involving sophisticated testing), then it would make sense to discuss the trial and the informed consent and even to have patients sign the informed consent before they are screened. Other examples could be described where Stage X comes earlier in the recruitment process, but in theory almost any trial could utilize this approach.

EFFICIENCY OF RECRUITMENT

The Funnel Effect of Recruitment

There is an almost invariable phenomenon whereby a pool of potential patients who are contacted about entering a clinical trial becomes progressively smaller as it passes through successive screens and the informed consent process. "Funnel effect" is proposed as a name for this phenomenon. Having a name for this concept is important because it allows discussion to occur more easily on methods to counter this effect, and encourages characterization and description of this effect in publications. Several actual examples of this phenomenon are shown in flow charts or graphically in Chapter 11. Lasagna (1979) describes in text format the funnel effect of over 8,000 potential patients being decreased to 100 for a clinical trial. Prout (1979) used a table to show the funnel effect. Chapter 12 on extrapolatability of data, indicates some of the limitations of a clinical trial that occur when the funnel effect is large.

The funnel effect illustrates the progressive shrinking of the patient population prior to enrolling in a trial. This phenomenon could be extended to include dropout and discontinuation of patients during the clinical trial, but these events are separate and relate to the clinical trial itself, and not to the process of patient recruitment described above. Listing the reasons for patient ineligibility to enter a clinical trial (e.g., Lee et al., 1980) does not illustrate the funnel effect, although that information is important to understanding recruiting patterns and the extrapolatability of data.

Chalmers (1982) presents what could be considered a corollary of the funnel effect. He states that such a small percentage of apparently suitable patients are actually randomized in most clinical trials that the control group can never be considered representative of that disease by practicing physicians.

Recruitment Yield

The end result of the funnel effect is the number of patients who enter the clinical trial. This number may be expressed as a percent yield of those screened or initially contacted. Recruitment yield for a specific trial may be given in table form (Table 1.2). This table breaks down the overall yield percent by indicating the yield from each source of patients used, illustrating how variable the yield may be. Table 1.3 presents the overall yield for many trials. The Lipid Research Clinics Program (1983) presents the data of 12 separate sites for (1) number of sources of patients, (2) number of initial contacts, (3) number of first protocol visits, and (4) number of entries, in addition to the percent yield for each site. The latter percents varied from 0.46% to 2.77% (average equals 0.87%). Table 1.4 presents references of major clinical trials whose recruitment experiences were published.

Corollary to Lasagna's Law

Although Lasagna's Law states a general loss of 90% of expected patients, data presented in Table 1.3 suggest that the screening yield probably depends on the type of trial population sought. The yield is primarily related to inclusion criteria of the

TABLE 1.2. *Yield of respective locating strategies for a pulmonary trial*

Patient-locating strategy	Persons assessed *n*	Persons confirmed for COAD *n*	Persons assessed and confirmed for COAD %	Confirmed cases not previously diagnosed *n*	Confirmed cases not previously diagnosed %	Strategy total yield[a]
Hospital records	75	63	84	NA	NA	7
Physician referral	352	247	70	94	38	27
Advertising campaign	475	204	43	104	51	22
Mailed questionnaire	932	409	44	198	48	44
Mean percent	NA	NA	50	NA	43	NA
Total	1,834	923		396		100

Reproduced from Barlow et al. (1984) with permission.
COAD, chronic obstructive airway disease; NA, not applicable.
[a] Indicates proportion of confirmed cases by strategy.

protocol plus the motivation of patients to enroll. Patients usually have less motivation to enter prevention trials than they do to enter treatment trials, and those requested to participate in follow-up trials are a select group who have already agreed and successfully participated in a clinical trial. Prevention trials generally have yields ranging from 1% to 6%, whereas medical care trials (excluding surgery) yield 20 to

TABLE 1.3. *Screening yields of various clinical trials[a]*

	Number of patients screened	Number of patients randomized	Percent yield
A. Primary prevention trials			
CPPT	436,679	3,810	0.87
MRFIT	361,662	12,866	3.56
HDFP	442,056	11,386	2.58
National Diet Heart	20,000	899	4.50
VA Mild Hypertension	120,000	1,012	0.84
SHEP	447,921	4,736	1.06
B. Secondary prevention trials			
BHAT	157,771	3,837	2.43
RTOG Lung Cancer	653	41	6.28
VA Epilepsy #118	4,985	681	13.66
VA Epilepsy #264	8,841	480	5.43
C. Medical care trials			
CAOD	5,538	1,015	18.33
CASS[b,c]	16,626	780	4.69
CLAS	719	188	26.15
POSCH[b]	11,976	838	7.00
NOTT	1,043	203	19.46
MIAMI	26,439	5,778	21.85
MILIS	9,450	985	10.42
TIMI (acute care)	1,159	316	27.26
DATATOP	6,146	800	13.02
D. Screening trials			
CARDIA	202,966	5,182	2.55
E. Follow-up trials			
NHS-2	1,191	477	40.05
CSSCD	5,021	3,241	64.55

[a] Abbreviations are indicated in Table 1.4.
[b] Surgical trial.
[c] Randomization was declined by 1,319 patients (7.93% of those screened).

TABLE 1.4. *Selected references that describe recruitment experiences in large clinical trials*

Clinical trial	Reference(s)
A. Single trials	
Aspirin Myocardial Infarction Study (AMIS)	Schoenberger (1987); and AMIS Research Group (1980)
Beta-Blocker Heart Attack Trial (BHAT)	Byington and the Beta-Blocker Heart Attack Trial Research Group (1984); Goldstein et al. (1987)
Bogalusa Heart Study	Croft et al. (1984)
Coronary Artery Surgery Study (CASS)	CASS Principal Investigators et al. (1983)
Cholesterol Lowering Atherosclerosis Study (CLAS)	Blankenhorn et al. (1987)
Cooperative Study of Sickle Cell Disease (CSSCD)	Gaston et al. (1987)
Coronary Artery Disease Risk Development in Young Adults (CARDIA) Study	Hughes et al. (1987); Orden et al. (1990)
Coronary Drug Project (CDP)	Schoenberger (1979)
Coronary Primary Prevention Trial (CPPT)	Agras and Marshall (1979); Benedict (1979); Agras and Bradford (1982); and The Lipid Research Clinics Program (1983)
Deprenyl and Tocopherol Antioxidative Therapy of Parkinsonism (DATATOP)	Parkinson Study Group (1989)
Hypertension Detection and Follow-up Program (HDFP)	Ford et al. (1987); Daugherty (1983); and Hypertension Detection and Follow-up Program Cooperative Group (1977)
Hypertension Prevention Trial (HPT)	Borhani et al. (1989)
Metroprolol in Acute Myocardial Infarction (MIAMI)	The MIAMI Trial Research Group (1985)
Multicenter Investigation of the Limitation of Infarct Size (MILIS)	Rude et al. (1983); Mullin et al. (1984); and MILIS Study Group (1986)
Multiple Risk Factor Intervention Trial (MRFIT)	Neaton et al. (1987)
National Breast Screening Study–Canadian (NBSS)	Baines (1984)
National Cooperative Gallstone Study (NCGS)	Croke (1979)
Natural History Study of Congenital Heart Defects (NHS-2)	O'Fallon et al. (1987)
Nocturnal Oxygen Therapy Trial (NOTT)	Williams et al. (1987)
Program on Surgical Control of the Hyperlipidemias (POSCH)	Buchwald et al. (1987)
Radiation Therapy Oncology Group (RTOG Lung Cancer)	Lee et al. (1980)
Systolic Hypertension in the Elderly Program (SHEP)	Vogt et al. (1986); Petrovitch et al. (1991)
The WHO European Collaborative Trial in the Multifactorial Prevention of Coronary Heart Disease	World Health Organization European Collaborative Group (1980)
Thrombolysis in Myocardial Infarction Trial (TIMI)	Knatterud and Forman (1987)
VA Cooperative Study of Surgery for Coronary Arterial Occlusive Disease (CAOD)	Detre et al. (1977)
B. Multiple trials	
National Heart, Lung, and Blood Institute (NHLBI) trials	Probstfield et al. (1987)
Veterans Administration Cooperative Studies Program (CSP) Trials	Collins et al. (1980)

27% of screened patients, and follow-up trials have even larger yields. We propose a corollary to Lasagna's Law:

Expect 1 in 5 screened patients to enroll if the trial offers benefit for an active medical problem.
Expect 1 in 40 screened patients to enroll if the trial offers the possibility of disease prevention.

Other Measures of Assessing Recruitment Efficiency

In addition to defining yield as the percent of patients enrolled of those screened, one may evaluate the efficiency of the recruitment process using other parameters. These include comparing the percent of patients enrolled to:

1. The potential total population targeted.
2. The total prevalence of the disease within the population screened.
3. The goal established for each center participating in the trial.
4. The number of patients at other points of the recruitment process than at the initial screen or those contacted.

Recruitment details of many medium and large trials have been published (Table 1.4) and are excellent sources of specific issues faced and lessons learned.

Trials That Failed Because of Recruitment Problems

Innumerable problems may lead to poor patient recruitment. Other chapters in this book discuss many of these problems. Several published trials have reported

TABLE 1.5. *Selected trials that were not completed because of low patient recruitment*

Patients	Major reason(s)	Reference
Very low birth weight infants	Change in medical practice during trial	Lumley et al. (1985)
Breast cancer–surgical treatment	Inclusion criteria, surgical judgment, and informed consent	Lucas et al. (1984)
Antidepressants in the elderly	High dropout and discontinuation rate	Waite et al. (1986)
Acute stroke therapy	Inclusion criteria	LaRue et al. (1988)
Ulcer surgery	Newly available oral medicine	Williford et al. (1987)
Antabuse for alcoholics taking methadone	Strict alcohol and substance abuse inclusion criteria	Williford et al. (1987)
Chronic brain syndrome	Inclusion criteria and definitions were very strict	Williford et al. (1987)
Contraceptive sponge	Clinic attendance decreased; Women satisfied with other methods	Kasse-Annese et al. (1989)
Yttrium and triamcinolone in rheumatoid arthritis	Patient numbers were overestimated because of a backlog who were treated initially	Arthritis and Rheumatism Council Multicentre Radiosynoviorthesis Trial Group (1984)

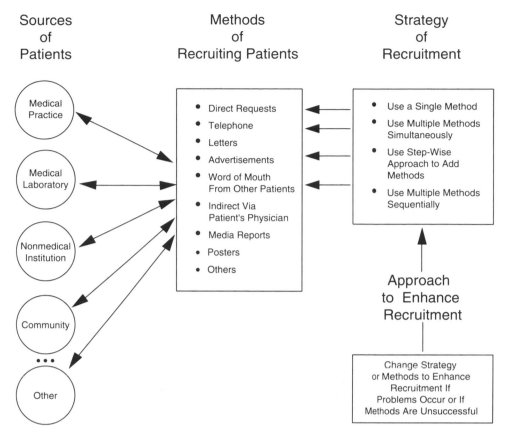

FIG. 1.10. Conceptual overview of the relationships between elements of recruitment and the approach to modify a strategy. Each of the four major categories shown is discussed in a separate chapter.

recruitment to be the primary reason that the trial was not completed. Table 1.5 lists some of these trials and the reason(s) for their inability to recruit a sufficient number of patients. The vast majority of clinical trials discontinued because of recruiting problems have never been published; such trials are believed, based on anecdotal evidence, to be quite common.

CONCEPTUAL OVERVIEW

Figure 1.10 illustrates the conceptual overview of recruitment used in this book. It illustrates the relationships of sources, methods, and strategies, plus an approach to enhance recruitment if problems develop. Each of these four topics is discussed in a separate chapter. Each of the four categories of sources contains numerous specific sources and examples of methods listed are also a highly incomplete list. Although strategies, sources, and methods tend to overlap in practice, it is generally useful to conceptualize them separately.

2

Perspectives of Patients, Physicians, and Staff About Recruitment

WHY EVALUATE PERSPECTIVES OF VARIOUS GROUPS?

The key to preventing recruitment problems lies in developing the most appropriate clinical trial design, protocol, and patient recruitment strategy. To do this success-fully, it is essential to understand the perspectives and motivations of all groups involved in a trial (Table 2.1). Failure to understand and consider these perspectives and motivations will make it difficult to achieve an adequate level of patient re-cruitment.

Every group described in this chapter has numerous and different perspectives about patient recruitment. For example, the issue for the investigator is primarily: "How can I enroll enough patients with the least effort and cost?" Questions relating to career, money, scientific interest, and other subjects may also be important, but

TABLE 2.1. *Groups whose roles and perspectives should be considered in developing a recruitment strategy for a clinical trial[a]*

1. Patients and their families
2. Treating physicians who refer patients
3. Principal investigator of the trial
4. Staff of the principal investigator
5. Additional staff helping to conduct the trial
6. Ethics Committees/IRBs
7. Data Monitoring Board
8. Regulatory authorities: reviewers, monitors, and directors
9. Sponsor's staff: monitors, statisticians, and managers
10. Coordinating center staff
11. Medical contractors
12. Other relevant groups

[a] Not all of these groups are necessarily involved in any one clinical trial.

are less related to patient recruitment. Patients and their family and friends are concerned with the essential question: "Should I (the patient) enroll or not in the clinical trial?" This question is usually addressed by answering two other questions: "What's in it for me?" and "How should the decision be made?" For the sponsor of a clinical trial, the major question relating to patient recruitment is: "Which investigators are best able to recruit patients and to conduct the trial successfully?" Secondarily, a sponsor may suggest techniques that investigators could use to achieve and maintain appropriate rates of patient recruitment. Regulatory authorities, data monitoring boards, and Ethics Committees/IRBs generally view patient recruitment with the question: "Are there any unusual or unethical recruitment practices that suggest the plan should or must be altered? For ongoing trials, the major question is: Does an exceedingly slow rate of recruitment necessitate termination or at least modification of the trial?"

REASONS PATIENTS ENROLL OR DO NOT ENROLL IN CLINICAL TRIALS

To develop and successfully complete an effective recruitment strategy it is imperative to understand what motivates patients to enroll or not enroll in a specific clinical trial (Table 2.2). Insight into these issues is not sufficient to assure adequate recruitment rates because many other factors may diminish patient enrollment. But, without knowledge about patient motivation, it is unlikely that patient recruitment will be successful. A knowledge of some of the benefits patients may expect from

TABLE 2.2. *Reasons why patients enroll in clinical trials*

1. Patients are not adequately treated with current therapy
2. Patients have adverse reactions to current therapy
3. Patients believe that their relationship with their physician would be jeopardized if they do not enroll
4. Patients desire free medical care
5. Patients desire remuneration
6. Patients want to help other patients with their disease receive better treatment
7. Patients seek attention to help alleviate their loneliness
8. Patients enjoy the special attention from physician and staff
9. Patients seek new challenges or changes in their life
10. Patients want to help their physician with his or her research

TABLE 2.3. *Benefits to patients from enrolling in a clinical trial*

1. Potential clinical improvement in the short-term, possibly with fewer problems than with current treatment
2. Potential influence on the long-term course of the disease
3. More attention is given to the patient's problems by professionals and more opportunities exist for discussions
4. More thorough evaluation of one's condition through laboratory tests and examinations, plus monitoring with repeated evaluations
5. Contact with more experienced medical staff
6. Full medical care and medicines provided at no or minimal cost, sometimes including the gift of a special device at the end of the trial
7. Payment for meals, transportation, or other out-of-pocket expenses may be provided
8. Payment for time spent and inconvenience may be provided
9. Contacts for future health care may be established
10. General humanitarian benefits exist for additional patients because of information/results obtained in the trial
11. Potential exists for early access to a new treatment
12. Having more complete information provided on their condition, as well as reports sent to their referring physician
13. Assistance with social services provided by the trial staff or by referral
14. Special clinic hours including evening and Saturday appointments to accommodate patients who work during regular clinic hours

enrolling in clinical trials is also helpful (see Table 2.3). Relevant factors that influence recruitment may differ for individual trials and for individual patients. Nonetheless, there are underlying principles and points that are common to most trials and which may be described.

Patient Attitudes

Patients who expect to improve their disease status on therapy are more likely to respond to medicine positively than those who rate other goals (e.g., pain relief, improved sleeplessness) as more important (Berry et al., 1980). Several surveys about patient attitudes toward clinical trials are flawed by the fact that the situations described are hypothetical. There is little assurance that patients can provide fully honest or accurate answers when they do not have to follow through on any decisions or comments expressed. Of course, the authors of such surveys are usually aware of many biases inherent in this type of study (Saurbrey et al., 1984, Cassileth et al., 1982).

Another type of survey conducted among the public assesses the public's views on clinical trials (Kemp et al., 1984). While there may be certain value in seeking this type of data, the results are even more suspect than those discussed above. The general public is not presently in a position to offer educated comments about randomized clinical trials of medical treatments (e.g., cancer). Cancer patients who are educated about a particular trial and asked to participate in a survey should provide better data. Barofsky and Sugarbaker (1979) came closest to this goal by interviewing both participants and refusers (i.e., patients who refused entry) in one of four randomized sarcoma trials. They observed that a number of factors relating to the treatments offered were the primary determinants of whether patients entered the trial (e.g., not wanting an amputation, not wanting to continue on chemotherapy).

"The greater the significance to the patients of treatment options determined by randomization, the greater the nonparticipation" (Barofsky and Sugarbaker, 1979). Other cancer trials have documented high resistance to enrollment by patients; the resistance was based on a wide variety of factors (Baines, 1984). Llewellyn-Thomas et al. (1991) reported that 100 cancer patients who received supplementary education about clinical trials were more likely to enter a clinical trial than those who did not receive additional information.

Another issue is whether people who do not accept an invitation to attend a screening clinic to assess whether they have a particular problem (e.g., hypertension, breast cancer, elevated blood cholesterol) have similar reasons to those who attend screening but do not enroll in clinical trials. The process of screening may or may not be directly linked to possible enrollment in a clinical trial (e.g., community screening versus screening for a specific clinical trial). Insufficient data exist to determine the correlation between nonattendees and nonenrollees. French et al. (1982) found that nonattendees at a breast cancer screening clinic tended to view it as a "place of risk" in that patients feared risk of detection and would rather adopt an "ostrich" approach. A much smaller percent of attendees had that fear.

McCusker et al. (1982) examined the records of 767 patients with lung cancer in a specific county in New York State, finding that 323 were eligible for entry into one or two protocols active at the time of the survey. Of this number, only 69 patients were actually enrolled. Three factors separated enrollees from those who did not enter the trials. The first factor related to the activity of the oncology unit at the local hospital. The more active that group, the greater the chance of patient enrollment. The second factor was the socioeconomic status of the patient. The higher the level, the greater was the chance of enrollment. The third factor was the length of time since diagnosis. The longer this period, the greater the chance of enrollment.

The concerns of the public and patients about clinical trials in oncology have been reviewed (Ganz, 1990). Croft et al. (1984) categorized nonparticipants in a large pediatric study as direct refusers, nonrespondents, and those whose parents consented but the children were absent from school when the examinations were performed. An interesting finding of this study was the different types of reasons given by children compared with adults (in other trials). Overall, 32% of Caucasian boys refused without giving any specific reason ("don't want to, don't have a reason"), 21% of Caucasian boys (10 to 14 years old) refused because of fear (e.g., doctors, undressing, examination). Their data point out the need to determine reasons for recruitment problems in each trial and that reasons for patient nonparticipation usually differ from trial to trial.

Mattson et al. (1985) interviewed patients who participated in two major clinical trials (BHAT and AMIS). They reported on the personal benefits patients felt they received as well as the perceived problems associated with participation. Reasons for enrollment were also given and a high percentage of both BHAT and AMIS participants gave altruistic reasons as a motivation. Data were collected from selected AMIS patients using open-ended questions in a structured interview format, whereas selected BHAT participants received a close-ended questionnaire. It is not possible to extrapolate these data to other trials because the methodology is flawed by the types of surveys conducted. In fact, that is the major limitation of most such surveys where patients are interviewed about their opinions. A trial offering a life-saving therapy will engender different motivations and perceptions in patients than

one offering therapy comparable to that already in existence. An additional discussion of patient perspectives about clinical trials is in Chapter 57 of *Guide to Clinical Trials* (Spilker, 1991).

Factors Influencing Patient Motivation for Volunteering for a Clinical Trial

Various studies have evaluated the specific factors encouraging patients to volunteer for clinical trials. The most important caveat is that the factors that are important for one group of patients (or volunteers) may be irrelevant to another group. For patients who enroll in clinical trials, the factors influencing their participation will depend on their background, medical experiences, degree of disease severity, philosophical beliefs, economic status, and other characteristics. Thus, if a particular survey of patients reveals that one or a few types of individuals predominated (e.g., stoic, hypochondriac, debilitated), the patient mix probably influenced the patients' list of reasons for enrolling. The primary reasons cited by 144 oncology patients for enrolling in clinical trials were (1) trust in the physician, (2) belief that the treatment would be beneficial, and (3) fear that the disease would worsen without treatment (Penman et al., 1984). Results of surveys about motivation to enter a clinical trial using the following groups would not be expected to be similar.

1. Medical students
2. College students
3. Alcoholics
4. Homeless people
5. Seminary students
6. Cross-section of a city's population
7. Staff of the investigator
8. Staff of the institution

Other groups could be identified, but the point should be clear.

Another important issue in some studies is whether patients (or volunteers) who did *not* enroll were also asked about the factors that influenced them. In this case it would be of great interest to know the factors (if any) that led them to decide not to enroll. The issue is that patient refusers (i.e., those who decide during the recruitment process not to continue) should be separated from patients who were disqualified for any reason during the screening period.

If a survey about patient motivation is conducted during a pilot run of a major trial or during the initial period of a trial, the results may be useful in tailoring the clinical trial's recruitment strategy so that it is more effective. For example, patients who live more than a certain distance may be encouraged to attend a clinic for screening, but none of them may enroll because of the great distance to be traveled for the frequent clinic visits that are required in the trial. In this situation, it would be best not to screen patients who live more than a certain distance (or time) from the trial site. Many other reasons for nonparticipation could be discussed with patients at an early stage of screening to avoid spending even more effort before learning that numerous patients would object to certain aspects of the trial.

Another caveat in accepting as valid results of motivational and decision-making surveys (either from questionnaires or interviews) has to do with the truthfulness and accuracy of the respondents. Many volunteers and patients believe at least some

of the questions to be private matters. Rather than refusing to respond, some people will not provide truthful answers.

Throughout most clinical trials, the accuracy of responses depends on the patients' understanding of the questions posed, which cannot be taken for granted among those with borderline intelligence, poor reading skills, or limited English vocabulary. Many people who are illiterate try very hard, often successfully, to hide this fact. There are many psychological reasons why patients who desire to be honest may not provide accurate answers to questions posed. These factors may be a major influence on the validity of the data obtained.

A special problem in many surveys about motivation and decision making in pilot and feasibility trials is that patients (or volunteers) are being asked their views of a hypothetical trial rather than a real one. If the trial has to be entirely conceptualized without first-hand knowledge and experiences of the procedures involved (e.g., colonoscopy, endoscopy), the responses given may be honest and accurate but ill-informed, and would be different if the patients underwent the trial described.

Characterizing the Population of Patients Who Enroll in Clinical Trials

Only a small proportion of potentially eligible patients enter clinical trials. One of the best ways to characterize those patients who enroll in a clinical trial is to compare them with those who do not. This may be done using a patient log. Hunter et al. (1987) evaluated the data of nearly 45,000 newly diagnosed cancer patients enlisted in the Community Clinical Oncology Program Physician's Patient Log for a 15-month period in the mid-1980s. They found that one-third of clinically eligible patients were entered into a clinical trial. Of interest is that a correlation was obtained between age and likelihood to enter the trial: younger patients were more likely to enter. The two major reasons why patients did not enter trials were physician's preference for an alternative treatment and patient refusal for protocol treatment.

Does Labeling of Patients as "Sick" or "At Risk" During Screening Create a Negative Psychological or Behavioral Impact?

Benfari et al. (1981) found that being labeled "sick" or "at risk" and participating in an intervention program has a beneficial effect on psychological scores for depression symptoms after the trial. The investigators evaluated 616 randomized participants from the Multiple Risk Factor Intervention Trial (MRFIT) conducted at the Harvard University site. Multiple interpretations are possible of the specific data they report and of the data reported by others (see their paper for references). The conclusion is based, however, on comparing scores for high-risk patients who entered the trial with low-risk patients who did not. At best, this topic is at an early stage of research and broad extrapolations are not possible.

PHYSICIAN PERSPECTIVES

Factors Influencing Physicians to Offer Clinical Trial Entry to Patients

A number of clinical trials have been widely discussed in the literature in which poor patient recruitment was attributed to the physicians' reluctance to offer enrollment to patients (see Langley et al., 1987, for references). Langley et al. (1987) studied the factors that influenced oncologists in deciding whether or not to offer enrollment in the trial. Nurses and family physicians also rated the factors. The need for a patient's primary physician to approve referral to a clinical trial also can be a roadblock to recruitment (Dicker and Kent, 1990).

Investigators' Attitudes About Treatments in a Clinical Trial

Investigators' attitudes about the treatments available in a clinical trial vary enormously. Whatever the specific attitudes of the investigators, these affect how they approach, recruit, and inform patients about entering a clinical trial. Some attitudes are more appropriate than others and some attitudes should preclude their participation in a multicenter trial or conducting a single site trial. When physicians do not feel that they can recommend treatment with one or more of the regimens allowed in a clinical trial, they cannot ethically encourage patients to enroll (see Chapter 5, Ethics). These physicians should not become investigators for that trial.

The most inappropriate attitude is, "I know what the trial will show and if it doesn't, the results are not believable." Another inappropriate, but somewhat common attitude is "I believe one treatment is preferable and I expect (or hope) that the trial will show this." This is inappropriate because the correct attitude for an investigator at the outset of a trial is "I do not know which treatment is superior and that is the reason I am performing the trial." An investigator who holds this last attitude can approach a patient with a clear conscience about enrollment in the trial and randomization to various treatments offered.

In a large randomized surgical trial of two methods for breast cancer resection, Taylor et al. (1984) found that numerous surgeons did not enter any patients. A questionnaire investigating the reasons why 66 of 91 surgeons did not enter all eligible patients revealed the following problem areas:

1. Concern with physician–patient relationship in a randomized clinical   73% trial
2. Problems with informed consent   38%
3. Dislike of discussing uncertainty with patients   23%
4. Conflict between their roles as clinician and scientist   18%
5. Practical problems with trial procedures   9%
6. Feeling personally responsible if treatments are unequal   8%

These data highlight numerous issues, including the importance of assessing and satisfying investigator qualms during *their* recruitment. If recruitment of investigators fails, it is unlikely that recruitment of patients can be successful. Investigators who are uncertain about their own commitment to a trial, are unlikely to successfully recruit patients.

Reluctance of Some Physicians to Enroll Patients in Clinical Trials

The common problem of slow or inadequate enrollment in clinical trials has led to a number of studies, over the last decade, exploring the reasons why physicians do not enroll eligible patients into clinical trials. Most of these studies have dealt with cancer trials, primarily breast cancer (Hellman, 1979; Schafer, 1982; Taylor et al., 1984; Mackillop and Johnston, 1986; Foley and Moertel, 1991). These authors discuss the physician–patient relationship and focus on the ethical conflict that physicians experience when they want to offer their patients the best treatment available. The physician is portrayed as caught in the dilemma of uncertainty that an experimental clinical trial is a reasonable choice, although most physicians accept some responsibility to support scientifically important clinical research. The evidence for this view comes from interviews and assessments of physicians (Langley et al., 1987; Hunter et al., 1987).

This interpretation could represent a self-serving explanation by physicians who chose not to enroll patients in a clinical trial. One has to wonder why most physicians, faced with the choice of recommending an experimental treatment or not, do not choose to recommend the treatment. Several important qualifications are necessary. First, most of the studies, editorials, and comments on this topic relate to cancer; second, many of the physicians involved are surgeons; third, breast cancer has been studied by several groups to understand why so few women enrolled in several of these clinical trials.

The causes of physician reluctance, probably, lie not so much in the ethical dilemmas of physicians struggling to justify the need for a clinical trial, but in several other areas. These factors, which are not listed in any order of importance, all could influence physician behavior in encouraging patients to enroll in clinical trials.

1. If surgical and medical oncologists referred all eligible patients to clinical trials, they would be giving up much of their patient base as well as their clinical role. More private practice physicians in oncology are asked to refer or enroll patients in clinical trials than in any other disease area. These trials are extremely large and lengthy (of necessity), and are usually regional or national. Private practice physicians in other therapeutic areas or disciplines are less often approached to enroll their patients in clinical trials. It is not surprising that some (or many) physicians are reluctant to enroll patients. Private practice physicians are less academically oriented, less motivated by academic advancement, and perhaps more motivated to maintain busy practices than their colleagues in academia. In addition, if the physician in private practice has or hopes to establish a long-term medical relationship with the patient, he or she does not want to send the patient elsewhere for treatment.

2. Surgeons have historically been less interested in conducting well-controlled trials to evaluate their surgery than nonsurgeons. In addition, for a surgeon to propose a trial to a patient suggests that he or she is not sure of the best treatment, and this may be interpreted by the surgeons as compromising their professional relationship with their patient and the respect they receive from patients and peers.

3. Some patients desire and even "need" authoritative decisions about their medical care made by physicians they trust. This is particularly true in many surgical areas. Current concepts about the surgical treatment of breast cancer have led many surgeons to offer choices to their patients. Unfortunately, this democratization of the medical process creates a dilemma for patients who participate in the decision to select their own treatment. For those needing radiation and/or chemotherapy, the dilemma continues if they are asked to consider enrolling in a clinical trial. The physician who senses that a patient needs an authoritative decision about treatment cannot be faulted for avoiding subjecting an anxious patient to choices that depend on technical information outside the patient's grasp.

4. The embarrassment and often personal discomfort in discussing a clinical trial will probably bother more physicians in a private practice setting than in a more impersonal clinic, where a physician may not see the same patient each time he or she attends clinic. A particularly uncomfortable moment is likely to occur when the patient must be told of the chance he or she might receive a placebo.

5. Some cancer trials are private practice based so the physician carries out the protocol in the private office and reports data to the coordinating center. The amount of paperwork and administrative details required in a clinical trial are substantial and may discourage physicians to participate.

6. Clinical trials require almost religious adherence to protocols. The ability to strictly adhere to a protocol is probably less in the private practice of nonacademic physicians, although most private practitioners fully realize the reasons for this need and understand the implications for the trial of not adhering to the protocol.

7. The primary authors and investigators in a small (or large) multicenter trial have a sense of ownership and involvement in the progress and outcome of a clinical trial. There is no way for many physicians in private practice who are asked to enroll or refer their patients to feel much allegiance or interest in the trial. They feel no need to enroll or refer patients if there is little benefit to them and perhaps none to their patients.

Although data to fully challenge the conventional interpretation of physician reluctance to enter patients into certain trials—the ethical argument—is not yet available, the ethical argument appears to be a post-hoc rationalization more than a sound interpretation, particularly when the common sense and frequently cited reasons for nonparticipation (described above) are considered.

Major Reasons Investigators Do Not Participate in Clinical Trials

Apart from a general lack of interest in conducting clinical trials, or a question about the scientific value of a proposed trial, there are some important reasons to consider why investigators may not be willing to participate in a trial they are interested in (Table 2.4).

TABLE 2.4. *Possible reasons for physicians' reluctance to participate in clinical trials as investigators*

1. Time consuming nature of many clinical trials
2. Inability to prescribe or treat outside the protocol
3. Expensive to conduct
4. Lack of time to spend on the trial
5. Poor experience in the past
6. Inability to obtain a grant
7. Inability to obtain third-party payment
8. An excessive number of centers involved so that his or her contribution to career enhancement is lost
9. Inability to discern how the trial will help his or her career
10. Belief that one of the treatments is superior
11. Fear that the trial would compromise the physician–patient relationship
12. Lack of staff to assist

Academic Priorities

Academic standing is of paramount importance to most investigators associated with medical centers and major hospitals. This issue particularly affects those who are not yet tenured. Many universities place greater value on basic science pursuits than on clinical research. Faculty are placed under subtle or overt pressure to emphasize the type of research that will result in primary authorship of publications in peer-reviewed journals, preferably one or more annually. Time spent in a clinic plus time required to complete forms and perform other clinical tasks, including patient recruitment, represents a major commitment that might otherwise be spent in one's laboratory or on a project of greater personal interest. In addition, the likelihood of being the primary author on the main publication of an important multicenter trial, or even on an auxilliary paper of the same trial, is small. Also, publications of clinical trials often do not appear for several or many years after the trial has begun and frequently only one publication describes the efforts of multiple investigators over many years.

These problems may be somewhat resolved for major multicenter trials by planning multiple manuscripts to be authored by a variety of investigators. Manuscripts describing the methodology used for the clinical trial are sometimes published prior to the conclusion of the trial. Investigators are often enticed to participate in a trial with the promise that all abstracts and manuscripts that emanate from the trial can be added to their bibliography. For some people this can become a lengthy supplement to an otherwise brief curriculum vitae, particularly for an investigator who has few other research pursuits.

Competing Clinical Trials

In contrast, Zimmer et al. (1985) list several reasons why university faculty and chronic care facility staff are motivated to establish clinical research programs (Table 2.5). Investigators who are well-known in a therapeutic area or who are interested in conducting clinical trials and have the reputation of conducting them well are

TABLE 2.5. *Examples of motivation for participants in university–nursing home relationships[a]*

Long-term care providers:
"We want medical students"
Desire to see needs for long-term care for elderly recognized by the university (geriatric priority)
Recognition of provider's status in the community
Assistance in recruiting capable medical director and physicians
Assistance in recruiting staff
Interest in research
University faculty:
Setting for clinical experience (clerkship or practicum) for students and fellows
Research opportunities; research support
Salary source for faculty
Interdisciplinary links
Better care for elderly in the community

From Zimmer et al. (1985) with permission.
[a] Listed in order of priority.

often asked by sponsors to participate in new trials. Therefore, when investigators are approached, many will be committed to one or more ongoing and future trials.

In the situation where two or more invitations to conduct trials occur at the same time, a choice may have to be made among them by the investigator. Some sponsors and organizers of clinical trials may offer the investigator a more tempting framework for their trial. These encouragements may include higher payments, more salary support for a trial coordinator, donation of a piece of equipment, a more convenient protocol, a more desirable therapy, annual meetings in resort areas, or an opportunity to work with experts in the field. A sponsor who wishes to counter the above inducements for an investigator to participate in a clinical trial should discuss both the specific and general benefits their trial offers the investigator.

Inadequate Numbers of Patients

It is unusual for an investigator to proclaim a paucity of eligible patients! Such honesty should be heeded. However, this response could mean that the eligibility criteria are far too strict or are misinterpreted. A careful review of the reasons why patients of the type needed are not seen at the site should alert the organizers to possible errors in the protocol. Investigators should not be pressured into participating in a clinical trial any more than patients, even though they do not sign an informed consent. Unhappy investigators can be expected to withdraw from or to neglect a clinical trial they are not motivated and committed to conduct. Some sponsors plan protocols with numerous sites but ask for a small number of patients to be enrolled by each investigator. This method circumvents some of the problems of an inadequate number of patients as well as the issue of competing trials that would otherwise utilize all the available patients at a site.

The American Medical Association (AMA) conducted a survey of 1,000 physicians in 1989, asking "Under appropriate conditions, would you be willing to participate as a clinical investigator in clinical trials or not?" Seventy-two percent (718) replied yes and 25% (248) replied no. "Responses according to specialty were uniform, ranging from 62% . . . to 77%." This survey was used as evidence by the American Medical Association Council on Scientific Affairs (1991) that there are many physicians in the community willing to conduct clinical trials. Another interpretation is that the physicians knew that "yes" was the desired answer, made them look better, and placed them under no obligation. Moreover, the question included the phrase "under appropriate conditions" and a physician could always claim that the conditions were not yet acceptable for him or her to conduct a trial. The major evidence in favor of our view are (1) the poor rate of patient enrollment in current oncology trials using community-based physicians (see Chapter 10 for a discussion on this specific point), and (2) the same 1,000 physicians were asked to identify the major inhibiting factors to participating and 76% identified lack of time, bureaucratic administration of trials, liability, or lack of interest, which are all factors that remain almost constant over time and are likely to be used by physicians as reasons not to become involved in a trial.

ROLES OF CLINICAL TRIAL STAFF

Although recruitment of patients into a clinical trial is an essential factor in determining whether a clinical trial is successful or fails, the recruitment strategy is often left to inexperienced junior level staff to implement. The administrative and management issues related to the recruitment process require careful attention during the planning and initiation process as well as throughout the duration of the clinical trial. All staff participants in a clinical trial should be cognizant of the entire protocol with particular emphasis on the inclusion criteria. Staff members may be considered emissaries for the trial, and some should constantly proselytize for trial candidates throughout the recruitment period.

Role of the Principal Investigator in Patient Recruitment

The principal investigator at each site is the most important person in the recruitment process. Whether that investigator is the trial initiator or a coinvestigator at a site, recruitment begins with the local investigator. It is up to the investigator to impart excitement about the trial in and a sense of urgency about the recruitment process and need for patients. Among colleagues, the investigators should stress the potential medical benefit of the trial for their patients as well as the scientific knowledge to be gained.

The investigator should make the initial contacts with colleagues and medical staff, after which trial coordinators can pursue details of recruitment. These physician-to-physician contacts should be repeated continuously throughout the recruitment period to reinforce the goals of the trial.

Not only during initiation, but also throughout the trial, the investigator should consider the feasibility of additional or alternate sources of patients. Expanding the screening process requires planning to reach new sources. As with all recruitment issues, the investigator must be the primary contact to establish new avenues for screening.

Responsibilities of the Investigator Regarding Patient Recruitment

Investigators have a variety of responsibilities, depending on the nature and scope of the trial. The following list includes typical investigator responsibilities.

1. Inform the medical community about the purpose and scope of the trial. This includes public relations efforts such as presenting lectures and writing journal articles or announcements.
2. Serve as the primary contact with physicians and other medical personnel (e.g., laboratories).
3. Plan the overall recruitment program, including review of advertisements, posters, letters, and script statements for staff to use in reponse to inquiries (e.g., for telephone screening).
4. Educate staff about the trial and how to approach patients.
5. Participate in the informed consent process.
6. Be available to answer any medical or procedural questions that arise during patient screening.
7. Review recruitment goals regularly and plan actions to initiate new sources for screening or new recruitment methods if necessary.

Role of the Recruitment Coordinator

Trials for which the funding includes the salary of a trial coordinator can divide the recruitment tasks between the investigator and staff. Some large-scale trials have the luxury of hiring several staff, one of whom can be designated as a part-time or full-time recruitment coordinator. The recruitment coordinator has the primary responsibility for screening and recruiting patients. If the trial has no centrally developed plan, the coordinator must work with the investigator to develop a system for finding patients to screen. Creativity and acceptance of new ideas and novel referral sources are assets in this role. Because the trial coordinator plays a central role in the recruitment process, a back-up person must be available to cover the trial during the coordinator's absence.

Several reports have emphasized the importance of designating staff to manage recruitment (Dunbar, 1982; Herson, 1980; Hunninghake, 1987; Mullin, 1989; Zifferblatt, 1976). Herson (1980) noted that the supervision and training of a specific person who is dedicated to recruiting patients who meet all entry criteria "can have a profound effect on the end product." Dunbar (1982) described the elaborate behavioral research system developed to advise Coronary Primary Prevention Trial (CPPT) groups about recruitment. She defines the major attributes needed by a recruitment coordinator as management, public relations, and interpersonal skills.

Responsibilities of the Recruitment Coordinator

1. Organize and carry out the recruitment plan.
2. Maintain records of the screening process listing all patients considered as potential candidates.
3. Identify areas for enhanced recruitment (e.g., alteration of inclusion criteria, adding new sources).
4. Assist the investigator with public relations efforts (e.g., placement of advertisements, choosing media announcements to be made to the public).
5. Train and supervise other staff who deal with patient inquiries. Maintain the accuracy and thoroughness of information provided throughout the recruitment process.
6. Maintain liaison with recruitment sources (e.g., laboratories, industries, lay groups).
7. Review recruitment goals with the investigator and undertake plans to initiate new sources if recruitment wanes.

Research staff in oncology programs often screen patients for several protocols simultaneously. Hunninghake et al. (1982) noted that the Coronary Primary Prevention Trial (CPPT) staff reviewed the patients screened for the Multiple Risk Factor Intervention Trial (MRFIT).

Roles of Other Trial Staff

Although a specific recruitment coordinator might be designated as the individual who is primarily responsible for screening, all other staff affiliated with the trial should be familiar with the screening process and inclusion criteria for the protocol. In trials with large staffs including a recruitment coordinator, a back-up system should be organized so patients can be screened and enrolled even if the designated staff person is unavailable. In small trials, a similar system can be organized that includes staff not directly associated with the trial (e.g., clinical staff) who are trained to serve as a back-up when the trial coordinator is unavailable (e.g., vacationing, ill).

Potential Problems in Staff Liaison with Recruitment Sources

All clinical trial staff and particularly the recruitment coordinator should carefully consider how to best integrate their approach and entry into clinics, organizations, facilities, and other sources of patients so as to cause the least disruption of the usual activities at that source. The impact of having a research team approach what they consider to be a good recruitment source can be disastrous if it is perceived as disruptive, burdensome, or in any way negative. "One should never underestimate the extent to which a seemingly minor change in procedure may be disruptive in a large, smoothly functioning organization" (Stern, 1982). The message provided by Stern is to use caution when recruiting, particularly in laboratories, clinics, or emergency rooms, where research staff might appear to be bothersome to the busy clinical staff. For example, the arrival of several researchers in the primary care area in a busy clinic might be considered intrusive if the clinic nurses are frequently interrupted to answer questions about where files are located, availability of examining rooms or work space, or use of scarce telephones. Similarly, even though permission has been granted to allow clinical trial staff to interview patients, exactly how this process can be integrated into the standard clinic or laboratory routine should be discussed with the clinic or laboratory supervisor and explained to those who work in the area before it is implemented. Research staff should do whatever is necessary to accomplish the goal of assessing suitable trial candidates without interfering with usual hospital or clinic procedures. Staff must beware of the difference between becoming a nuisance while checking emergency department and clinic records, and serving as a resource person who can help other medical staff with referrals to the specialty clinic.

One approach to overcoming this problem is to make clear that the motivation for searching for specific types of patients is to provide patients with a special opportunity to try a new medication at no cost, or to receive free diagnostic testing, or whatever is available as a patient benefit from the trial.

Utilization of Other Personnel

Laboratory technicians, including ECG, EEG, and blood laboratory staff are sometimes excellent sources of patient referrals. They can screen patients during testing or use their knowledge of inclusion criteria to assess eligibility based on a test requisition. House staff and emergency room staff should be educated regularly about the purpose of the trial and the general inclusion criteria. They usually need frequent reminders to refer patients because of their numerous other priorities. Not all staff have the same motivation as the investigator or trial coordinator! Being unfamiliar with clinical research and the need for discipline within a research protocol, they may be reluctant to screen with specific inclusion criteria in mind. Simple referral to the recruitment coordinator or trial staff is adequate.

ROLE OF THE DATA MONITORING COMMITTEE

Large trials initiated in academia often have a data monitoring committee that oversees trial activities and approves changes recommended by the principal investigator or an executive committee. Although the duration of the recruitment period is usually designated in the protocol, the process of recruitment often is not well defined. When the organizers of a trial are faced with a shortage of enrollees, they generally initiate discussions to consider altering inclusion criteria, extend the recruitment period, add more sites, or otherwise maneuver to increase recruitment. The data monitoring committee must usually approve the plans. Requests that require increased funding also must be reviewed by the committee so that they can make a recommendation to the funding agency about the appropriateness of their making an additional investment in the trial.

The central roles of the committee are to assess whether the changes in recruitment are likely to result in randomization of a sufficient number of eligible patients, or whether the trial should be terminated because of inability to achieve statistical power. The sponsor (if any) plays a role in this decision, particularly if extra funding is an issue. As documented in Chapter 6, extensions of time and additions of sites are both costly procedures. The committee can use randomization rates and screening logs to review the effect of various recruitment strategies on the entire trial and on individual sites. In smaller, single-site trials, the investigator must play the devil's advocate in assessing trial status.

RECRUITMENT ISSUES IN COOPERATIVE GROUP CLINICAL TRIALS

Large cooperative group clinical trials usually receive referrals after diagnosis is made by other physicians (e.g., in oncology). Recruitment in these trials is complicated by issues not commonly found in most other clinical trials. The foremost issue is that patient recruitment is not controlled by the principal investigator at each site, but he or she is dependent on cooperation of the staff physicians. The motivation for the referring physicians to collect data is usually low because they do not directly benefit from their efforts, either academically or by authorship. Lee et al. (1980) suggested that a specific staff physician at each site should be responsible for recruitment and made a coinvestigator and author on publications, enhancing this person's sense of participation in the clinical trial. Cancer trials are largely reliant on referrals from other physicians to whom the concept of the clinical trial must be "sold" (Lee and Breaux, 1983). Herson (1980) describes patient registration in cooperative oncology groups where the coordinator must wait and see what patients are referred for screening. These large-scale clinical trial groups have numerous advantages in terms of recruitment over specific trials established to evaluate a specific issue. These advantages stem from the fact that the central staff of the cooperative group remain constant from trial to trial and can apply their experiences to future trials in ways that optimize patient recruitment.

3

Sources of Patients for Clinical Trials

Inclusion criteria in a clinical trial protocol are designated to identify a specific population of patients who are eligible for entry into the trial. The investigator and staff must consider where eligible patients can be found. The major sources of patients for recruitment into a clinical trial are discussed in this chapter.

It is important to distinguish between *sources* of potential patients (i.e., where to look for patients) and *methods* used to approach one or more of those sources (i.e., how to look for patients) in an attempt to enroll patients in a clinical trial. These are separate recruitment elements in a recruitment strategy, and are best understood when viewed separately, although the concepts are not totally independent (see Fig. 1.10). Additional elements of a recruitment strategy include ethical issues, economic issues, and a variety of other topics listed in Table 3.1 (e.g., when, who, how much will it cost?, are there quotas?). When all of these elements are considered and a plan is developed to recruit patients, then that plan constitutes the recruitment strategy (Fig. 3.1).

The investigator is responsible for developing a recruitment strategy to be imple-

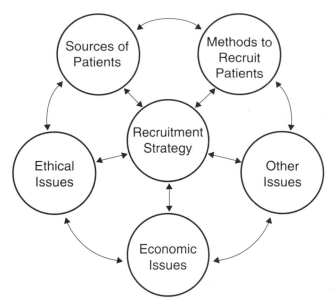

FIG. 3.1. Interactions among all elements of recruitment, as well as the ramifications of each must be considered in developing the core recruitment strategy.

mented alone or with assistance from others. He or she uses various methods to contact the sources of patients, either directly (Fig. 3.2A) or indirectly via other professionals (Fig. 3.2B), or using medical records (Fig. 3.2C).

TYPES OF SOURCES

A summary of various sources of patients is presented in Table 3.2 and an illustration of the distinction among sources, methods, and strategies is given in Table 3.3.

TABLE 3.1. *Major elements of patient recruitment[a]*

1. Sources of patients
2. Methods to use to reach patients
   a. Direct
   b. Indirect
3. Ethical issues
4. Economic issues
5. Staff to conduct recruitment activities
6. Protocol design and requirements for the trial
7. Protocol inclusion criteria
8. Importance of the trial for investigator, medicine, and science
9. Importance of the trial for patients and their families
10. Competing activities and timing considerations
11. Regulatory issues

[a] Some of these may be minor for a specific trial and others may be major in one or more situations.

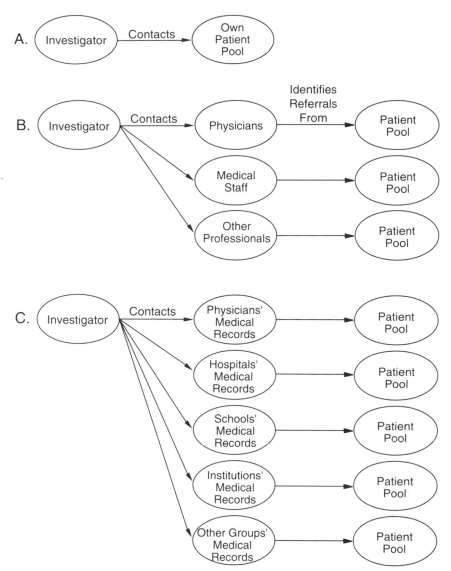

FIG. 3.2. Selected approaches for identifying prospective patients. In panel A, the investigator directly contacts his or her own patients. In panel B, the investigator uses other professionals as the source of patients by requesting referrals. In panel C, the investigator searches medical records of various sources to identify referrals.

The Investigator's Own Medical Practice

The traditional first step in seeking patients for a clinical trial is to look at the investigator's own practice. Whether the investigator is in a primary, secondary, or tertiary care setting; in a health maintenance organization (HMO), preferred provider organization (PPO), or other type of medical environment, his or her own practice is often a potential pool of eligible patients.

Referrals from Medical Sources Within the Community

Clinical trial patients can be recruited from sources within the local medical community. Table 3.2 lists the types of health care providers who should be evaluated as potential sources of patients for a specific trial. This judgment initially should be based on the likelihood that appropriate patients are or will be seen by the medical provider (e.g., physician, emergency medical technician) or at the specific medical facility (e.g., blood laboratory). The interrelationships among sources of patients, methods of recruitment, and the strategies for recruitment are listed in Table 3.3. Sources for special populations based on age are listed in Table 3.4. These include both medical and nonmedical sources.

Referrals from Nonmedical Sources Within the Community

Other groups to consider are nonmedical sources within the community, particularly lay medical organizations. Use of an appropriate method to enlist assistance

TABLE 3.2. *Types of sources used to recruit patients*

A. Referrals from medical sources
    1. Physicians (colleagues and others including private practitioners)
    2. Health care personnel at medical centers and in the community
    3. Prepaid provider organizations [e.g., health maintenance organizations (HMO)]
    4. Emergency rooms
    5. Mobile intensive care units (e.g., ambulances)[a]
    6. Medical laboratories (e.g., blood, ECG, radiology)
B. Referrals from nonmedical sources
    1. Family and friends of patients
    2. Professional societies (e.g., American Cancer Society)
    3. Lay groups (e.g., National Organization of Rare Disorders)
C. Screening medical records
    1. Clinic rosters
    2. HMO members
    3. Nursing home or residential institution
    4. Hospital admissions (using ICD or other codes)
    5. Hospital discharges (using ICD or other codes)
    6. Laboratory requisition or report
    7. Radiology requisition or report
D. Targeted sources
    1. Mailing lists (i.e., specific and general)
    2. School registrants or alumni lists
    3. Catchment areas (e.g., postal or zip code, or district)
    4. Social service or welfare recipients
    5. Specific minority groups
    6. Industrial sites
    7. Worker or union groups
    8. Credit unions
    9. Military groups (e.g., recruits, hospitalized patients, families)
    10. Community groups
E. Self-referral from:
    1. Poster notices
    2. Lectures and talks
    3. Media stories
    4. Advertising
F. General sources
    1. Community screening

[a] See Schroeder (1989) for details of this source.

TABLE 3.3. Interrelationships among strategies, sources, and methods of recruitment

Strategies	Sources	Methods
Use a single method	Medical practice or clinic	Medical
Use multiple methods	Investigator	Physician contacts
Stepwise	Colleagues	Other health care provider
Sequentially	Other physicians	contacts
Simultaneously	HMO, VA hospital	Medical lectures
	Medical facility or laboratory	Nonmedical
	Emergency room	Poster
	Ambulance	Mail
	Blood drawing laboratory	Telepone
	Cardiology laboratory	Advertisements
	Radiology department	News story
	Nonmedical institution	Radio
	Union or worker group	Television
	Factory or private company	Newspaper
	School	Newsletters
	Military	Lectures to groups
	Lay medical interest group	Talk shows
	Clubs and associations	Other
	Community	
	Catchment area	
	Zip code or telephone area	
	Tax or registration list	
	Pension or welfare list	
	Other	

from these groups is an important step in identifying patients who are eligible for the trial.

Referrals from Medical Sources Outside the Community

Regional and national medical organizations are potential sources of referrals to clinical trials (e.g., state medical society, American Academy of Pediatrics). Trials that take place in tertiary care centers benefit from the existing referral network for the medical center that usually reaches beyond the local area.

Referrals from Nonmedical Sources Outside the Community

Regional and national lay organizations and organizations that interact with patients are potential sources of referrals for clinical trials (e.g., American Cancer Society, national organizations for patients and families). Clinical trials for selected diseases can benefit from well organized lay groups that serve as a source of patients outside the local community.

TABLE 3.4. Sources for special populations based on age

Target	Source
Infants, toddlers	Pediatricians, day-care centers
Children	Pediatricians, schools, camps, clubs
Teenagers	Adolescent medical doctors, schools, clubs, athletic groups
Adults	Family doctors, unions, employers, churches, clubs
Elderly	Family doctors, senior centers, churches, clubs, nursing homes

Medical Records as a Source of Patients

Many clinical trials seek to enroll patients who have an established diagnosis or specific characteristic(s) in their medical history. For such trials, examining medical records can be an excellent way to identify eligible patients. Table 3.5 lists the major types of medical records, requisitions, and reports that can serve as sources of information. Reviewing medical records is a screening procedure discussed in Chapter 4.

Patient Registries

Selected medical organizations maintain registries of patients who have a specific diagnosis (e.g., end-stage renal disease patients who are eligible for a kidney transplant). These registries can sometimes be used to identify potential patients for a clinical trial. A more extensive type of computer data base is maintained by some medical centers (e.g., Mayo Clinic); patient records are stored in a system that can retrieve information on all patients who have a specific disease or have undergone specific diagnostic testing. As more medical centers develop data bases, this sophisticated type of chart screening will become a more important source of locating patients for certain clinical trials.

The General Clinical Research Center (GCRC) at Vanderbilt University (Nashville, TN) maintains a directory of protocols seeking patients with uncommon disorders. The data base includes trials ongoing at GCRCs all over the United States. Information in the directory is added to the Rare Disease Data base of the National Organization for Rare Disorders (NORD), put on-line in the NORD Services section of CompuServe, and publicized through *Orphan Disease Update*, a NORD newsletter mailed to more than 30,000 people three times a year. Patient advocate organizations (e.g., gay rights advocates for AIDS, women's rights groups for some obstetric or gynecology trials) also may maintain registries of patients that may be used for clinical trials.

Entire Populations as Sources

A community can be targeted, either as a whole or in segments, to screen for appropriate patients. There are several well-known epidemiological studies (e.g., Framingham, Massachusetts) that have used this approach. Alternatively, a specific group within a general population can be targeted (e.g., people over the age of 70 who are not being treated for diabetes). Table 3.6 lists several target sources that can be used for screening special populations.

Self-Referrals as Sources

When a clinical trial receives significant positive press coverage, and when the problem to be treated is relatively common, self-referrals may be an adequate source of patients for a clinical trial. A variety of methods are available for reaching the community to encourage patients to evaluate their interest in, and eligibility for a clinical trial.

TABLE 3.5. *Types of medical record sources*

1. Charts
   a. Hospital
   b. Clinic
2. Requisitions or reports from tests or procedures
   a. Laboratory services (e.g., chemistry, hematology, urinalysis or other tests)
   b. Radiological services (e.g., x-ray, CT, MRI, ultrasound tests)[a]
   c. Physiological tests (e.g., ECG, cardiovascular stress, EEG, Doppler, pulmonary function tests)
   d. Pathology services (e.g., Papanicolaou smear, biopsy, autopsy)
   e. Surgical services (e.g., procedures, anesthesia)
   f. Therapeutic procedures (e.g., radiation or chemotherapy, physical therapy)
3. Prescriptions
4. Special medical orders (e.g., no food by mouth, physical therapy)
5. Special diet orders
6. Requests for a specific consultation (e.g., ophthalmology, dietetics)

[a] CT, computerized tomography; MRI, magnetic resonance imaging.

TABLE 3.6. *Sources for national recruitment campaigns*

1. Regional labor unions
2. National labor unions
3. National news services
4. Chains of retail stores (e.g., food markets, fast food, pharmacies)
5. Rehabilitation units in hospitals
6. Bank displays
7. Fraternal organizations
8. Utility bills
9. Health maintenance organization (HMO) members

Mass Screening in a Community

Mass screening in a community is sometimes used to recruit patients to a clinical trial. It differs from the other approaches in that it neither targets known medical problems, nor is it passive in expecting eligible candidates to refer themselves for screening. A typical mass screening (1) highlights a specific disease (e.g., high blood pressure, high cholesterol, colon cancer, breast cancer), (2) advertises the availability of testing (usually free) to determine whether the asymptomatic person has the disease, and (3) screens the general population. The usual method for reaching community sources (e.g., testing in health fairs, a booth in a shopping mall, a mobile van equipped for testing) utilizes a marketing approach (see Chapter 4).

PRACTICAL APPROACHES TO USING SOURCES

Characterizing the Sources

To modify the recruitment focus during an ongoing clinical trial as well as to choose sources for a future trial, it is useful to characterize both the usefulness of and the types of patients obtained from each source used thus far. The Lipid Research Clinics Program (1983) characterized the eight types of sources they used in several ways. Table 3.7 describes the productivity of various sources used to recruit patients with elevated cholesterol levels. The decline in numbers of patients who progressed

TABLE 3.7. *Source characteristics*

Source	Volume of Initial contacts	Volume of Entries	Ratio of entries to initial contacts	Effort level required
Blood banks	High	High	Low	Low
Clinical laboratories	Moderate	Low	Moderate	Low
Clinical studies	Low	Moderate	High	Low
Community screenings	High	High	Low	High
Mass mailings	Moderate	Low	Low	Moderate
Mass media	Moderate	Moderate	Moderate	Moderate
Medical referrals	Low	Low	High	Low
Occupational screenings	High	High	Low	High

Reprinted from the Lipid Research Clinics Program (1983) with permission.

TABLE 3.8. *Percentage of eligibles[a] who were excluded because of unwillingness to proceed to the next evaluation visit*

Source	Initial contact	Protocol visit 1	2	3	4	5
Blood banks	36.3	11.6	3.3	4.7	7.7	1.7
Clinical laboratories	44.0	10.2	3.5	3.4	3.9	1.4
Clinical studies	36.2	12.3	2.4	3.5	6.4	0.7
Community screenings	33.9	9.0	3.2	4.0	10.0	2.9
Mass mailings	9.7	8.3	5.4	3.4	5.1	3.6
Mass media	6.8	9.1	3.8	3.2	4.1	1.1
Medical referrals	11.6	10.6	3.9	2.2	1.2	0.0
Occupational screenings	30.6	14.8	5.2	5.0	9.2	1.4
Mean	28.5	11.3	3.8	4.1	6.9	1.5

Reprinted from the Lipid Research Clinics Program (1983) with permission.
[a] Participants who were eligible but unwilling to enter the study.

TABLE 3.9. *Efficiencies (proportion of initial contacts proceeding to the first protocol visit) and proportions of first protocol visits proceeding to entry, categorized by source[a]*

Source	Initial contact to first protocol visit Number of centers	Efficiency (%) Median	Efficiency (%) Range	First protocol visit to entry Number of centers	Percent proceeding Median	Percent proceeding Range
Blood banks	8	2.4	0.9–4.3	7	22.8	12.8–34.2
Clinical laboratories	7	7.8	1.5–12.8	7	21.3	12.9–41.0
Clinical studies	5	35.9	22.2–51.3	5	22.9	16.6–36.1
Community screenings	8	2.9	1.6–3.9	7	19.6	14.4–25.6
Mass mailings	3	4.9	4.5–5.0	3	14.6	14.3–28.0
Mass media	8	10.9	6.2–27.1	7	19.0	14.2–36.1
Medical referrals	9	30.3	27.3–99.2	7	29.0	20.0–38.9
Occupational screenings	9	3.5	1.7–4.2	9	16.7	12.2–30.2

Reprinted from the Lipid Research Clinics Program (1983) with permission.
[a] Data are presented for centers accounting for at least 4.25% of the source total.

TABLE 3.10. *Characteristics of those attending screening visit categorized by recruitment source[a]*

Source	n	(%)	Percent >70 years	Percent male	Percent black	Percent employed	Percent college educated
Senior community sites	12,841	(50)	65	25	29	7	15
SHEP clinic	7,534	(30)	42	47	3	20	41
General community sites	2,508	(10)	55	30	15	14	28
Industry	1,616	(6)	35	44	4	26	23
Medical record/referral	1,003[b]	(4)	46	53	16	19	34
All sources	25,502	(100)	55	35	15	13	25

[a] There were 1,697 persons screened for whom recruitment source is unavailable—these are not included in the table. Reprinted from Vogt et al. (1986) with permission.

[b] Although medical records were reviewed on more than 15,000 persons, few of those reviewed were actually invited to screening. This row refers to those persons originally identified through such reviews, who were subsequently invited to and attended the screening visit.

through eligibility screening visits based on sources is shown in Table 3.8. The efficiency of each source based on the ratio of patients proceeding toward entry is described in Table 3.9. Characteristics of patients recruited from different sources in the SHEP trial are shown in Table 3.10. If the information in these tables is generally known or surmised prior to a trial, the process of choosing sources to use, or at least to evaluate, will be enhanced.

Questions to Pose When Estimating the Number of Patients Available from Each Source

The following questions should be posed and answered before estimating the availability of patients.

How current are the data and records used to create the pool of patients and the degree of their problem?
How likely is it that the individual patients in the pool will be willing to enroll and comply with the protocol requirements?
Are there competing protocols or projects currently underway or during the same time frame that will compete with this trial for patients.

Planning a clinical trial includes an estimate of how useful each source will be in providing appropriate patients. Tables 3.2, 3.4, and 3.6 list many of the sources that can be approached. Given this large variety and number of choices, investigators want to know how and where to look for patients at each possible source they consider, as well as the advantages and disadvantages of each source.

Investigator's Medical Practice

Where and When to Look for Patients in an Investigator's Medical Practice

The first place to look for potential participants for a clinical trial is within the immediate resources of the initiating investigator (i.e., the medical practice and clinic roster). The clinician and staff might start the process by trying to think of specific patients whose medical history is appropriate for the proposed trial. If only a dozen patients are needed (e.g., for a pharmacokinetic trial), this type of instantaneous recall approach might be sufficient to obtain full patient enrollment. A data base that lists patients by diagnosis, type of problem, severity of problem, medications, and other factors is an ideal tool to use in initial screening. More commonly, a chart review is necessary. Starting the search for eligible patients in the group best known to the investigator is appropriate for most trials, but simultaneously searching for patients in other sources is usually necessary. In a VA Cooperative Study of epilepsy (Mattson, 1985), one of the sites leading in recruitment found most of their eligible patients in the investigator's private clinic. When the private clinic was closed, recruitment dropped sharply.

Advantages and Disadvantages of Using the Investigator's Own Practice as a Source of Patients

A clinical trial limited to patients well-known to the investigator has several advantages besides simple convenience. Time is saved by not having to perform extensive screening examinations and chart reviews because most information is available to the investigator. Even a chart review is simplified because seeing the patient's name can trigger recall of substantial medical information that enables the investigator to mentally perform a rough screen without a detailed chart review. However, many investigators overestimate the number of patients who meet inclusion criteria for a trial. This is the origin of Lasagna's Law (see Chapter 1). Depending on the number of patients needed and the desired rate of recruitment, the number of appropriate patients in one's own medical practice is usually inadequate.

Colleague's Medical Practice

Where and When to Look for Patients in a Colleague's Medical Practice

As described above, if a data base is available, that is an ideal primary source to screen for eligible patients. Otherwise, a chart review by the investigator or research staff is needed. It may be possible to meet with colleagues for an informal discussion of potential patients in hopes of eliciting recall of specific patients in the practice who might be eligible. Collaboration-based relationships with colleagues in nearby offices is an appropriate and convenient source to consider in patient recruitment.

Advantages and Disadvantages of Recruiting Patients from a Colleague's Practices

Expanding the screening phase beyond one's own practice into groups of patients well-known to colleagues could fulfill the needs of small or moderate-sized trials. On the other hand, assisting your recruiting efforts may not be a high priority for your colleagues, and waiting for them to consider potential patients or to conduct chart reviews can cause extensive delays. If a sufficient number of referrals are not forthcoming within the period of time agreed at the outset, and the investigator does not wish to jeopardize his or her friendships or professional relationships with colleagues, other sources should be screened. Waiting for someone who has already failed to meet the schedule could delay a trial significantly. Frequent reminders could antagonize the colleague.

Colleagues who see similar types of patients may be able to help each other with special clinical projects. It may be necessary to educate your colleagues that even though it may seem like a nuisance for them to refer patients to someone else's trial, it is anticipated that the courtesy and favor will be reciprocated. Colleagues can serve as informal advisers by helping to review and critique aspects of the trial design or comment on questions that arise during the trial's conduct, whether or not they contribute patients. In fact, asking their advice may encourage them to refer patients.

Medical Center Clinics

Where and When to Look for Patients in a Medical Center Clinic

As the number of patients needed for a trial exceeds the available pool in the investigator's clinic and those of colleagues, the next logical step usually is to seek patients in the local hospital or medical center clinic(s). Screening in specialty medical clinics will identify patients with medical problems in either that general therapeutic area (e.g., cardiology, neurology, psychiatry, rheumatology), or in the specific disease treated (e.g., arthritis, epilepsy, hypertension). Primary care clinics at major medical centers have rosters that include patients who visit the medical center for general medical problems. The choice between specialty and general clinics as a source for patients depends on the likelihood that inclusion criteria would be met by patients seen at each clinic. For example, refractory hypertension is more commonly seen in a hypertension specialty clinic than in a primary care clinic, but newly diagnosed untreated hypertension is seen more frequently in the latter type of clinic.

Most of these clinic sources are duplicated in hospitals and medical centers that are affiliated with but geographically separate from the academic institution that is organizing a trial. The patient population from the affiliated hospitals is usually referred to the major academic medical center for specialized treatment. The informal or formal affiliation between regional medical centers and the academic center may be sufficiently organized to allow access to patients at the remote site. If not, the links can be established or strengthened with staff who are used to working in conjunction with the referral center. Recruitment considerations will influence the types of relationships established, if they do not already exist in the desired format. Gaston et al. (1987) described how to establish access to patients in rural locations by organizing satellite centers 100 miles from the main site, where staff traveled as needed.

Advantages and Disadvantages of Using a Medical Center's Clinic(s) as Sources of Patients

Recruitment of patients who are accustomed to receiving their medical care at a major medical center is eased by the simple transition from one clinic to another during entry into a trial; at the conclusion of the trial, patients are referred back to their original physician. A major concern when screening patients whose primary medical center is distant from the trial site is the ability and willingness of those patients to attend the research clinic. This often serves as a barrier to patient recruitment. If this is anticipated as a problem, establishing a satellite clinic for this trial at the other hospital might help recruitment. If referrals are important for the trial, then the investigator should visit relevant physicians and administrators at each affiliated hospital, discuss the clinical trial and explain the procedures for returning referrals back to their original hospital clinic. Recruitment of patients for a follow-up trial was simplified by using medical center records of patients who had cardiac surgery as children (O'Fallon et al., 1987). Locating patients was accomplished by a careful system of mailings to selected patients.

Private Practice Sources

Where and When to Look for Patients in a Private Practice Source

Since most clinical trials are initiated within academic centers, turning toward private practitioners for referral of trial candidates is a special step that must be taken cautiously. Data base listings by diagnosis are rare, usually making a chart review necessary. Nevertheless, the same approach used with other colleagues might provide recall of the names of selected appropriate patients for screening.

If the investigator has established a relationship with local physicians in private practice, they should be approached early in the recruitment phase. Those who frequently refer difficult to manage patients to the academic medical center may be prepared to provide a list of potential patients. Other physicians or appropriate health care professionals should be informed about the referral procedure in case an appropriate patient appears. It is important that local physicians be informed about the trial before any publicity is disseminated to the general public. If a patient learns about the trial and calls his or her private doctor for advice about whether to participate, it is usually awkward for the physician to be unaware of ongoing research at a nearby medical center. If the investigator approaches the physician after this event has occurred it will be much more difficult to convince the physician to refer other patients.

Some medical contractor organizations have established networks of private clinics and are able to provide sponsors (e.g., pharmaceutical companies) with ready-to-use sources of patients. Because many types of patients are more prevalent in such settings than in hospitals, this approach often is an efficient one to use.

Advantages and Disadvantages of Using Private Practice Sources of Patients

Private practice physicians referred few patients to the Lipid Research Clinics trial, averaging only six patients weekly nationwide (Little, 1982). However, patients referred by their private physician are more likely to meet the trial's eligibility criteria than self-referred patients because of the prescreening that occurs in the referral process. Access to a therapeutic trial often assists physicians with the care of severely ill or refractory patients for whom all standard treatments have failed.

Physicians in private practice are often reluctant to refer patients for research projects primarily because of concern about losing control of the care of that patient, and concern that the patient might not return to their private practice at the termination of the trial. Some of these concerns are economic. Other factors reflect the physician's concern about the general well-being of the individual patient, their continuity of care, and possible concerns about the scientific basis (and possible clinical value) of the specific clinical trial. Recruitment in the Beta Blocker Heart Attack Trial suffered from physician's strong positive and negative attitudes about the use of beta-blockers post-infarction (Goldstein et al., 1987). The physician may be sceptical about the value of the trial, because even if the patient benefits from treatment, they often can remain on therapy only for a relatively short period. Other concerns may relate to the possibility of the patient's receiving placebo instead of active medicine. These issues are discussed in Chapter 2. The Aspirin Myocardial Infarction Study sought post-infarction patients who were in the care of physicians local to the sites. Unfortunately, physician referral was ineffective, resulting in only 16% of enrolled patients. Circumventing the physicians, the trial successfully appealed directly to patients through advertising (Schoenberger, 1987).

Do Physicians Refer Patients Willingly to Clinical Trials?

Relatively few clinical trials have found private practitioners to be a secure source of patient referrals. One of the authors (JAC) and B. DeVries (*personal communication*) have had experiences where sending letters to several dozen local physicians resulted in fewer than a half-dozen calls describing patients, most of whom were clearly ineligible based on information already outlined in the letter. Numerous papers on recruitment activities in large clinical trials have concluded that anticipating a significant portion of patients from referring physicians is a major pitfall to be avoided [e.g., Program on Surgical Control of the Hyperlipidemias (POSCH) (Buchwald et al., 1987); Canadian National Breast Screening Study (Baines, 1984)]. However, the opposite conclusion was reached by Schoenberger (1979), who stated: "The chief lesson that we learned from the Coronary Drug Project was that the required number of participants for a large multicenter clinical trial could successfully be recruited in a reasonable time with support from the medical profession." Each recruitment planning group must assess this issue in the context of their own trial.

Prepaid Health Plans

Where and When to Look for Patients in a Prepaid Health Plan

A prepaid health plan (PHP) should be approached through its management. These organizations commonly use electronic data bases to record a significant amount of information on patients. These data bases can be used to generate lists of patients by diagnosis or possibly by major symptoms. Individual physicians within prepaid health plans should be approached similarly to private practitioners. Contacts with a prepaid health plan should be initiated prior to, or early in the course of the trial: it could take several months to gain permission to recruit patients, and to develop a system of identifying and screening patients.

Advantages and Disadvantages of Using Prepaid Health Plans as Sources of Patients

Prepaid general medical care is based on the premise that increased attention to preventive medicine will reduce the number of serious medical problems requiring intensive medical attention. The cost consciousness focus of these plans might suggest an eagerness to refer patients to qualified physicians who offer free care, so long as it is medically appropriate. Nevertheless, clinical trial investigators have not generally found prepaid health plans to be good sources of patients. This could be partly attributed to the PHPs focus on care for the entire patient, which may translate into reluctance to relinquish part of that care to an outside organization. Various other explanations also are possible.

The conduct of a clinical trial entirely within a small or large (e.g., Kaiser-Permanente, Puget Sound) HMO or other prepaid group is a separate issue. Many trials have been conducted in this way, particularly if the clinical trial is operating within the organization to evaluate part of its standard medical care system. Such an arrangement is not only cost-effective for the group plan, but also provides careful screening and recruitment opportunities throughout its entire population. Sclar et al. (1991) conducted a trial of health education in promoting prescription refill compliance at several independent HMOs around the United States. They used pharmacy and medical records to identify eligible patients. Similar trials are readily conducted in areas with a national health care system (e.g., Canada, United Kingdom) or centralized records (e.g., Mayo Clinic).

Department of Veterans Affairs (VA) Medical Centers

Where and When to Look for Patients in VA Medical Centers

Many academic centers are affiliated with VA medical centers, where a large population of patients is cared for by academic physicians. These patients are an excellent source of recruitment for clinical trials at the academic hospital, particularly if a secondary site can be established at a VA medical center. The close liaison and proximity between university and VA hospital makes the process both efficient and convenient. Single-site and multicenter trials should consider recruiting adult male patients from the population of veterans whenever the demographic scope of the trial allows. If the principal investigator is not affiliated with the VA medical center, a colleague might be able to establish a satellite site by serving as a coinvestigator. Williford et al. (1987) and Collins et al. (1980, 1984) describe a sample of the variety of clinical trials undertaken by the VA Cooperative Studies Program. VA medical centers are usually the sole source for patients in these trials, but arrangements can be made to enroll nonveterans or to collaborate with other medical institutions.

Other federal and state hospitals in the United States can be approached in similar ways. These include Public Health Service hospitals; state hospitals designated for veterans; and mental health, rehabilitation, and residential centers for the physically handicapped and mentally retarded. Comparable groups of hospitals exist in other countries and their advantages and disadvantages must be carefully evaluated on an individual basis.

Advantages and Disadvantages of Using VA Medical Centers as Sources of Patients

Multicenter clinical trials conducted within the VA system can utilize the efficient, centralized communications systems of the VA system to enhance recruitment to clinical trials. Announcements distributed nationally that describe the planning or initiation of special trials often bring large numbers of inquiries from VA hospitals throughout the nation. In addition, the VA Cooperative Studies Program sponsors multicenter clinical trials similar to those organized by the National Institutes of Health (NIH) and industrial sponsors at academic centers. Cooperative study sites usually are geographically scattered across the United States to allow for regional screening of eligible patients. Transport of selected individuals for follow-up at regional VA sites is a convenience for the investigator as well as for a remote site that encourages patients to participate in special research programs.

Single-site trials of all sizes can take advantage of the nearby population of veterans, many of whom are well-known to the investigator or colleagues who attend VA clinics. Similar to prepaid health plans, VA patients usually receive all their medical care at a single medical center, and have a complete medical chart on file at that location. This is in contrast to the fragmented care received by many patients in the United States who are followed by a variety of physicians for individual problems. European practices differ widely, but nationalization of health care delivery makes centralized files more likely.

Utilization of veteran patients can be awkward if the veterans must travel to the academic medical center for follow-up visits. Conversely, if the trial and research clinic are based at the VA medical center, nonveteran patients often are reluctant to attend visits there. In addition, separate informed consents from each patient are needed if two independent institutions are involved in a single clinical trial and one patient attends clinics or undergoes testing at both sites.

Industrial Sites

Where and When to Look for Patients in an Industrial Site

Many large-scale clinical trials, particularly preventive trials, seek patients who are not yet diagnosed with a disorder but whose medical history of risk factors suggests greater than average probability of their developing such a disorder. Such trials must identify large pools of patients to screen to be able to enroll an adequate number of patients. The industrial setting is a prime source for patients who are not severely ill or disabled, as well as for volunteers. The principal investigator must contact various companies in the community to seek their cooperation. If they agree, then it is necessary to arrange for screening of employees, enrollment, and follow-up of subjects entered in a trial. Initial contacts should be at the highest level in the industrial organizations, preferably from the site investigator to the senior medical personnel or chief executive officer at the target company. It is often helpful to describe the benefits of trial participation in terms of free medical benefits for employees.

Advantages and Disadvantages of Using Industrial Groups as Sources of Patients

The Multiple Risk Factor Intervention Trial (MRFIT) trial used industrial screening to take advantage of the convenient logistics in screening large groups of potentially eligible men at the same location (Neaton, 1987). Approximately one-fourth of the initial contacts for the Lipid Research Clinics trials came from private industry occupational screening (Ogilvie et al., 1982) and another 11% came from screening government employees (McKeown, 1982). Arranging screening at an industrial site can be inexpensive to the company if staff are provided by the trial organizers. This minimizes the time commitment and involvement of company medical personnel, although employees usually are providing a large total number of hours to the endeavor. Various accommodations might have to be made with the industry representatives to allow screening on-site, or even for them to allow publicity about the trial on-site. For example, exclusion of people of certain ages or sex might initially appear to be discriminatory to some individuals. General screening of all employees, but selection only of appropriate age and sex mandated eligible candidates might circumvent the potential problem of bias against ineligible candidates who do not have the opportunity for a free medical test or other screening benefits. Nonetheless, this approach is not advocated. An open and honest statement of the trials's objective(s) should satisfy employees about the basis for and the motives for patient selection. An interesting approach to eliciting greater worker cooperation would be to include their spouses in the screening. An example might be the inclusion of spouses of male employees for mammography screening that would otherwise be limited to female employees. To avoid discrimination against female employees, industrial screening in one trial allowed screening and reporting of cholesterol levels for women even though inclusion in the trial was limited to men. The advisability of this approach may be questioned.

Unions or Workers Groups

Where and When to Look for Patients in a Union or Workers Group

An alternative to liaison with the company executives, as described in the previous section, is to work with union or workers group representatives. The recruitment appeal can be made on the basis of a free medical benefit with the possibility of a selected group of members receiving free medical care during the course of the trial. This is in addition to the perceived benefit of generosity and altruism of the union group toward medical science.

Advantages and Disadvantages of Using Union or Workers Groups as Sources of Patients

Unions and employee groups often work at multiple companies within a community. The economy of scale is apparent if enlisting the aid of a single union allows access into several companies for screening (Neaton, 1987). Some screening programs must function during off-duty hours (e.g., lunch break, before or after shifts) so as not to interfere with the company's work schedule. Workers may also need special accommodations for follow-up appointments that do not interfere with their work schedules.

Military Populations

Where and When to Look for Patients Using Military Sources

Individual military bases or hospitals as well as military-wide appeals can be used to recruit patients and volunteers for clinical trials. Sites that are in the vicinity of a military installation can work directly with base headquarters to establish screening on-site. Initial contact should be made at the highest level (e.g., from the chairman or site investigator to the base commander), with subsequent liaison established at the base hospital or dispensary. Depending on the nature of the trial, arrangements can be made to screen not only active duty military personnel but also their dependents and any retired personnel who visit the base. These groups expand the age range and gender distribution beyond that of a typical military population. Asymptomatic patients, or relatively well patient groups, are likely to be found in the military. Military hospitals also have large numbers of patients with diseases not commonly found in the United States (e.g., tropical diseases) because of troop exposure to disease in other countries and relatively centralized hospitalization inside the United States after troops are returned home.

Clinical trials conducted within Department of Defense hospitals can utilize the unique resources of a large military population to screen potential patients. Working with Department of Defense headquarters, it is possible to solicit a request to certain bases for volunteers or patients who might be willing to participate in a trial. Such volunteers might be transported to a central research facility (e.g., Walter Reed Army Medical Center or the Bethesda Naval Hospital) for trials that require special facilities. Other trials might be conducted at multiple regional military bases, similar to the conduct of multicenter clinical trials in the civilian community.

Advantages and Disadvantages of Using Military Sources of Patients

Most active-duty military staff are in excellent health, so that few will be eligible for clinical trials except as normal volunteers. However, epidemiological studies might find this population to be a good source. If the military administration encourages participation in the trial, participants may be allowed to take the necessary time for clinic visits during the workday. On the other hand, military personnel move frequently, preventing long-term follow-up at a specific site. Military recruits may be used as a cohort during their training, particularly when it is important to have relatively complete control on factors such as diet, exercise, and life-style. Recruits are housed together and a large number can undergo standard procedures or exposures. They can be used to evaluate an antidiarrheal, antitussive, or various other medicines, for conditions commonly observed in crowded housing conditions.

A Community

Where and When to Look for Patients in a Community

Large-scale clinical trials that seek to enlist thousands of patients often have to appeal to entire communities to screen adequate numbers of patients. The community can be approached in a variety of ways, including telephone, mail, radio, newspaper, and television. Telephone call appeals can be established by designated area code or geographic location in order to cover every family in that section or may use a random selection of telephone numbers. Similarly, mail screening can cover every household in a zip code or specified area, or cover a randomly selected subpopulation. The Lipid Research Clinics used community screening to achieve a high volume of initial contacts although this approach required a high level of effort by staff (Melish, 1982). Schrott and Meredith (1982) described the experiences of the Iowa site to approach small and large communities.

Screening can be defined according to demographic characteristics of the community. For example, a search for hypertensive black males might be done in one area of a community, whereas a mixed population of white and black patients of both sexes may be sought using a more general appeal. A commonly used approach is to establish booths in shopping centers or mobile vans to attract casual observers to come in for a screening interview or blood test. The High Risk Utah Pedigree Trial conveniently screened the local Utah population using the detailed genealogical files available in the community (Williams, 1987). Recruitment of an elderly population was effectively accomplished by approaching residents of retirement villages with leaflets and posters, followed by lectures on the purpose of the trial (Silagy et al., 1991).

Advantages and Disadvantages of Using Community Sources of Patients

Recruiting from a community for a large trial usually requires a major commitment of staff and sufficient funds for advertising, telephoning, mailing, and other methods to contact and screen potential participants. On the other hand, specific community sources might easily reach an appropriate population for even small trials. For example, self-help and support groups as well as lay organizations include patients or their families so that a single contact with the group could provide a high yield of eligible patients for a trial. The Hypertension Detection and Follow-up Program focused recruitment efforts on communities using entire geographical areas (e.g., census tracts, housing projects) or the random sample of all census tracts in an area (Ford et al., 1987). This approach resulted in screening 85–95% of enumerated people aged 30–69 years.

Island Populations

Groups of people living on isolated islands may represent an ideal source of patients for a clinical trial, particularly if a prophylaxis or treatment trial is to be conducted on a prevalent disease. The island's population could be divided into two or more groups, or alternatively the results of the islanders could be compared with those of a control island's population. A third possibility is to perform a community trial of all island inhabitants. An excellent example of this last approach is the study conducted by Taplin et al. (1991). These investigators studied the prevalence of scabies in Kuna Indians in the San Blas islands of the Republic of Panama for more than 3.5 years, before and after treating the population with 5% permethrin cream (Elimite). Their results illustrate well how outside influences (e.g., invasion of Panama by forces from the United States) influenced the prophylactic protection of their study population. Permission for the study was given by (1) the village council, (2) the local health committee, and (3) the regional director of health.

Prisoners

Prisoners are no longer a suitable source of volunteers or patients because of their inability to provide a freely given informed consent. Nonetheless, there may be special circumstances under which prisoners could participate in a clinical trial. These trials must be discussed with an Ethics Committee/IRB on a case by case basis.

CRITERIA FOR CHOOSING SOURCES OF PATIENTS

There are a number of general factors to consider prior to choosing the specific sources for patient recruitment.

1. Size of referral population
2. Geographical location relative to trial site
3. Reputation of the individual or institution
4. Prior experience with specific source
5. Willingness of the leaders at the source to assist with patient recruitment
6. Competing trials being conducted or planned at the source
7. Liability issues for the source

The choice of sources is dependent on the methods used in a trial, ethical issues that arise, economic questions, plus a large number of other practical factors (e.g., importance of the trial, availability of staff, trial design). Using the published literature of characteristics and yields of various sources may be informative, particularly if the trial design and population are similar. Various characteristics are shown in Tables 3.7 to 3.10. Yield from the study whose sources were shown in Tables 3.7 to 3.9 are given in Table 3.11. All of these elements must be considered *in toto* when the question of choosing sources is addressed. This topic is discussed more extensively in Chapters 7 and 8.

Silagy et al. (1991) used three sources for elderly patients for an aspirin trial. Although the recruitment yield was highest from general practice sources (18.2%) compared to electoral rolls (5.7%), and community-based (3.4%) sources, the community-based approach was most efficient in terms of staff time (13.3 hours per

TABLE 3.11. *Recruitment outcomes by source*

Source	Number of				Entries
	Individual sources	Initial contacts	First protocol visits	Entries	Initial contacts %
Blood banks	19	113,020	2705	574	0.51
Clinical laboratories	102	12,234	958	217	1.77
Clinical studies	28	4,869	1589	438	9.00
Community screenings	376	90,151	2583	535	0.59
Mass mailings	28	26,355	1252	212	0.80
Mass media	125	19,270	1933	437	2.27
Medical referrals	21[a]	1,139	555	161	14.14
Occupational screenings	1135	160,307	5057	904	0.56
Other/unknown[b]	23	9,334	1381	332	3.56
Total	1857	436,679	18,013	3810	Mean 0.87

Reprinted from the Lipid Research Clinics Program (1983) with permission.
[a] At each LRC, referrals from individual private physicians were reported together as coming from a single source.
[b] One LRC combined several sources in reporting its data. These are included in the category "Other/Unknown," and represent 3,969 initial contacts, 584 first protocol visits, and 169 entries.

TABLE 3.12. *How to select a clinical trial site based on its potential for recruiting patients*

1. Contact potential sites (twice as many as are needed)
2. Request an estimate of the number of patients followed and how many might be eligible
3. Divide the number of potential eligible patients by ten to estimate the number likely to be screened
4. Ask the site to perform an informal pilot screening for 3 months
5. Divide the number of patients identified during the pilot screening by five to estimate the number likely to be entered
6. Review the date of diagnosis of patients identified in the pilot screening. If all were previously diagnosed, assume a limited pool
7. Consider the proportion of newly diagnosed patients to represent the number of new referrals that will be found after the core pool is screened
8. Ask the investigators about ongoing or planned participation in other trials that seek similar patients
9. Select sites based in part on overall patient pool, likely number of eligible patients, and the mix of core patients and new referrals

enrollee) compared to electoral rolls (24 hours) or general practice (18 hours) sources. Their pilot trial found that retirement villages were the most cost-effective sources for identifying appropriate elderly patients.

The selection of clinical trial sites for a multicenter trial depends on many factors (e.g., experience and interest of the investigator, work load of investigators and potential competing trials, availability of skilled staff). The size of the catchment area is not necessarily a key factor in determining the pool of eligible patients; some sites in small cities enjoy a large referral population because of their special expertise. Instead of making judgments based on the local census, the potential for recruiting patients for a specific clinical trial can be estimated using the steps listed in Table 3.12.

4

Methods for Recruiting Patients

In the early days of clinical trials (approximately 1948 to 1970), investigators would write a protocol and then begin to think about how to enroll patients. A specific recruitment strategy was rarely designed in advance of the trial; different approaches to recruiting patients were usually tried as needed and as ideas about recruitment occurred to the investigators or staff. This type of random approach to patient recruitment is still widely practiced, but the state-of-the-art has progressed far beyond this "primitive" unplanned approach. This chapter describes various methods that may be incorporated into the recruitment strategy. The methods include seeking referrals from physicians and nonphysicians, advertising, and community screening. As discussed in Chapter 7, the plan for a specific trial may be to use: (1) a single method; (2) a series of methods in a sequential manner; (3) a stepwise, cumulative addition of methods; or (4) multiple methods simultaneously for patient recruitment. For example, the Lipid Research Clinics Program (1983) used a progressive cumulation of methods. Beginning with medical referrals from local physicians and laboratories, the various sites later progressed to mass screenings. The specific methods used included mass media appeals, blood bank donor screenings, occupational industrial screenings, and community screenings, used additively in a stepwise manner (see Figs. 7.20 and 7.22).

Many methods described in this chapter may be utilized more efficiently if various aspects utilize computers. The use of computers in recruitment varies so greatly between trials, and even as used by various sites in a single trial, that these approaches are not generally described in this book. Johnson and Lieford (1990) discuss this topic.

This chapter also includes a discussion of how to choose methods and how to use the methods chosen. Recruitment methods used in many large clinical trials are

TABLE 4.1. *References to specific methods of recruitment[a]*

A. Medical methods	
Recruitment in a nursing home	Lipsitz et al., 1987
Using pharmacists for postmarketing survey	Facklam et al., 1990
Using pharmacists for postmarketing survey	Borden and Lee, 1982
Inpatient screening of very sick patients	Koenig et al., 1989
Medical records	Quick et al., 1989
Blood bank referrals to the CPPT	Stern, 1982
Clinical trials as a source of referrals for the CPPT	Hunninghake et al., 1982
Clinical laboratories referrals to the CPPT	Little, 1982
Inpatient screening for the AMIS trial	Schoenberger, 1987
Inpatient screening for the BHAT	Goldstein et al., 1987
Inpatient screening for the TIMI trial	Knatterud and Forman, 1987
Clinic screening for the POSCH trial	Buchwald et al., 1987
Clinic screening of geriatric patients	Williams and Hunt, 1987
Clinic screening for the NOTT	Williams et al., 1987
B. Mailing methods	
Mail invitations for the SHEP trial	Petrovich et al., 1991
Mail questionnaire for self-eligibility	Albanes et al., 1986
Mail and telephone follow-up	Baines, 1984
Mail less effective than advertisement or poster	Burns et al., 1990
Mass mailings for the CPPT	McDearmon and Bradford, 1982
Mail follow-up trial	O'Fallon et al., 1987
Mass mailing for prevention trial (HPT)	Borhani et al., 1989
C. Telephone methods	
Toll-free telephone number	Parkinson Study Group, 1989
Ask to donate blood	Ford and Wallace, 1975
Community screening for the CARDIA trial	Hughes et al., 1987
D. Media: Television, radio, newspaper methods	
Announcement for cancer chemoprevention	Arnold et al., 1989
Media announcement for CPPT	Levenkron and Farquhar, 1982
E. Paid advertisement methods	
Self-assessment advertisement for symptomatic volunteers	Brauzer and Goldstein, 1973
Self-assessment advertisement for symptomatic volunteers	Covi et al., 1979
High yield from advertisement	Burns et al., 1990
Advertise for symptomatic volunteers	Mitchell et al., 1988
F. Community-screening methods	
Multiple types of screening for the CPPT	Melish, 1982
Screen entire community for the CPPT	Schrot and Meredith, 1982
Private industry occupational screening for the CPPT	Ogilvie et al., 1982
Government employee occupational screening; CPPT	McKeown, 1982
Various community screenings for the MRFIT trial	Neaton et al., 1987
Household screening for the HDFP trial	Ford et al., 1987
Leaflets and talks at retirement villages	Silagy et al., 1991

[a] Abbreviations are described in Table 1.4.

discussed in detail in the literature (Table 4.1). Chapter 7 discusses recruitment methods in the context of a specific recruitment strategy, whereas only the methods are discussed in this chapter.

INFORMING PHYSICIANS DIRECTLY ABOUT A TRIAL

The sequence of activities undertaken to inform physicians about a trial is based on the degree of convenience and simplicity desired. Even small trials often are open to patients who are not part of a principal investigator's private clinic. Informal and formal discussions with colleagues within the investigators subspecialty is the simplest way to communicate the general entry criteria for the project and solicit referrals. It is often possible to learn about a patient who may be appropriate for a trial during the time a clinic is ongoing and the patient is being seen by a colleague. Screening as well as an invitation to participate in the trial is sometimes accomplished in the same day. When colleagues are too busy to review patient histories during their practice hours, the investigator or an assistant can review charts of patients scheduled for the next day, so that files can be tagged to remind the colleague that this patient might be a potential candidate for a specific protocol. It is important to note that most colleagues who are interested in clinical research, have their own priorities and tend to be too busy to remember the trial and its inclusion criteria, or to take the time to help a colleague enroll patients, particularly during the hectic clinic schedule. It is important for soliciting investigators to provide staff and other assistance to their colleagues to minimize their burden when making referrals for the trial.

One must determine whether recruiting activities that go beyond the immediate subspecialty area and into general medical departments or primary care areas are likely to identify a sufficient number of patients. If so, personal discussions with every potential referring physician are desirable; thus the enthusiasm and commitment of the principal investigator will be demonstrated. Introduction of the trial coordinator, referring centers, and physicians, is important. It enables that staff person (e.g., recruitment coordinator) to review charts in other clinics subject to the approval of appropriate physicians and possibly administrators. Recruitment problems are likely to arise if the trial coordinator visits various clinics and requests permission to search charts without the investigator having first discussed the issue with other physicians or section chiefs.

Use of Lecture Presentations to Medical Staff

Various types of lectures, seminars, and presentations are used in all types of medical practice, and some of these offer opportunities to introduce professionals to a clinical trial. This is a notoriously poor recruitment strategy but useful to inform peers, particularly for small clinical trials. Investigators may wish to participate in one or more of these lectures or presentations to seek referrals, but their motivation could be strictly educational. This latter motive is most common after a trial is completed and the results are being disseminated. In a talk, present the background and objectives of the proposed (or ongoing) trial, the anticipated medical benefits to patients, and the potential for advancing clinical and scientific knowledge. This presentation may be given formally at grand rounds, departmental seminars, professional meetings, or at medical society meetings. Informally, the presentation may be given at almost any meeting. The message may reach many potential referral sources in addition to those in attendance at formal medical meetings because of the wide publicity usually given to the title of the talk in lecture schedule bulletins at medical centers, agendas of the professional society, or medical society newsletters.

Special brief lectures should be arranged in many departments. For example, emergency department and primary care clinic staff may hold weekly or monthly conferences to discuss staff and quality assurance issues. Request time to present a brief overview of the trial to the staff. It is often appropriate to bring the trial coordinator who may help describe the chart reviews desired, so that interested individuals will know who to request further information from, and to whom referrals should be made (in addition to the investigator).

How to Approach Physicians and Other Medical Personnel About Patient Referrals

1. The investigator should contact the other physicians and the chief of the medical department in which recruiting is proposed. Initial contacts can be made by visit or by letter. Letters should be followed by a telephone call or visit by the investigator. The investigator should personally establish lines of communication at the senior level of each source to be used.

2. The initial contact should include a brief outline of the trial with emphasis on desired patient characteristics (i.e., inclusion criteria).

3. The investigator should explain how recruitment may (or will) impinge on the daily routine at the prospective source (e.g., how much time and effort is involved, what type of interference with the office or laboratory routine is likely to occur).

4. The investigator should explain the scope of any assistance (in terms of staff) that would be provided to the referring physician for recruiting activities. Introduce the trial coordinator (if any) at this time, explaining his or her role. Indicate any benefits to the referring physician as a result of his or her participation.

5. Ask the referring physician or medical staff to designate a specific contact person (e.g., medical office staff member, laboratory head, appointment secretary, nurse, technician) for the investigator or trial coordinator to use as a communications link.

6. A description of the clinical trial and the types of patients desired for referral should be given to as many staff as possible at each recruitment source. Discussions about the trial should be planned to occur during changes of shift for hospital staff, and at regular staff meetings. Reminder posters for the bulletin board or a procedures manual left at each referral source are useful supplements. Describe the types of patients needed for the trial to colleagues, interns, residents, nurses, and other professional staff who may come in contact with the types of patients desired.

7. Write letters to colleagues and other physicians in the community describing the types of patients sought. Three examples of letters sent to physicians requesting referrals are shown in Fig. 4.1.

8. Prepare a poster (approximately 25 × 40 cm), geared to potential patients listing essential characteristics desired in patients referred to the trial. List whom to contact and how (e.g., telephone numbers to call 24 hours a day). List the investigator and the research staff who can answer questions about the trial. Post

Text continues on p. 68.

DEPARTMENT OF VETERANS AFFAIRS
Medical Center
950 Campbell Avenue
West Haven CT 06516

In Reply Refer To:

April 12, 1991

John Smith, M.D.
Department of Neurology
Yale University School of Medicine
333 Cedar Street
New Haven, CT 06510

Dear John,

Dr. Mattson and I are initiating a study of compliance with antiepileptic drug regimens. You have heard us talk about a special pill bottle with a microprocessor in the cap that records the date and time of each opening. Data can be retrieved from MEMS units (Medication Event Monitor System) using a specially adapted computer. Data are displayed on screen and on a paper print-out in two forms:
1. Calendar format of the number of doses taken daily
2. Listing of the dates and times of every dose.

We would like to recruit patients to use the MEMS bottles longterm. All that is required is to use only the MEMS bottle for all doses and to visit me at the VA Hospital at months 1, 2, 3, 4, 6, and quarterly thereafter. Visits last 10 minutes with *no* waiting. To benefit the patient, drug levels will be done at no cost. For your information, attached is a copy of the consent form that I will use.

All I ask of you is to discuss with patients the concept of monitoring doses to see how their compliance pattern relates to seizure or side effects, and to learn how to improve their compliance. Please give patients my card and ask them to call me for further information and an appointment. I will pick up from there. Of course, I will let you know how your patients are doing.

Thank you for your assistance with our research.

Sincerely,

Joyce A. Cramer
Project Director
A Epilepsy Research

FIG. 4.1A–C. Three examples of letters sent to physicians requesting referrals for a clinical trial. The last enclosed a plastic card to serve as a reminder (C1 and C2). Such plastic, paper, or plastic-coated cards are commonly used, sometimes with calendars attached. All are reprinted with permission.

Figure continues on next page.

𝔇uke 𝔘niversity 𝔐edical 𝔆enter

DURHAM, NORTH CAROLINA 27710

DEPARTMENT OF SURGERY   TELEPHONE (919) 684-6133
BOX 3873

Dear Colleague:

The Duke University Multidisciplinary Breast Oncology Clinic seeks patients who are at high risk for breast cancer by virtue of a strong family history to participate in a protocol designed to more accurately assess risk. Several studies reveal that women with a family history who also have atypical epithelial hyperplasia on breast biopsy have a life-long risk for breast cancer as high as 50%. Although these studies are retrospective reviews of breast biopsies done for benign disease, the finding of atypical epithelial changes is a potent risk factor. In contrast, if *no* such changes are found, breast cancer risk is much less. We propose to offer women with strong family histories a blind incisional breast biopsy in a prospective study of cancer risk. The institutional review process at Duke has granted permission to perform biopsies after informed consent. Although third parties carriers will be billed, total coverage cannot be guaranteed. The following women will be eligible for this study:

1. **Women over the age of 39**

2. **Family history of documented breast cancer in — and only in — mothers, sisters, and daughters**

3. **Primary relatives with breast cancer must have been diagnosed prior to their 55 year birthday**

4. **Patient willingness to submit to biopsy under local anesthesia and after informed consent to participate**

The biopsy will be done under local anesthesia in the operating room through a one inch incision in the upper-outer quadrant of either breast. Pathology review will be performed in a three tier system which will include routine review and reporting, specialized review by Dr. Allan Tucker who is our clinic pathologist, and outside review by Dr. David Page at Vanderbilt University. This process will take approximately two weeks and results will be given to patients and their physicians. The Multidisciplinary Breast Clinic will offer patients in depth counselling about risk of breast cancer and options available to reduce risk. Under most circumstances, we have discouraged prophylactic surgery as a means to reduce risk but will assess and recommend on a case-by-case basis.

If you have questions, wish a copy of our protocol, or have referrals, please call me directly at 919-684-6133. The Multidisciplinary Breast Clinic number is 919-684-2995.

Sincerely,

B   J. Dirk Iglehart, M.D.

FIG. 4.1. *Continued.*

𝔇uke 𝔘niversity 𝔐edical ℭenter
DURHAM, NORTH CAROLINA
27710

DIVISION OF NEUROLOGY

P. O. BOX 2900
TELEPHONE (919) 684-5963
(919) 684-6274
FAX   (919) 684-6514

May 10, 1991

Dear Colleague:

On April 1, 1991, we began a new study to investigate the use of tissue plasminogen activator (TPA) in patients with acute stroke. This is a very important study, since brain reperfusion has the potential to reverse many of the deficits caused by an acute ischemic stroke. However, to be safe and successful, this therapy must be started within **6 hours** of symptom onset.

The aim of this study is to determine the safe and effective dose of TPA for acute stroke patients. The enclosed study card has a summary of the inclusion and exclusion criteria. All patients undergo an angiogram before and after the administration of TPA to determine if the occluded vessel has reopened following therapy. Patients are then admitted to the Stroke Acute Care Unit and carefully monitored for neurologic changes and any bleeding complications.

Since most stroke patients do not seek medical care immediately, we need the help of our colleagues in ascertaining patients immediately after they present to their local hospitals, clinics, and emergency rooms. The enclosed study card and this letter include toll-free numbers that can be called for referrals or questions. A study neurologist is available 24 hours a day to assist in screening patients for the study.

The study will pay for the special tests associated with the protocol, but it will not pay for the standard costs of being hospitalized due to a stroke. When a patient completes the protocol, we will certainly send them back to the referring physician with a full report. We wish to maintain excellent relations with our referring physicians, and will do everything possible to make transfers and communications proceed smoothly.

Thank you for your cooperation and assistance with this very important study. If you have any questions, please do not hesitate to call me.

PATIENT REFERRAL
DUKE LIFE-FLIGHT: IN STATE — 1-800-362-5433
OUT OF STATE — 1-800-524-5433
OR
CALL DUKE 919-684-8111, BEEPER 7025

Yours very truly,

Mark J. Alberts, MD
Assistant Professor
Division of Neurology
Director, Stroke Acute Care Unit

C

FIG. 4.1. *Continued.*

Figure continues on next page.

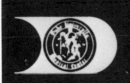

THE DUKE STROKE ACUTE CARE UNIT
announces a new clinical trial
"TISSUE PLASMINOGEN ACTIVATOR IN ACUTE STROKE"
sponsored by Burroughs Wellcome, Co.

PURPOSE

To evaluate the safety and efficacy of various doses of tissue plasminogen activator (TPA) given intravenously following angiography to patients with acute thrombotic or thromboembolic stroke.

INCLUSION CRITERIA

— Over 21 and under 80 years old
— Acute stroke within **8 hours** of expected treatment time
— Clinical syndrome consistent with large vessel thrombotic or embolic stroke
— No significant neurologic impairment prior to the new stroke
— Normal PT and PTT

EXCLUSION CRITERIA

— Significantly altered level of consciousness
— Complete hemiplegia, forced eye deviation, or locked-in syndrome
— Pregnancy or within 28 days post-partum
— Prior stroke within 6 weeks of new stroke, or prior intracerebral hemorrhage
— Malignant hypertension (BP>200/120 on 3 readings)
— Septic embolus
— Recent surgery, trauma, GI/GU hemorrhage, inflammatory bowel disease, or coagulopathy

FOR REFERRAL OF PATIENTS OR QUESTIONS, PLEASE CALL:

DUKE LIFE FLIGHT
in state   **1-800-362-5433**
out-of-state   **1-800-524-5433**

DUKE LIFE CARE
in state   **1-919-681-2273**
out-of-state   **1-800-422-3393**

— OR —

C1

FIG. 4.1. *Continued.*

66

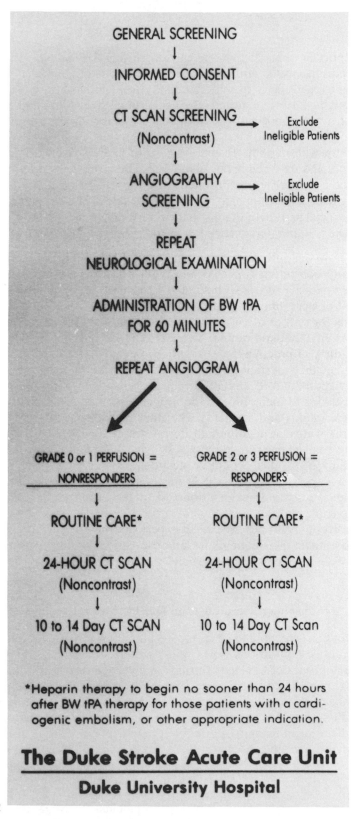

GENERAL SCREENING
↓
INFORMED CONSENT
↓
CT SCAN SCREENING ——→ Exclude
(Noncontrast)   Ineligible Patients
↓
ANGIOGRAPHY ——→ Exclude
SCREENING   Ineligible Patients
↓
REPEAT
NEUROLOGICAL EXAMINATION
↓
ADMINISTRATION OF BW tPA
FOR 60 MINUTES
↓
REPEAT ANGIOGRAM

GRADE 0 or 1 PERFUSION =	GRADE 2 or 3 PERFUSION =
NONRESPONDERS	RESPONDERS
↓	↓
ROUTINE CARE*	ROUTINE CARE*
↓	↓
24-HOUR CT SCAN	24-HOUR CT SCAN
(Noncontrast)	(Noncontrast)
↓	↓
10 to 14 Day CT SCAN	10 to 14 Day CT Scan
(Noncontrast)	(Noncontrast)

*Heparin therapy to begin no sooner than 24 hours
after BW tPA therapy for those patients with a cardi-
ogenic embolism, or other appropriate indication.

The Duke Stroke Acute Care Unit

Duke University Hospital

C2

FIG. 4.1. *Continued.*

notices in important areas at the referral source (e.g., in heavily trafficked areas, near chart recording areas) after permission to do so is obtained.

9. Frequent repetition is usually necessary to maintain awareness of the types of patients sought. Posters fade into the background over time, and even the daily appearance of a trial coordinator may no longer be associated with patient recruitment.

10. Follow-up with periodic telephone calls to likely sources to determine their levels of activity and also their levels of interest. These calls may provide information that the source is unlikely to be productive.

11. In some trials it is essential to be prepared to screen and enroll patients quickly.

12. Provide a call or note of thanks to the referrer. A standard letter may be stored in a word processor and personalized with the referrer and patient names.

No matter how well-intentioned referring physicians and other medical staff are, they have many competing concerns and other priorities that diminish their motivation to refer patients to trials conducted by others. Many people simply forget. Bulletin board posters quickly blend in with the wallpaper and lose their stimulus; reminder cards for staff to use are quickly lost. House staff respond well to positive stimuli such as gifts, but still require frequent reminders. It is much easier to follow one's usual course of practice than to bother to evaluate for eligibility (even superficially) a patient they are talking to, to briefly describe the trial, and then to refer the patient to appropriate trial staff. Frequent reminders and often incentives are generally necessary to maintain the recruitment issue at a sufficient level in their minds. Medical interns and residents who interact with patients in the emergency room and in the wards are a potential referral source for some trials, but these staff are unlikely to remember protocol details or have sufficient motivation to refer patients. For many of them, it would be desirable if referred patients went off their service and to a special unit or ward. If this is not done, then the protocol requirements for special tests and examinations guarantees that many staff will not refer anyone to the trial.

Dicker and Kent (1990) describe their experiences in approaching physicians for permission to contact their patients for an observational study. Permission was denied to 8% of 243 subjects. Their article reprints the letter they sent requesting permission.

Expanding Recruitment to Outside Medical Centers

When expanding screening to other medical facilities, private practice physicians, and group practices of various types (e.g., preferred-provider organizations), the same general approach of having the principal investigator initially contact the chief of the organization should be followed. Again, short presentations about the nature and importance of the clinical trial to staff are most appropriate. Some private physicians attend grand rounds in a medical center and might hear of the trial at a lecture there, and others might listen to a brief overview while on rounds in the hospital or at medical society meetings.

Model Clinic Format

The Program on Surgical Control of Hyperlipidemia (POSCH) (Buchwald et al., 1987) developed a model clinic format after the failure of recruitment by physician referral. The model clinic recruitment approach can be outlined in ten phases.

1. Identify the population of patients desired.
2. Determine the potential patient population in the catchment area.
3. Identify patients in the hospitals who meet the eligibility criteria and the names of volunteers obtained from media efforts.
4. Establish a primary physician contact especially for hospital-based patients and obtain permission to contact the patient.
5. Screen for eligibility and subject interest by telephone contact.
6. Log and assign referral numbers to individuals who agree to attend an appointment for further screening.
7. Conduct comprehensive screening in the research clinic after review of medical records and analysis of mailed-in cholesterol sample.
8. Determine final eligibility for all patients.
9. Perform a secondary screening for eligibility of patients.
10. Conduct randomization.

These investigators stress the importance of using a standardized approach at each site of a multicenter trial (e.g., the model clinic format) rather than allowing autonomy at each local clinic, although this standardized approach is not suitable for all clinical trials.

Reiterating the Recruitment Message

1. Weekly verbal reminders to referring physicians and medical sources help counteract the natural tendency to forget about the trial. Care must be taken to do this in a positive, nonjudgmental tone or the recipient of the message may become upset and purposely neglect the trial or decline to refer any more patients.

2. In long-term trials lasting several years, the process of engaging the attention of resident physicians, laboratory staff, should be repeated periodically (e.g., at least annually) or whenever the professional staff change (e.g., residents change in July in the United States).

3. Food may be used as a positive association factor for the clinical trial. An occasional box of cookies or candy will draw medical staff to the trial coordinator who can then reiterate the recruitment message. Sandwiches, pizza, or snack foods can be considered if the budget allows.

4. Distribute small purse or wallet-sized cards to interns and residents that briefly list essential information about the trial (e.g., inclusion criteria, telephone numbers).

5. The research assistant or trial coordinator should identify himself or herself by the name of the specific clinical trial in contacts with medical personnel, patients, and patient families to keep the topic of the trial at the forefront of discussions.

6. If a logo or acronym can be devised for the trial (Fig. 4.2), the investigator and research staff should wear a button or tag with that identifier whenever walking through the hospital. This logo should be added to posters, stationery, and other materials that will create more publicity. It also serves to display an image of professionalism about the trial that is greater than simple handwritten or typed notices.

7. Mail or distribute cards to put in Rolodex telephone indexes. Each card should have the disease or trial name at the top, depending on whichever is easier to remember. Also include the names and telephone numbers of the investigator(s) and trial coordinator. This card may be printed in a bright color.

8. Print information about the trial on pads of paper or sticky sheets and give pads to physicians for their use.

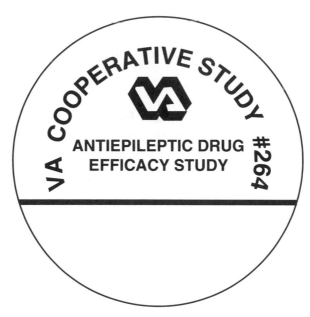

FIG. 4.2. Example of a clinical trial logo. The design was imprinted on buttons (2 inch diameter) that were worn by trial staff while talking with potential sources in the hospital and during clinic visits with patients. Each staff person's name and title was typed on a label affixed to the button to serve as an identifier for the trial. The logo was also used in newsletters and posters.

APPROACHING PATIENTS ABOUT ENROLLMENT IN A CLINICAL TRIAL

Approaching Patients Directly

The general steps used to approach patients can be systematized, if desired. The exact order of these steps may be changed to suit each trial or each patient within a trial. Investigators or staff should discuss with prospective enrollees:

1. Shortcomings of the patient's present treatment or problems the patient is having with their disease.
2. Alternative treatment options, both older established approaches and experimental ones.
3. The investigator's role in evaluating a particular treatment.
4. The possibility of individual patients enrolling in the trial.
5. Advantages and disadvantages of the treatment for the individual patient.
6. What would be involved if the patient decides to enroll in the trial.
7. The process that the individual patient can follow to make up his or her mind about participating in the trial.
8. Their willingness to answer questions so that the patient will make the best decision for himself or herself.

Various direct approaches that can be used with patients are shown in Fig. 4.3.

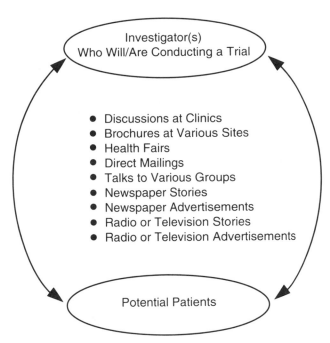

FIG. 4.3. Direct approaches to reach participants for recruitment into a clinical trial. Any one or more of the methods shown with bullets may be used.

Approaching Patients Indirectly

If there are too many potential patients for the investigator to approach patients directly, it may be preferable to design an alternative indirect approach. Such as one of the following (see Fig. 4.4):

1. Have the clinic nurse or trial coordinator discuss the trial initially with the patient.
2. Send prospective enrollees literature to read about the trial and ask for volunteers, or approach them directly at a later time.
3. Ask their referring physician to discuss the trial with them.
4. Discuss the potential benefits of a new treatment before mentioning that a clinical trial is to be conducted and they will be invited to be screened for entry.

Typical Responses to an Invitation To Be Screened

In Clinical Trials

In certain large clinical trials, it is necessary to invite many patients to be tested for possible qualification for entry. In the MRFIT trial (Multiple Risk Factor Intervention Trial of the National Heart, Lung, and Blood Institute), it was necessary to screen healthy men for their heart disease risk. Each of the 22 centers that participated in this trial used their own approach to recruiting patients. Greenlick et al. (1979) described the experiences of the Portland, Oregon center. They reviewed

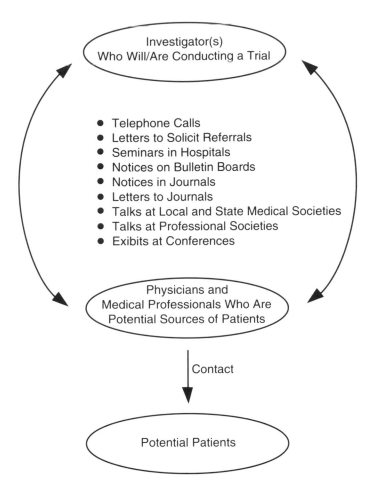

FIG. 4.4. Indirect approaches to reach participants for recruitment into a clinical trial. Any one or more of the methods shown with bullets may be used.

18,872 medical records for known risk factors and invited 12,646 men to be screened. Of those, 6,241 (49.3 %) accepted the invitation to be screened. Social, economic, demographic, medical, and risk factor characteristics were compared between groups of men screened and those not screened. Results were generally consistent with those of other similar trials: people who were not likely to accept the offer of screening were (1) older, (2) had more dependents, (3) were more likely to see physicians, and (4) had a higher socioeconomic level.

General Medical Care (i.e., Outside of Clinical Trials)

Published reports of various clinical trials describe the public's response to appeals to attend medical screenings at hospitals or clinics that are not part of the trial. For example, Kirscht et al. (1975) discuss the different responses of the public to threats and to positive appeals to encourage enrollment in a clinical trial. One sentence from the threat message said: "You may be feeling fine, but that doesn't guarantee that you are really healthy." One of the sentences from the positive message was:

"Everyone wants good health and our new clinic can help you stay healthy." Women reacted more favorably to the positive letter than did men. Both the positive and negative letters drew more attendance at a health screening from men than did a neutral letter.

Other references that discuss public responses to direct recruiting for screening programs include:

1. *Hypertension screening program in Atlanta, Georgia* (Wilber et al., 1972). Door-to-door screening and mobile van screening were the most effective methods.
2. *Hypertension screening program in five areas of Indianapolis, Indiana* (Stahl et al., 1977). They found that "home visits by community members trained to take blood pressure measurements" uncovered a larger number of newly diagnosed patients than did letters inviting people to attend screenings or gift offers.
3. *Mammography screening for breast cancer in a single group general practice in Manchester, United Kingdom* (Hobbs et al., 1990). These authors reported a higher attendance by older women (65 to 79 years) at the clinic than by younger women who were approached in the same way.

For Epidemiological Studies

Epidemiological studies differ from clinical trials in several important ways that alter recruiting strategy. It is usually relatively easy in a clinical trial to maintain a screening log and evaluate (if desired) whether trial enrollees differ from nonenrollees and in what ways the two groups differ. This depends of course on collecting the appropriate data. In an epidemiological study, it is often extremely difficult to collect accurate information on the group that is not involved or refuses to participate in the study. Given the large number of patients and limited data collected on each patient in epidemiological studies, it is often difficult to collect enough data on participants, particularly in retrospective studies. Some Ethics Committees/IRBs require investigators to obtain permission from the physicians of potential participants (Dicker and Kent, 1990).

Contacting Patients After They Are Identified from Medical Records

The most conservative approach to contacting patients after they are identified from their medical records is to contact the patient's physician and request permission to contact the patient directly or to have the physician contact the patient. If the latter method is used, then suitable materials must be prepared in advance so that the physician who is asked to contact his or her patient has sufficient information about the clinical trial to provide to the patient.

In other cases, it may be acceptable for the principal investigator to contact the appropriate Ethics Committee/IRB to request permission to contact patients directly. In this situation, the materials that will be mailed to the patient, or the information to be presented (or read) over the telephone, should be preapproved. The letter or telephone call should not pressure the patient in any way to be screened or enrolled. One way to do this is to inform the patient that he or she may be suitable for a specific trial and that the patient may request more information if desired. A self-addressed stamped card from the site may be provided for the patient's use.

Excellent sources of recruitment include lay groups that encompass patients, families, nonprofessionals, and professionals interested in the specific medical disorder being studied in the trial. Larger, disease-oriented organizations such as the American Cancer Society, Jimmy Fund, American Lung Association, Epilepsy Foundation of America, and others, have national staff as well as regional and local chapters. Their public relations and publicity departments can assist investigators by informing members about the clinical trial through newsletters and bulletins. Local investigators usually are welcome to speak at group meetings where they can explain the general scope of the trial and specific details of the clinical trial entry criteria.

Approaching Nonmedical Sources of Patients

Outlined below are six steps to take when contacting nonmedical groups for potential patients to enroll in a clinical trial.

1. Identify which community organizations and lay groups may be interested and able to assist with recruitment.

2. Define the scope of involvement and resources to be requested from the nonmedical sources (e.g., publicity, assistance with screening, direct recruitment of group members, volunteer office work such as stuffing envelopes or making telephone calls).

3. Contact the group director or leader of each organization and explain the trial's objectives, what is being asked of the group, and present the request identified in item 2.

4. Develop a timetable for implementation of the planned group liaison. If the group is in the midst of an annual fund-raising or education campaign, their resources might be too strained to assist with the trial. The investigator should determine if a shift in time would be reasonable, or to simply withdraw so as not to delay trial schedules.

5. If nonmedical people serve as volunteer staff during screening or recruitment processes, everyone must be carefully trained. Training should include education about the (1) objective and design of the trial, (2) reasons for establishing specific inclusion criteria, (3) procedures for answering patient questions, and (4) questions that should be referred to trial staff. Volunteers should be asked *not* to offer medical advice, but to focus solely on logistical and social issues.

6. Formal appreciation should be extended to the group as a whole and to every lay volunteer who assists with recruitment for the trial. In long-term trials, accolades should be provided annually.

Direct Recruiting of Patients Through Lay Organizations

Patients and families who attend lectures or other events and receive notices or other direct invitations to participate in a trial usually are outside their sphere of medical care. Even if they are interested in the trial, many patients will wish to discuss it with their personal physician before, during, or after being screened, but definitely before consenting to participate. The investigator should contact the patient's physician and explain potential benefits and risks for the individual patient. If the other physician concurs that the trial might be beneficial, it is helpful for the patient to hear the approval from his or her own physician.

Auditorium Presentations

In recruitment activities within various types of institutions, it may be possible to address large numbers of potential enrollees at the same time. Investigators may address school children, prison inmates, or employees of a company or other organization in an auditorium. Groups of patients with a disease or their families may be assembled by organizations dedicated to that disease. Investigators should use these opportunities to reduce potential stress about the clinical trial and to emphasize the pros and cons of the trial from the relevant perspectives (e.g., that of the patient, the institution, medical practice, and society).

Drawbacks to Nonmedical Recruitment

Two major drawbacks of direct recruiting through lay organizations are (1) the fact that entry is restricted to only specific individuals meeting entry criteria must be explained and emphasized, and (2) patients and families are often tempted to ask personal medical questions. The liaison investigator or staff must explain from the outset that questions about individual medical problems cannot be discussed at this public venue. The occasional, persistent lay questioner must be carefully requested to desist to allow adequate time for discussion of the primary topic, particularly during a public lecture.

A comparison of three methods of recruitment was made by Breckenridge et al. (1985) who compared three referral sources of patients. The "traditional" group were patients referred from typical medical sources. The "semi-traditional" group were recruited by contacts and publicity to patients within the medical center community. The "non-traditional" group included patients who heard about the trial from the media. The characteristics of the three groups did not differ although two-thirds of the patients were essentially self-referred through the media. This report demonstrates the effectiveness of newspaper, radio, and television methods in (1) approaching patients, (2) allowing them to determine their general eligibility for a trial, and (3) encouraging them to contact the investigators. The fact that a single newspaper story elicited 489 of the 725 referrals in this trial suggests that the individuals preferred a lengthy description of the background and purpose of a trial in written format, giving them time to peruse the information before deciding to contact the investigators.

SPECIFIC METHODS OF RECRUITMENT

Posters

Posters are a well accepted and widely used "firstline" method of advertising for clinical trials. Posters can be prepared using commonly available computer software designed to generate simple designs and text (see Fig. 4.5). The posters illustrated

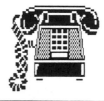

SEIZURE STUDY

WE NEED YOUR HELP

We are looking for patients with

NEW ONSET SEIZURES

OR

KNOWN SEIZURE DISORDERS

TO ENTER A STUDY OF

ANTIEPILEPTIC DRUGS.

IF YOU SEE ANY LIKELY CANDIDATES

PLEASE CALL US AT extension 123

Dr. John P. I.

Principal Investigator

or

Jane S. A.

Study Assistant

After hours call ext.456

to leave a message for us.

A

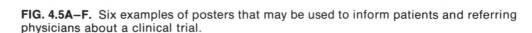

FIG. 4.5A–F. Six examples of posters that may be used to inform patients and referring physicians about a clinical trial.

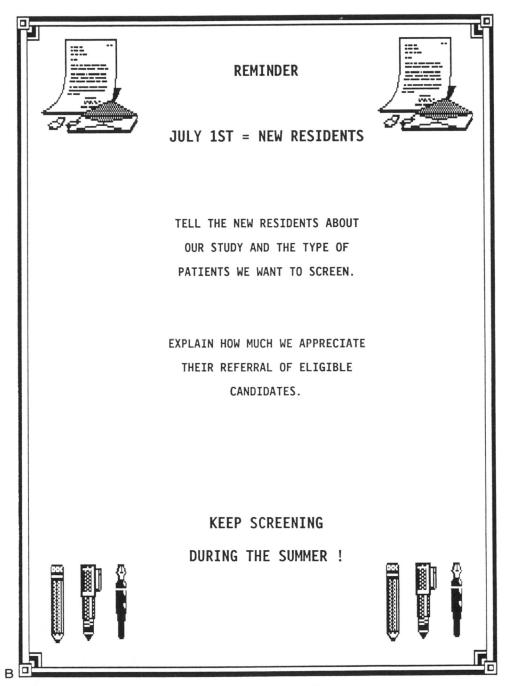

FIG. 4.5. *Continued.*

Figure continues on next page.

PATIENT RECRUITMENT IS YOUR TOP PRIORITY

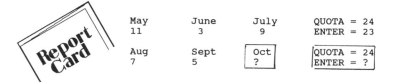

**WE NEED TO ENTER 12 PATIENTS IN OCTOBER
IN ORDER TO MEET OUR QUARTERLY GOAL.**

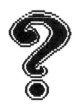

May	June	July	QUOTA = 24
11	3	9	ENTER = 23
Aug	Sept	Oct	QUOTA = 24
7	5	?	ENTER = ?

**DON'T LET POTENTIAL CANDIDATES SLIP THROUGH YOUR NET.
ACTIVELY SCREEN ALL OVER THE HOSPITAL EVERY DAY.**

*CALL JOYCE TO FIND OUT HOW AN EARLY CLOSE-DOWN OF ACCESSION COULD
AFFECT THE STUDY AND YOU.*

C

FIG. 4.5. *Continued.*

in Fig. 4.5 present various messages geared to internal hospital or institutional staff. Posters directed to patients are not illustrated but can contain any message and amount of information desired. This is discussed in the next section. The first poster in Fig. 4.5 provides an introduction to a new clinical trial that is being initiated. If the trial is to be an extremely large and important one then it makes sense to put posters in relevant places up to one or two months before the trial is to start, as long as Ethics Committee/IRB approval has been obtained. For medium and small size trials, posters should only be distributed after the investigator is ready to screen and enroll patients. The next five posters in Fig. 4.5 encourage physicians to refer patients to the trial using a variety of approaches and messages. Table 4.2 lists types

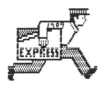

CS# 264

SPECIAL DELIVERY MESSAGE

We entered only 3 patients
in March, all GTC.
That **DOUBLES** our task
for April.
CPS patients are in short
supply. Be on the lookout
for them during screening.

D

FIG. 4.5. *Continued.*

Figure continues on next page.

E

FIG. 4.5. *Continued.*

<u>CS #264 PARTICIPANTS</u>

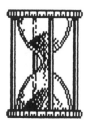

We are rapidly approaching April 26th –
the CSEC review date.

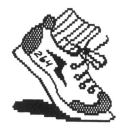

Every Investigator and Study Assistant
must quicken the pace in
search of new patients.

Nothing is a certainty. Renewal of the study is not a
sure bet.

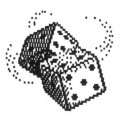

<u>Investigators:</u> Keep in touch with Dr. M   about
recruitment schemes at your center. How often do <u>you</u>
remind residents (VA and university) about the
study?

<u>Study Assistants:</u> Call Joyce weekly with an update
of your screening activity. How often do you
visit the emergency room, walk-in clinic area?

Most importantly, keep calling (anytime) to discuss
entry of a new patient.

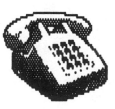

F

FIG. 4.5. *Continued.*

TABLE 4.2. *Types of inexpensive advertising posters[a]*

1. Poster for medical center bulletin boards
2. Poster for local stores (e.g., supermarkets)
3. Poster for distribution at shopping centers
4. Poster for placement on cars in parking lot (e.g., shopping center, movie theater)
5. Small poster included with commercial or civic mailing (e.g., included with utility bill, church newsletter)

[a] Generally printed or photocopied on white or colored paper sheets.

of handmade posters and where they can be used. More elaborate posters can be prepared by commercial artists. Once the master format is designed, it can be re-produced by photocopying or offset printing, depending on the quantities and uses planned. A single poster on a bulletin board is an easy way to start the advertising process.

Features to Consider when Planning Posters for Recruitment

Telephone Reminder Slips

When a poster is placed on a bulletin board that will be seen by many people, it is helpful to provide multiple tear-off slips listing the clinical site's or contact's telephone number and the name of the trial. The larger the tear-off slip, the less likely it is that it will be lost or mutilated. Rather than cutting slips along the edges of the poster, one may use a small pad of slips attached to the poster (e.g., stapled to a corner of the poster). Although preparation of a stack of slips is more tedious, and printing a pad of slips is more expensive, it allows for larger size reminder slips.

Multiple Posters

Instead of relying on a single poster remaining intact and visible as reminder slips are torn-off, multiple full-size posters or additional quarter-page reduced versions of the poster could be available for individuals. This system allows each person to take the entire message home for consideration. A stack of full or partial-size versions of the poster can be attached to a slightly larger cardboard backing that is mounted on a bulletin board.

Multiple Formats

Changing the style or color of the poster on each bulletin board at periodic intervals renews the stimulus for people who walk by bulletin boards regularly. Alternatively, a variety of posters can be merely rotated at intervals among the bulletin boards used.

Style

Use of different size type and the addition of graphic designs add visual interest. However, these should not overwhelm or obscure the message. This is a relevant issue to discuss with artists or advertising personnel.

Location

Keep records of where posters are placed. Check each location periodically (e.g., weekly) to assess poster impact by the number of tear-off slips or copies removed. Replenish the supply of slips or pads at each location or seek a more heavily trafficked location for the poster. Tables 4.2 and 4.4 list a number of possible locations.

Materials

Heavy cardboard may be used, though it is more difficult to mount on some types of bulletin boards and often does not stay taped to wall surfaces as well as lighter weight paper.

Advantages of Bulletin Board Posters in Medical Centers

Posters are particularly effective for the recruitment of normal volunteers because many medical center staff are interested in clinical research and willing to participate in trials, particularly if a fee is paid. People walking through a medical center who see the poster are an important group to target because they are probably familiar with the medical center and at least some of the facilities. Posters placed in staff areas can be designed to remind residents and others about the trial and the importance of referring patients for screening.

Chart Reviews

Chart reviews are not fruitful to use in most trials, but remain a standard method to be considered during recruitment planning. Use of medical charts to screen patients for an ophthalmic medicine trial was attempted by Quick et al. (1989). Names of potential patients were derived from outpatient clinic records, medical staff, and clinic staff. Although 1,388 charts were reviewed, the yield was incredibly low: only 15 patients were randomized (1%). This time-consuming chart review method led to the immediate exclusion of 86% of potential candidates based on clinical notes.

Mail Campaigns

Information about a trial can be disseminated to potential patients using standardized form letters or notices, each designed to elicit interest from specific groups

(Table 4.3). This technique is useful for trials of all sizes, easily repeatable, and readily assessed for effectiveness.

Major types of mail approaches include:

1. Letters requesting assistance mailed to physicians, staff, and others at referral sources.
2. Letters of invitation to attend the clinic for screening mailed directly to potential candidates.
3. Informational notices mailed directly to potential candidates or to a general medical list.
4. Informational notices mailed to the general public.
5. Purchasing lists of people to send the letter to.

The key aspect of a successful mail campaign is the procurement of appropriate mailing list(s). Sources include: (1) state motor vehicle administration lists (e.g., vehicle registration, driver's license), (2) voter registration lists, (3) Health Care Financing Adminstration (HCFA) lists.

Properties of an Efficient Recruitment Letter

1. Begin with an explanation of the purpose of the letter. This informs the reader about a forthcoming assessment of a new treatment for a particular disease.
2. Explain the objectives of the clinical trial (e.g., evaluation of an experimental medicine, efficacy comparison of two widely used medicines, long-term health status assessment after surgery).
3. Briefly define the inclusion criteria for the trial.
4. Include an invitation to be screened if it is a direct appeal to patients who are identified as likely candidates for enrollment.
5. Explain the screening process (e.g., patients visit the clinic for a half hour interview and blood tests at no cost to them).
6. Indicate the positive aspects of the trial for patients and for society.
7. List the names, telephone numbers, and addresses of the investigator and trial staff, and the best times for calling. Indicate whether an answering machine will be used to record caller information after usual office hours.
8. Include a brochure describing the trial, clinic, staff, and other details. See examples in this chapter (Fig. 4.13).

TABLE 4.3. *Contents of a recruiting notice*

1. Name of clinical trial
2. Sponsoring institution and department
3. Type of patient sought
4. Condition to be treated
5. Investigational nature of the treatment
6. Advantages for patients (e.g., free care and evaluation)
7. Honorarium or fee, if any
8. Name, address, and telephone number to call
9. Time(s) to call for more information

Practical Pointers

A few of the practical aspects to consider include:

1. Tailor the tone and sophistication of language in the mailing to the level of the group who will receive it. Have an expert in language skills assess the material and redo any text or material that is written at too low or high a level.
2. Make the material visually interesting. An art department can provide valuable pointers and advice in this regard (e.g., designs, logos).
3. Use colors on postcards, envelopes, and elsewhere to gain attention.
4. Enclose postpaid (i.e., stamped or metered mail) return envelopes. Do not expect prospective patients to pay to return an envelope or card.
5. Address letters to individual patients. Computers are readily able to do this.
6. Have the appropriate physician personally sign each letter.
7. Repeat the mailing a second or third time to those who have not returned a card or otherwise contacted the clinical trial site.
8. Follow mailings with telephone calls or possibly with visits, depending on the particular trial and amount of resources available.
9. Adhere to the KISS rule (Keep it short and simple). Do not be verbose.

How to Assess the Efficiency of Mailing Campaigns

Comparing the number of pieces of mail sent to the number of responses received defines the method's efficiency. However, rarely is a single recruitment method used in isolation. Patients who contact the site or undergo screening should be asked where they heard about the trial, as described in the chapter on screening logs. If mailings are sent to several groups and potential patients are asked to return a sheet in a prepaid envelope, then the sheet they complete may be easily coded to identify which mailing they received (e.g., that sent to group A, B, or C; the first, second, or third letter to that particular group).

It is possible to review the names of responders to identify which source(s) provided the greatest yield of patients for screening and for enrollment into the trial. For example, notices to lay groups might result in a 50% response rate in terms of people calling for information. However, if only 10% of the calls lead to screening, and only 60% of screening visits lead to consent to participate, the actual yield is only 3%. On the other hand, direct invitations to a small number of patients known to the investigator might result in 50% participation.

Baines (1984) described the special problems in recruiting women for a breast cancer screening program. Thousands of form letters of invitation were sent to women teachers and nurses; a low yield of volunteers resulted. A second approach was attachment of a pamphlet describing the trial to Canadian Department of Health and Welfare checks going to all families with children. Some "adverse events" resulted from this method because women living outside the region where centers were located were unable to participate. Some women also were critical of the federal agency for allowing distribution of material describing the trial because of their opposition to low level ionizing radiation used in mammography. The third method was an individually addressed letter sent to every woman of appropriate age on a school list maintained by the City of Toronto. Women were invited to participate or call to learn more details, resulting in 858 appointments. Telephone follow-up to nonresponders achieved an additional 1,081 appointments. This method raised another issue: some women were concerned about how the investigators had access to their name and address and knew that they were of eligible age. In addition, although the follow-up phone call yielded a large number of appointments, this group had a lower rate of patient enrollment and randomization. The authors characterized patients for whom a repeated effort must be made as "reluctant" participants.

Use of Telephones

Calling Patients Directly

Telephone calls *to* prospective patients are sometimes made as a recruitment tool. These calls depend on obtaining names and telephone numbers of prospective enrollees. If they are within the investigator's own practice, then there is no problem in discussing the trial and inviting them by telephone or letter to participate by being screened. If the prospective enrollees are not within the investigator's own practice, a number of issues must be considered.

Before telephoning or mailing information to patients about a trial, the following issues should be discussed with the Ethics Committee/IRB, in addition to discussions among the clinical trial staff:

1. Are the patients likely to be under another physician's care for the disease being evaluated and are those physicians likely to object to the telephone calls or letters?
2. Is it likely that the patients will know whether they have the problem being sought?

Combined or sequential use of mass mailing and telephone follow-up is costly but will increase the yield in terms of patient enrollment.

Media: Radio, Television, Newspapers, and Magazines

Two types of media publicity are helpful in recruiting patients: stories and advertisements. Both news stories and paid advertisements draw attention to a clinical trial and serve to supplement the initial request for referrals from within the medical community. Although the opportunity for a free announcement via a news story usually occurs only once (at best) for a trial, the image of the trial may sometimes be maintained through paid advertisements thereafter.

Information about a clinical trial can be broadly disseminated using a variety of media reports and paid advertisements that can be designed to reach the local community or the entire nation. These methods can be scaled up or down for use in trials of virtually all sizes. However, engaging the attention of the media is neither simple nor readily repeatable, and paid advertising is generally too expensive to repeat frequently.

News Story

Medical reporters often welcome the opportunity to interview an expert clinician and learn about important clinical research being conducted in their area and its implications for advancing medical treatment. If the newspaper, radio, or television station does not have an ongoing medical program, arrangements can be made for special coverage. Whether the trial is ongoing at a single institution with one physician, or is part of a multicenter clinical trial, the news focus is invariably on the local community, particularly if patients are expected to benefit from a new treatment. Even if the local hospital is one of dozens of sites, it becomes the center of attention for the local media. Several newspaper articles about clinical trials being conducted in the community are shown in Fig 4.6. Talk shows on radio stations or on-the-air interviews are particularly helpful because they allow the opportunity for telephone questions from the audience that help clarify issues beyond what the physician can present in a brief, formal overview of the trial. This method was used by some of the Lipid Research Clinics (Levenkron and Farquhar, 1982). The drawback is that, as with lectures to lay groups, some questions are likely to relate to personal medical problems. Keeping to the central issue is vital. Television news comments reach a wide audience but are invariably short and often do not indicate whom to contact about the trial. Methods using media are listed in Table 4.4.

Sanders et al. (1990) developed an entire clinical trial around a television recruitment plan. They announced a diet trial on television, inviting viewers who wanted to lose weight and were willing to participate in a research project to write for information. Respondents who met the inclusion criteria were randomized to one of eight diet plans and were weighed at their local television station before and after the 6-week diet plan. At the conclusion of the trial, results were announced on the television program, including an explanation of why a control group was used.

Magazine stories are only useful as a recruiting tool if the trial is continuing for a relatively long period and if patients are reached by the magazine. Certain magazines are closely linked to the target patient population (e.g., DAV magazine for veterans). An example of a letter requesting a story be written is shown in Fig. 4.7.

Develop a Series of Message Points for Interacting with the Press

Develop a series of message points that present the heart of your story in a succinct manner. For example, you could say:

A clinical trial is underway in the area and will help local patients with disease X.

Disease X causes pain and suffering for Y patients nationally and Z patients in the metropolitan area.

Disease X is caused by A and is characterized by symptoms B,C, and D.

The clinical trial is evaluating a new medicine to treat disease X.

This medicine has already been tested in F patients and has shown G, H, and K.

If patients know they have this disease and are between the ages of L and M, and N, O, P, then they could call telephone number R for more information.

People who want to know more about this disease should also call telephone number R.

UMC seeking children to participate in new chicken pox drug study

The University of Mississippi Medical Center in Jackson is searching for children between the ages of two and 18 to participate in the study of a new drug that promises to ease the discomfort and decrease the rash of chicken pox, one of childhood's most contagious illnesses.

UMC is one of 10 medical centers in the country chosen to evaluate a liquid form of the drug acyclovir, or zovirax, for the treatment of chicken pox in normal, healthy children. A preliminary study done last year at the University of Minnesota indicated that children who receive the drug within 24 hours of initial outbreak experience a shorter lighter episode of the illness.

According to Dr. Sandor Feldman, professor of pediatrics at UMC, the study revealed that not only was the duration of the illness cut in half for those children who received the drug, but the number of chicken pox lesions also was markedly decreased.

In practical terms, he adds, that implies that not only do youngsters return to school faster, but working parents don't use as many sick or personal days to care for their ailing children.

Dr. Feldman urges parents who would like their children to participate in the evaluation to contact UMC within the first 24 hours of outbreak. Children are seen daily in emergency room for five days, the length of treatment. UMC provides Tylenol for pain and fever and Benadryl for itching, as well as the drug acyclovir, which Dr. Feldman says is proven to be safe and causes no serious side effects.

Half the 100 participants needed to complete the evaluation will be given acyclovir, while the other half will receive a placebo. Parents will be notified at the end of the study whether their child received the drug or the placebo.

"There is no cost to the patient," stresses Dr. Feldman, adding that parents will be reimbursed $50 per child for travel expenses. So far, 28 children have participated, some traveling from as far as Columbus.

According to Dr. Feldman, a child exposed in the household to chicken pox for the first time has a 90 percent chance of contracting the disease, which has a two-week incubation period. The child is contagious the day before outbreak begins, and remains contagious as long as there is fluid in the lesions, about five days.

Acyclovir in tablet form has been used for the past 10 years to treat herpes in adults. It also has been used successfully in intravenous form to treat pediatric cancer patients suffering with chicken pox.

"We already know the drug is effective," says Dr. Feldman, noting that a chicken pox vaccine is only two to five years away. "The liquid form needs to be evaluated to receive Food and Drug Administration approval."

Interested participants should contact Leila Parker, R.N., or Dr. Sandor Feldman at UMC, 984-5206.

A

FIG. 4.6A–D. Examples of newspaper articles written about clinical trials being conducted in the local area. The first is from the Yazoo City Herald with permission, the second from the Minneapolis–St.Paul Star Tribune with permission, the third from the Houston Chronicle with permission, and the fourth from the Chapel Hill Newspaper with permission.

These may be presented in a news release, cover memorandum, or may be mentioned during interviews with investigators and staff.

Advertising

The major questions regarding advertisements as a means of increasing recruitment are (1) Is the advertisement conducted in an ethical manner? (2) Does it lead to enrollment of the types of patients desired? (3) Is it initiated during the clinical trial or from its outset? If advertising is initiated after a clinical trial is in progress, a different population of patients could be enrolled yielding results different from those that would be obtained from patients enrolled before the trial was initiated. Thus, the data of the two groups (i.e., patients enrolled via advertisements versus others) should be analyzed separately and compared prior to being pooled and combined.

Drug may aid chicken pox recovery

By The Minneapolis-St. Paul Star Tribune

A University of Minnesota medical researcher is heading a 10-city national study to see if a drug commonly used to treat genital herpes can also speed children's recovery from chicken pox.

The chicken pox virus is a member of the herpes family of viruses. There are tantalizing clues that the drug acyclovir may be able to play a widespread role in combating this illness, said Dr. Henry Balfour. He is a professor of pediatrics and medical director of the study that will include 1,000 patients.

The study is sponsored by the Burroughs Wellcome Co., which makes acyclovir.

Chicken pox causes a blistery, itchy rash along with fever that typically keeps a child out of school for three days to more than a week. Complications can range from bacterial infections of the sores or ear infections, which may occur in 5 percent of the cases, to pneumonia or encephalitis (inflammation of the brain).

About 5,000 American youngsters are hospitalized annually with the more serious complications. And virtually every youngster gets chicken pox sometime while growing up.

Here's why Balfour said he is encouraged that acyclovir will turn out to be valuable:

• Acyclovir has proven its ability to work against another illness caused by the chicken pox virus. It helps speed recovery from shingles, a painful rash in adults. Shingles occurs when the chicken pox virus, which remains in the body after the childhood illness, reactivates many years later.

• As part of a broader study of acyclovir at several medical centers, children who had leukemia were given the drug when they developed chicken pox. Chicken pox can be particularly severe in such children. The drug appeared to reduce the number of complications, but the study was too small to prove anything more, Balfour said. And those patients got the drug by infusion into a vein, which would be an impractical method for widespread use.

• In a pilot study, oral acyclovir was given to 50 Minneapolis area youngsters with chicken pox in 1987. No side effects were detected in those participants, Balfour said. The drug still may cause headaches and other minor symptoms in some people. But this study clearly showed that the drug is safe to give youngsters who have chicken pox.

But did the drug help against chicken pox?

Balfour said those results won't be announced until they've been reviewed by outside experts. He said different dosages were used in different patients, making analysis tricky with such a small group of patients. But the larger study now under way should provide definitive results.

Balfour said that acyclovir potentially could save millions of dollars nationally by reducing complications and by reducing the time that some parents now have to miss work to care for their ill children.

Balfour offered this advice to parents whose children have chicken pox:

• Don't give aspirin to a youngster who has chicken pox. One of the rare complications of chicken pox is Reye's syndrome. Studies indicate that aspirin use while a youngster has chicken pox (or some flu strains) can increase the risk of Reye's developing. Tylenol and similar nonaspirin pain relievers don't carry this risk.

• While it's best not to scratch the itchy blisters, it's hard to keep children from scratching some of them. So keep fingernails short and scrubbed clean, to reduce the risk of germ-carrying dirt getting into the sores.

• Keep the ill children out of the sun, since sunlight can aggravate chicken pox.

• Check with a doctor if the child has a temperature of 101 degrees (by mouth) for 48 hours or longer, is complaining of a headache or vomiting or has other complications.

• "Kids tend to get sicker as chicken pox goes through a family." Experts aren't certain why, but it may be that larger doses of the virus are picked up from a sibling than typically occurs when the child picks up the virus from a playmate.

FIG. 4.6. *Continued.*

General Use of Advertising

To maximize the benefit of a news story, paid advertisements in the newspaper should follow. Advertisements should be placed in the news section, rather than in the classified section. Advertisements should describe the general inclusion criteria as briefly as possible so as not to confuse readers but rather encourage inquiries.

Figure continues on next page.

Briefs

Volunteers sought for study

Baylor College of Medicine researchers are looking for volunteers to participate in a study of an anti-viral drug to treat childhood chicken pox. The drug, acyclovir, will be tested by Baylor's dermatology department on children ages 2-18 who have chicken pox. Acyclovir is commonly used now to treat oral and genital herpes and has been used to treat chicken pox in children with chronic illnesses. The Baylor study will seek to determine if the drug lessens the length and severity of illness in normal children. Volunteers must have been diagnosed with the disease within 24 hours of entering the study. Those who have received an experimental chicken pox vaccine cannot participate. For more information, contact Cyndee Lisenbe at 794-2508.

C

FIG. 4.6. *Continued.*

The copy for advertisements should be reviewed by the Ethics Committee/IRB for comment on the ethical acceptability of the approach. It must be decided how to indicate (if appropriate) that a fee will be paid to participants.

When is Advertising Appropriate?

There is an apparently simple answer to this question. When an insufficient number of patients have been obtained through other recruitment methods (e.g., one's own practice plus those of colleagues, friends, and other referral centers), advertising should be considered. If it is known at the outset of a trial that an insufficient number of patients are likely to be enrolled, then advertising could be an important consideration from the start. Budgetary and other factors will greatly influence whether this approach can be followed.

Where Should Advertising be Placed?

The choice of media (e.g., radio, television, newspapers, magazines) depends on several factors.

Doctor studying new shingles drug

By UTE FINZEL Correspondent

Chapel Hill Dermatology, under the direction of Dr. Robert S. Gilgor, is testing a new, as yet unnamed drug for the treatment of herpes zoster, a viral disease also known as shingles.

Shingles is an often painful outbreak of skin sores, which is caused by the same virus that causes chicken pox. This means that everyone who has had chicken pox has the potential to develop shingles. But the risk and the severity of the attacks increase with age.

The chicken pox viruses lie dormant in certain sensory nerves below the skin. Reactivation is more likely to occur among people with a weakened immune system, such as elderly people, cancer patients and people with immunodeficiencies such as AIDS.

"I believe it's a safe drug," said Gilgor. "It's very exciting for me to be involved in the study. If you have the opportunity of looking at a new drug that can help ease someone's pain and make people feel better, it's very exciting and very gratifying."

According to Jean D. Pons, a nurse helping to coordinate the study, the incidence of herpes zoster might be slightly elevated in Chapel Hill, given the high number of elderly residents.

"Chapel Hill has seen an influx of retirees into the area. It stands to reason that we should see more cases of shingles," said Pons.

"What is very important to us is to make the elderly aware what shingles is," said Gilgor. "Oftentimes, by the time they find out it's shingles, it may be too late to treat it. It has to be treated within 48 hours after the onset of the rash."

Unlike the more common herpes simplex, which causes cold sores around the mouth, and herpes genitalis, which affects the genital organs, herpes zoster typically affects the trunk or the waist areas, although it can also can affect the facial area.

There are about 300,000 cases of shingles in the United States each year. "In the last year, our office saw over 30" zoster patients, said Gilgor. "That's one every one and a half weeks."

The sores heal in two to six weeks. Usually the rash erupts only once in a lifetime. The recurrence rate is 7 percent or less.

But shingles can cause severe pain as a consequence of the damage caused to the nerve cells. The pain might last for years and can cause serious emotional problems.

There is no way to prevent the outbreak of the disease. It is, however, possible to reduce the severity of the active stage and to minimize nerve damage.

People who have not had chicken pox might develop it upon contact with open blisters, but they won't contract zoster. "You cannot 'catch' the disease [zoster] as such," Pons said. Anyone who has not had chicken pox — infants, young children and pregnant women in particular — should avoid contact during an active shingles outbreak.

Burroughs Wellcome Co. developed Zovirax, the first antiviral drug for the treatment of herpes simplex, about five years ago. Now, the company has contracted with almost 20 dermatology centers across the United States to conduct studies of the new drug, which has shown good potential as a shingles therapy.

Volunteers are needed to take part in the study.

There will be two age groups, one involving patients between 18 and 49 years of age, the other one involving people 50 years and older.

Patients in the lower age group will receive either the new drug or a placebo. Patients over 50 will receive either Zovirax or the new drug.

Patients will be evaluated daily for seven days and again on days 10, 14 and 21. Over a period of 20 weeks after the initial treatment, patients will be contacted weekly to evaluate the course of the illness and the recovery process. Participants will receive free treatment and a one-time compensation of $100.

Individuals or their doctors interested in the study can contact Gilgor or Pons at 942-3106.

FIG. 4.6. *Continued.*

1. Whether special rates for medical topics are available.
2. The extent of financial resources available for advertising.
3. The availability of media suitable to reach the target population of patients. Cable television may be an effective means of targeting potential enrollees in a specific catchment area.
4. Which media (i.e., radio, television, magazines, newspapers) are expected to reach the largest number of potential patients for the least amount of money? It may be possible to calculate an approximate cost to reach each potential enrollee using different media approaches.
5. Which types of each medium will reach potential patients in a cost-effective manner? For example, *Modern Maturity*, the magazine of the American As-

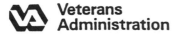

Medical Center   3801 Miranda Avenue
Palo Alto CA 94304

COOPERATIVE STUDIES PROGRAM COORDINATING CENTER

In Reply Refer To: 640/151K

September 23, 1988

Frank R. Norberg
Editor
DAV Magazine
807 Maine Avenue, S.W.
Washington, DC 20024

Dear Mr. Norberg:

The Veterans Administration is currently conducting a multi-hospital study of stroke prevention in patients with nonvalvular atrial fibrillation. Although there are sixteen participating VA medical centers, it is possible that non-participating VA medical centers might become aware of eligible patients who could be referred to the study. We would not only like to try to recruit eligible patients from VA facilities, but would also like to reach out to the veteran population that does not necessarily use VA hospitals.

We are looking for a large population and an article in your magazine about the study would be appreciated. The study potentially can be of benefit to veterans with nonvalvular atrial fibrillation who are at a higher risk of developing a stroke. Enclosed is a brief description of the study.

Your assistance in this matter would be greatly appreciated. If you do decide to publish a brief article, we would greatly appreciate you sending a copy of it for our information. If you have any questions, I can be reached at (415) 852-3252.

Sincerely,

KENNETH E. JAMES, Ph.D.
Chief, Palo Alto Cooperative Studies
Program Coordinating Center

Enclosure

KJ/pl

A   *"America is #1 — Thanks to our Veterans"*

FIG. 4.7A and **B.** Example of a letter written to a magazine requesting that a story be written about a clinical trial. Information about the trial is included. Reprinted with permission.

VA'S COOPERATIVE STUDY ON
STROKE PREVENTION IN NONVALVULAR ATRIAL FIBRILLATION

The Veterans Administration is currently conducting a multi-hospital cooperative study of stroke prevention in patients with nonvalvular atrial fibrillation. The study is being sponsored by the Cooperative Studies Program of the Medical Research Service, directed by Daniel Deykin, M.D.

Nonvalvular atrial fibrillation affects as much as 5% of the elderly population and is most common in individuals with ischemic heart disease or hypertension. Nonvalvular atrial fibrillation is a risk factor for stroke, causing at least 10% of all strokes. For patients who develop *chronic* nonvalvular atrial fibrillation, the lifetime risk of stroke probably exceeds 30%.

Long-term oral anticoagulation is the logical therapy for stroke prevention in nonvalvular atrial fibrillation, but to date it has not been widely employed except in patients with a history of prior stroke. Even in that circumstance, the treatment is hardly universal. Reluctance to anticoagulate can be attributed to the risk of hemorrhagic complications. Recent evidence has indicated that lower doses of anticoagulation can yield a substantial reduction in hemorrhagic complications in the treatment of venous thromboembolism.

Appreciation that nonvalvular atrial fibrillation poses a greater risk than once thought, and that effective anticoagulation may be achieved more safely than previously thought, has resulted in widespread interest in the prospect of randomized trials to resolve the issue of whether or not such patients should be chronically anticoagulated.

The Cooperative Studies Program is conducting a study to assess the effect of low dose anticoagulation for the prevention of stroke in patients with nonvalvular atrial fibrillation. Approximately 1100 patients will be entered into the study over a three-year period. Medical treatment and the study medication will be provided at no charge to the patient. Veterans do not have to be service connected to enter the study. Patients will be followed very closely by a medical research team.

The Co-Chairmen are located at the VA Medical Center in West Haven, Connecticut and are faculty members at Yale University School of Medicine. Samuel L. Bridgers, M.D., Co-Chairman, is Director of the Stroke Unit and Neurovascular Laboratory. Michael Ezekowitz, M.D., Co-Chairman, is Director of the Echocardiography and Cell-Labelling Laboratory. The study is being coordinated by the Cooperative Studies Program Coordinating Center at the VA Medical Center, Palo Alto, California, under the direction of Kenneth E. James, Ph.D.

Veterans will be entered by sixteen participating VA Medical Centers: Ann Arbor, Michigan; Baltimore, Maryland; Boston, Massachusetts; Cincinnati, Ohio; Hines, Illinois; Little Rock, Arkansas; Long Beach, California; Minneapolis, Minnesota; Newington, Connecticut; Northport, New York; Roseburg, Oregon; San Diego, California; Seattle, Washington; Tampa, Florida; Washington, D.C.; and West Haven, Connecticut.

Any veteran of military service in the Armed Services of the United States who has nonvalvular atrial fibrillation and who is interested in being considered as a candidate to participate in the study should write to or phone Kenneth E. James, Ph.D., Chief, VA Cooperative Studies Program Coordinating Center (151-K), VA Medical
B Center, 3801 Miranda Avenue, Palo Alto, California 94304, telephone (415) 852-3252.

FIG. 4.7. *Continued.*

TABLE 4.4. *Methods for advertising a clinical trial*

1. Posters for bulletin boards or handouts left at:
   Supermarkets
   Pharmacies
   Hospital waiting rooms
   Churches
   Libraries
   Community centers, senior centers
2. Talks given at:
   Community events
   Radio shows and interviews
   Television talk shows
   Medical grand rounds
   Medical society meetings
3. Stories published in:
   Newspapers
   Magazines
   Newsletters
   Program books at special events
4. Advertising and Public Service Announcements in:
   Newspapers
   Radio
   Magazines
   Newsletters
   Bus or subway

sociation of Retired People (AARP), is expensive to advertise in, but it reaches approximately 30 million people and therefore may be cost-effective for recruiting enrollees to certain clinical trials.

6. The emotional and professional comfort level of the investigator and sponsor, if any, with each of the media. Utilizing television or radio to advertise for patients is not a reasonable alternative for every investigator to consider.
7. The appropriateness of the media chosen for a particular trial.
8. The type of patients expected to be recruited by each medium and each specific station or newspaper. The *New York Times* and the *New York Daily News* reach quite different groups of patients, as do classical music and rock music radio stations.
9. Try to have stories about a trial or advertisements placed on page three of a newspaper to achieve maximum benefit.

Types of advertising are listed in Table 4.4. A comparison of three media techniques on recruiting patients for a major trial is shown in Fig. 4.8.

How Should Advertisements be Created?

In some cases a substantial budget will be available for creating advertisements, and professionals may be hired to produce them. This is particularly relevant for television advertisements, although it is possible for a single individual to read a script without anything more elaborate being done. Script writers or others could be asked to prepare material for a 30-second or 1-minute recorded message, or to prepare copy for a newspaper advertisement. Whatever approach is used, a suitable plan should be developed to attract the attention of patients, their families, or friends and to encourage them to consider enrolling in the clinical trial.

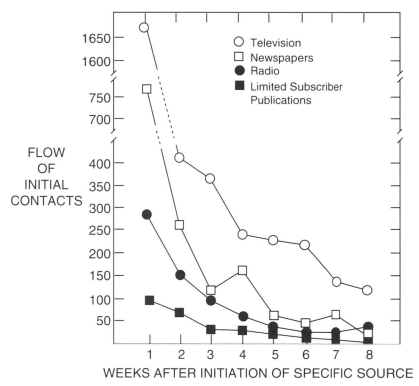

FIG. 4.8. Flow (number per week) of initial contacts over time since initiating recruitment from individual sources. Results presented for radio exclude data from the Toronto LRC because it was atypically effective. Reprinted from Levenkron and Farquhar (1982) with permission.

The newspaper advertisements in Fig 4.9 illustrate a wide variety of approaches to interest patients in enrolling in clinical trials. In general, smaller size advertisements are solely prepared using text, but with as large size type as possible. Larger size advertisements have the possibility to include a drawing or photograph to add visual interest. This is often provided by a human figure, but a variety of approaches are shown.

A letter from the Food and Drug Administration (FDA) discussing United States policies on advertising for research subjects is shown in Fig. 4.10. An advertisement must convey the concept of the trial and where to obtain more information. Flow charts for the use of newspaper or other advertisements are shown in Figs. 4.11 and 4.12.

How Large a Budget is Needed for Advertising

Advertising may be incredibly expensive. On the other hand, many imaginative uses of advertising can achieve a great deal of publicity with limited resources. This can be achieved through:

1. Utilization of radio or television "public service" advertisements that promote the trial.

DEPRESSION

FREE EVALUATION AND
INVESTIGATIONAL MEDICATION
FOR QUALIFIED SUBJECTS
IN A MAJOR RESEARCH STUDY

CLINICAL STUDIES CENTER

DEPRESSED?

Eating or Sleeping Poorly?
Lack Energy? Feeling Hopeless?

If you are suffering from the symptoms of depression and are 18 and over, you may be eligible
for a FREE program. This research study offers a general health assessment (physical exam,
routine lab tests) and treatment with investigational medication AT NO COST. Care provided
by physicians and other health professionals. If you believe you are eligible call:

_____ .

HELP
DO YOU FEEL DEPRESSED OR ANXIOUS

Test yourself to determine if you may need a free evaluation.

Do you have trouble sleeping?	Y	N
Do you feel anxious or fearful?	Y	N
Do you feel tense, keyed up or unable to relax?	Y	N
Do you have reduced interest in daily activities?	Y	N
Do you feel low in energy?	Y	N
Do you feel depressed, sad or blue?	Y	N

If you answered yes to 2 or more of these, you may be suffering from depression or anxiety
and you may qualify to participate in a research study concerning depression.

The _____ is offering a free evaluation
for people suffering from anxiety or depression. As part of a research study, those who qualify
may receive a medical evaluation, EKG, and investigational medication, all at no charge.

A Call: _____

FIG. 4.9A–R. Examples of actual newspaper advertisements used to recruit patients for
clinical trials.

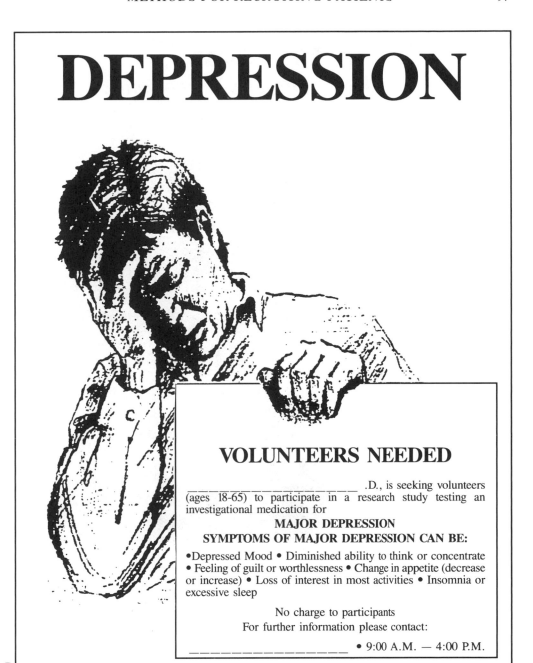

FIG. 4.9. *Continued.*

Figure continues on next page.

DEPRESSION

There is a way out . . .

At some time in their lives, 15 out of every 100 adults suffer from a crippling medical illness. Treatment is available, but often not sought. Frequently, the symptoms go unrecognized, and appropriate treatment is delayed or never begun. The illness is depression.

Common symptoms of depression are:
— sadness
— low energy
— difficulty sleeping
— loss of pleasure

If you have some of these symptoms, you may be suffering from depression triggered by a biochemical imbalance. Studies show that seven out of ten people who suffer from depression never get the right help. Understandably, many people feel embarrassed to seek help or are reluctant to enter into lengthy or expensive treatment. Even when they do, such treatment may not be effective. The _____ _____ may be able to help you. The_____ offers completely **free** evaluations and investigational medication.

One of our doctors will help you decide if our program is right for you. Your progress will be closely monitored in private and confidential surroundings. Funded by research grants, _____ _____ _____ has helped thousands of _____ residents.

The _____ progressive professional staff functions under the direction of_____M.D., who is a leader in the treatment of clinical depression in the United States. He has done pioneering work in depression and related problems for over twenty years, and is associated with area hospitals and medical schools.

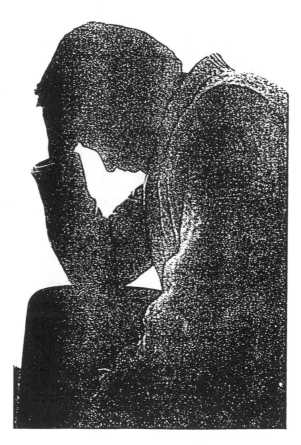

For information or to see if you qualify, call

_____
_____

FIG. 4.9. *Continued.*

2. Having the investigator be interviewed as a part of the news or as a part of a talk show on a local television or radio program.
3. Printing newspaper advertisements in less expensive newspapers or newsletters (e.g., community, college, or neighborhood newspapers, or those targeted to a specific group).
4. Placing many signs in conspicuous places throughout hospitals and the communities involved.
5. Send press releases on a periodic basis to newspapers to print as stories, or news.

DEPRESSION

The_____Clinic needs volunteers with mild to moderate depression, ages 18 and over, to participate in a study comparing an investigational drug with placebo in the treatment of depression. If you feel depressed but don't know if it is serious enough to be considered for a study, please give us a call.

The symptoms include:

☐ Crying spells
☐ Loss of interest
☐ Feeling hopeless and helpless
☐ Weight gain or loss
☐ Fatigue
☐ Increased or decreased sleep
☐ Guilt feelings
☐ Indecision
☐ Poor concentration
☐ Increased health problems

Suitable volunteers will receive a physical examination, EKG, Lab work and weekly psychiatric visits with a physician.

If interested please call _____ 9:30-10:00 a.m., or 2:00-5:00 p.m.

FIG. 4.9. *Continued.*

Balancing the Size or Length Versus the Number of Advertisements

It is natural to wish to place large size or long advertisements at frequent intervals in whichever medium is chosen. Nonetheless, money and convenience usually force a choice between placing a smaller number of large (or long) advertisements and placing a larger number of small (or shorter) ones. The conventional wisdom in this context is that it is usually preferable to choose size or length over frequency. Too often, a small advertisement is overlooked and thus has less impact, even when

Figure continues on next page.

Is Someone You Know Having Memory Problems?

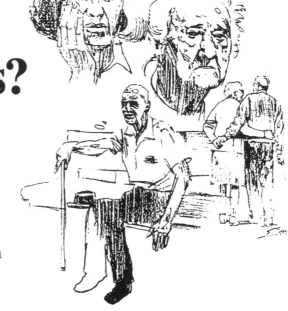

Do you, or a member of your family, have difficulty remembering what day it is or events which happened recently?

If you, or someone in your family, fits this description, you may be qualified to become a volunteer in a very important Alzheimer's Disease study being conducted by _____ M.D. in _____

Individuals with memory problems or with a diagnosis of Alzheimer's disease are sought to participate in an outpatient research study which will continue for up to one year. Volunteers will receive a series of physical and neuropsychological tests. These tests, in conjunction with the patient's medical history, will provide valuable information to those studying memory loss. There is no charge to the subject.

For more information, please contact _____ **before**
E _____ at _____ Tuesday through Friday, 9:00 a.m. to 4:00 p.m.

FIG. 4.9. *Continued.*

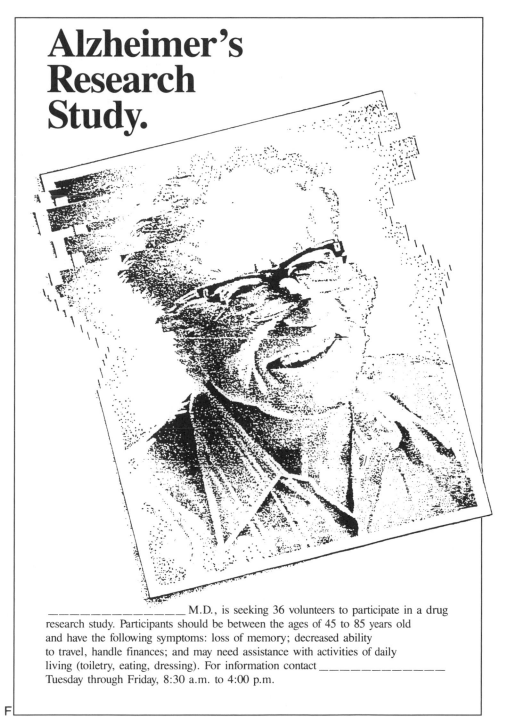

Alzheimer's Research Study.

_____ M.D., is seeking 36 volunteers to participate in a drug research study. Participants should be between the ages of 45 to 85 years old and have the following symptoms: loss of memory; decreased ability to travel, handle finances; and may need assistance with activities of daily living (toiletry, eating, dressing). For information contact _____ Tuesday through Friday, 8:30 a.m. to 4:00 p.m.

FIG. 4.9. *Continued.*

Figure continues on next page.

FIG. 4.9. *Continued.*

repeated on a number of occasions. There may be times when frequency is more desirable than size, but there should be specific reasons for making this choice.

How to Judge Results of Advertisements?

The outcome of one or more advertisements may be simple, complex, or virtually impossible to judge. If advertising is the only way that patients are recruited, then it is a relatively straightforward matter to evaluate its overall success. Comparison with other methods, however, is likely to be difficult or impossible. If a variety of types of advertisements or different recruitment methods are used, it will be more difficult to assess the value and results of each advertisement. The Cholesterol Lowering Atherosclerosis Study (CLAS) (Blankenhorn et al., 1987) determined that a relatively small advertisement (4 inches high × 3.25 inches wide) in the *Los Angeles Times* averaged 76 telephone inquiries each time it was run. These contacts resulted in an average of 19 screening visits and randomization of five patients from each advertisement, a 6.6% yield.

The evaluation of a particular advertisement's effectiveness can be made easier in a few ways. Patients may be asked to send in a form from the newspaper to be eligible for screening. These forms should have a code to identify the name as well as the date of the paper in which it was printed. Patients who telephone a site to request information on a specific trial may also be asked where they saw information about the trial (e.g., television or newspaper).

**NORMAL VOLUNTEERS NEEDED
FOR LUNG STUDIES AT**

Healthy nonsmoking subjects between the ages of 20 and 70 are needed for standardization of a lung function test. Testing requires inhalation of a very small, nontoxic concentration of test gases (0.3% carbon monoxide, acetylene and methane) and having the uptake of these gases measured during the following exhalation. The test is performed at rest and at a low level of bicycle exercise. Standard lung function tests will also be performed. The tests should take one hour. Reimbursement is $10.00, and a parking pass will be provided. Contact Dr._____, Beeper_____, for details.

PROBLEMS with STRESS or ANXIETY?

Physically healthy volunteers with stress, panic disorders, or tension are needed for a research project on a new anti-anxiety medication at the_____University Medical Center. Psychological consultation, testing and treatment will be provided free of charge. For appointment please call _____ .

Paid Volunteers Needed

1. Individuals 18 years and older with frequent runny nose needed for a research study on a new nasal spray. $350.00 paid incentive if qualified to participate.

2. Individuals 12 years and older with asthma on daily inhaled steroids needed for research study. $800 paid incentive if qualified to participate.

    Contact:_____
    _____

H

FIG. 4.9. *Continued.*

Figure continues on next page.

DO YOU HAVE ANXIETY ATTACKS? PANIC ATTACKS?

— Fear
— Dread
— Heart pounding
— Dizzy or faint
— Trembling
— Short of breath
— Anxiety
— Chills
— Sweating
— Fear of losing control

If you
— Have 4 or more symptoms per attack
— Have at least two attacks per week
— Are age 18 to 65
— Avoid or fear certain situations

You may qualify to participate in a research study of an investigational anti-panic and anti-anxiety medication.

For further information call _ _ _ _ _

I

Menopause Study

Learn About The Benefits of Hormone Replacement

Healthy women are needed for a _____ Medical School research project with _____ M.D. Blood sugars and cholesterol will be studied over 1 year. Study candidates must be 12 months without a period, not have had a hysterectomy and not have used hormones for 3 months.

Volunteers will be placed on hormones. Blood samples obtained and free supervision for study year provided. Call Dr. _____ at _____ .

J

FIG. 4.9. *Continued.*

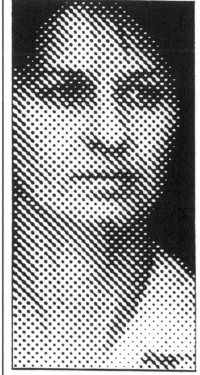

Can hormone therapy relieve menopausal symptoms?

STUDY VOLUNTEERS NEEDED

If you are a woman 40 or older who is experiencing numerous hot flashes and have:

☐ **had your last menstrual period within the past five years.**

☐ *not* **taken any hormone supplements in the last three months**

☐ *not* **had a hysterectomy**

then you may be eligible to participate in a four-month study evaluating various hormone supplement regimens for the treatment of menopausal symptoms.

Study medical tests and medication at no cost. As a study participant, you receive free physical examinations and a complete diagnostic evaluation of your current health status including blood tests, mammogram and Pap smear.

For further information, please call:

FIG. 4.9. *Continued.*

Pitfalls of Advertising

Attracting Different Types of Patients than Originally Enrolled

This problem is more likely to occur when advertisements are initiated while a trial is in progress. This problem would be greatly compounded if the inclusion criteria were broadened at the same time that advertisements were initiated. Before the results of a trial are pooled, the statistician(s) should ensure that comparable data were obtained from patients recruited from advertising and those recruited by other methods (see Chapter 12 on extrapolatability of data).

Figure continues on next page.

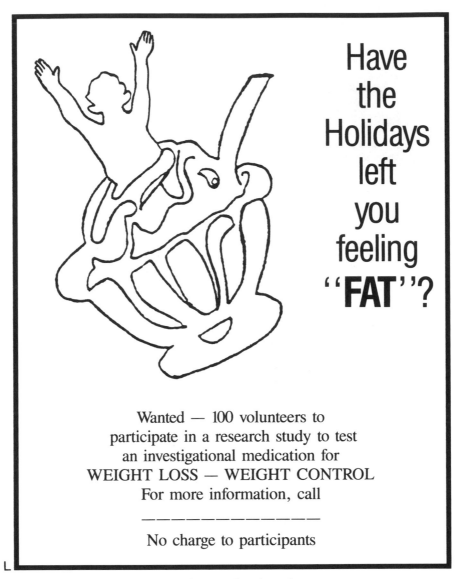

FIG. 4.9. *Continued.*

The Advertising has No Effect on Patient Enrollment

   To avoid this potential problem, it may be possible to conduct a pilot trial to assess whether or not advertisements will be successful. This pilot phase could provide information suggesting that (1) the message should be modified or changed totally, (2) the size (or length) of the advertisement should be increased, (3) a different medium should be used for the advertisement, (4) a different geographical area should be targeted, or (5) advertising is inappropriate for the particular trial.

WOULD YOU LIKE TO STOP DRINKING? The _____ University Department of Psychiatry is conducting a study combining psychotherapy with a promising new medication for the treatment of alcohol abuse. Treatment will be provided free of charge to individuals who volunteer and are eligible for the study. **Call _____ 9:00 a.m. — 4:30 p.m.**	Drug Research Study **ACNE** We are seeking men & women age 13-35 with Acne of the face to evaluate a new external Antibiotic Lotion. Volunteers will be evaluated by Dr._____ who has performed many such studies. Patients will be paid, and treatment is free. Please help us, and help yourself. Patients must qualify. Call for further information. **For information and qualifications call:_____**
Drug Research Study **TINEA VERSICOLOR** **(spotty body)** We are seeking men ages 18-70 to participate in a study to evaluate a new oral medication for the treatment of a white spotty fungus infection of the upper body which is called Tinea Versicolor. Women who are surgically sterile may also participate. Volunteers will be evaluated by Dr._____ who has performed many such studies. Patients must qualify. Call for further information. **For information and qualifications call:_____**	_____ **University** **OBESITY** **RESEARCH STUDY** Searching for healthy female subjects 18-55 years old, who need to lose a range between 40-70 lbs. Subjects must be available for hospitalization for 5-6 consecutive weeks. *No cost to those subjects who qualify.* **Call_____**

M

FIG. 4.9. *Continued.*

The Advertising Policy is Too Expensive

A strict limit should be established for the amount of money to be spent during the initial period of advertising, until results can be evaluated. Rather than commit all of one's resources to a single comprehensive advertising plan that is untested, and possibly ineffective, it is wise to establish a cut-off point for advertising campaigns.

The Advertisement May Attract Many Inappropriate Responders

If the text prepared for the advertisement does not carefully define the type of patient or volunteer sought, many readers will consider themselves or others as probably eligible for the trial. The result could be a large number of telephone calls in response to the advertisement, but a low yield of appropriate candidates. Investigators are generally concerned about possible selection bias if too many protocol details are listed in an advertisement and often use very broad statements to attract many responses to be screened by telephone. Shtasel et al. (1991) found that half of the callers in response to an advertisement for healthy people were ineligible

Figure continues on next page.

HIGH BLOOD PRESSURE

Volunteers either currently on or off treatment, needed for hypertension study. Men or women, 18-60 years old in otherwise good health. All examinations, blood testing, EKG's, and investigational medications are free.

You will be paid up to $300 for participating.

Board Certified Internist _____ Call _____

HIGH BLOOD PRESSURE?

Volunteers Needed
FOR HYPERTENSION STUDY

All examinations, laboratory testing, EKG's and research medications free. Enrollment limited, so call now. Qualified volunteers will be paid for their participation.

Call Nancy or Amy

_____

_____

MON.-FRI. 9AM-5PM

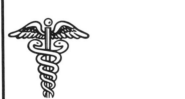

FIG. 4.9. *Continued.*

because of medical problems and 23% were not interested when the trial was described. Although the telephone screening efficiently reduced the number of secondary screening visits needed from 1,670 to 462, the recruitment process might have been more efficient if some items for self-assessment were included in the advertisement.

Publicity Campaigns

Publicity campaigns vary from some informal efforts by trial staff to large and formal campaigns conducted by professional groups (Tables 4.5 and 4.6).

HIGH BLOOD PRESSURE?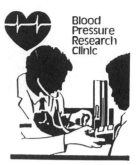

We need research volunteers with high blood pressure to participate in ongoing investigational medication studies.

Blood Pressure Research Clinic

Benefit from Free Medication,
Counseling, and Medical Care.

Call _____ Out of Area 1-800
_____ MD, F.A.C.P.

Did you know that hypertension is called the "silent killer" and can lead to strokes, heart and kidney disease, and death? Volunteers with high blood pressure are needed to participate in a nationwide trial of an investigational medication for hypertension. Patients with high blood pressure will be seen in Fresno, and those who meet the criteria will not be charged for office visits, blood pressure checks, labs, EKGs, Chest X-rays, or medication. In fact, patients will receive up to $200.00 for time and travel expenses.

O For more information please call _____ .

FIG. 4.9. *Continued.*

Preparation for Calls After Publicity

Trial staff should be prepared for a deluge of telephone calls after any lecture, media presentation, or advertisement. The investigator and staff should be prepared to handle the following:

1. Have a sufficient number of people available to talk with prospective enrollees. People who are knowledgeable about the clinical trial's inclusion criteria and who

TABLE 4.5. *Activities to consider that utilize public relations firms*

1. Conduct community screening at athletic events, entertainment events, shopping centers
2. Request public figures and celebrities to endorse the trial and recruitment activities at major events through public service radio and television announcements
3. Create attractive pamphlets about the trial and have mailing companies send to purchased lists of potential enrollees
4. Request a city's mayor or state's governor to issue a proclamation about the trial and then advertise this event widely
5. Prepare a series of different newspaper, radio, or television advertisements
6. Issue press releases and background material about the disease or the medicine being studied from which reporters can create stories and heighten public awareness
7. Place an investigator on a radio or television talk show
8. Contact media representatives. The advantage of having public relations people do this is that they have more experience and knowledge in (1) who to contact, (2) what time of day is best to contact them[a], (3) what to say to them, and (4) how to deal with them most effectively

[a] It is best to contact radio reporters immediately after a show airs, television reporters from 10 AM to noon for the evening news, and newspaper reporters from 10 AM to noon for the next morning's paper.

Figure continues on next page.

Do You Suffer From Angina?

_____ is conducting a clinical trial of a new investigational medication for treatment of chronic stable angina.

Participants must be 21 years or older and have at least a three-month documented history of chronic stable angina triggered by physical effort and relieved by rest or nitroglycerin.

Participants who qualify will receive:

☐ **Free medication**
☐ **Free physical exam**
☐ **Free electrocardiogram (ECG)**
☐ **$100 compensation**

If interested please call

_____
_____

P

FIG. 4.9. *Continued.*

TABLE 4.6. *An example of an incremental approach to the public relations process*

1. Pretrial announcement
2. Startup announcement
3. Contacts with department physicians
4. Letters to local physicians and clinics
5. Press release to public and local lay groups
6. Advertisements in local media
7. Calls to local physicians and clinics that have referred patients to encourage continuing referrals
8. Community screening

DOCTORS _____ **IN**
RHEUMATOLOGY
ARE SCREENING VOLUNTEERS
FOR PARTICIPATION IN
CLINICAL RESEARCH TRIALS WITH
INVESTIGATIONAL ARTHRITIS MEDICINES
FOR THE TREATMENT OF
RHEUMATOID ARTHRITIS, OSTEOARTHRITIS

AGES 18 THROUGH 70   CALL: _____

DO YOU HAVE HEARTBURN
3 TO 10 TIMES A WEEK?

If the answer is yes and you
would like to participate in a
Research Program with marketed
medications, contact us at:

_____

_____

You will be compensated for time & travel

Q

FIG. 4.9. *Continued.*

are generally capable of discussing the medical disorder should handle contacts with potential participants.

2. Be prepared for queries unrelated to the trial. Many calls will relate to issues not pertinent to the trial from patients and families anxious to make contact with an expert in that disease. These contacts must be handled with particular care and concern without interfering with the ongoing relationship between the patient and their regular physician.

Figure continues on next page.

OSTEOARTHRITIS OF THE KNEE

VOLUNTEER PATIENTS NEEDED FOR INVESTIGATIONAL DRUG TRIAL WITH SAN ANTONIO RHEUMATOLOGIST. MEDICINE, LABORATORY TESTING, PHYSICAL EXAMINATION AND MEDICAL SUPERVISION ARE FREE TO ELIGIBLE PERSONS. PLEASE CALL _____ 9:00-12:00 OR 1:45-5:00 FOR FURTHER INFORMATION.

Diabetes Research.
is conducting several research studies on Diabetes. The studies are particularly for adult-onset (or Type II) diabetes which is controlled by **insulin only**. Volunteers need to be diabetics who are 25 years or older and are not taking oral medications for their diabetes. Participants will receive physical examinations, diet counseling, EKGs and lab tests; and a stipend for their time and effort. For more information, call _____ and ask for either _____ R _____ .

FIG. 4.9. *Continued.*

3. Information about the investigational status of the trial. Whether or not medical benefit is expected, the status of the investigational medicine or device should be revealed to potential participants. Scrupulous honesty about the risks involved in a trial is mandatory at all stages but particularly during the initial screening so that patients are not led to believe that the medicine is thoroughly safe and without risk. Some patients experience shock and letdown when they read full details in the informed consent.

4. Screening appointments. Although most initial telephone contacts are used as a means to quickly screen for potentially eligible participants, not all callers are willing to leave their name. A plan should be established whereby the recruiter or person answering the call can make a nonthreatening request for follow-up information. As an example, the recruiter could say: ''I understand that you are not prepared to make an appointment to discuss the trial with the doctor, but would you kindly give me your name and telephone number so that I can call you in a few weeks, after you have had time to think about the clinical trial?'' or, ''May I have your name and address in order to send you some material describing the clinical trial that you can look over and discuss with your family or your doctor?'' Telephone bank operators are usually not medically trained but can perform well with simple telephone skills training.

5. Briefing material. Prepare a small booklet describing the details of the trial that can be sent to interested callers (as described above). This should be more detailed than the poster. A simple method to ensure that adequate and accurate information is included is to abstract the information in the informed consent form. This approach is not generally suitable for small trials. Trials sponsored by the National Heart,

DEPARTMENT OF HEALTH & HUMAN SERVICES   Public Health Service

Food and Drug Administration
Rockville MD 20857

February 1989

ADVERTISING FOR STUDY SUBJECTS

Institutional Review Boards (IRBs) are responsible for ensuring the equitable selection of research subjects (21 CFR 56.111 (a) (3)). In fulfilling this responsibility, IRBs should review the methods that investigators use to recruit subjects. One method of recruiting subjects is through advertisements. Advertising for research subjects is not in and of itself an objectionable practice. However, when advertising is to be used, the IRB should review the information contained in the advertisement, and the mode of its communication, to determine that the procedure for recruiting subjects affords adequate protection.

FDA requires that an IRB review and have authority to approve, require modifications in, or disapprove all research activities covered by the IRB regulations (21 CFR 56.109). FDA expects an IRB to review all the research documents and activities that bear directly on the rights and welfare of the subjects of proposed research. The protocol, the consent form, and the investigator's brochure have consistently been cited as specific examples of documents that the IRB should review.

Advertisements used to recruit subjects should be seen as an extension of the informed consent and subject selection processes. (See 21 CFR 50.20, 21 CFR 50.25, and 21 CFR 56.111 (a) (3).) Institutions should, therefore, require IRB review of such advertisements. IRB review is necessary to ensure that the information is not misleading to subjects, especially when a study will involve persons with acute or severe physical or mental illness or persons who are economically or educationally disadvantaged. The IRB is responsible for assuring that appropriate safeguards exist to protect the rights and welfare of research subjects (21 CFR 56.111 (b)).

Generally, FDA believes that any advertisement to recruit subjects should be limited to:

1. the name and address of the clinical investigator;

2. the purpose of the research and, in summary form, the eligibility criteria that will be used to admit subjects into the study;

3. a straightforward and truthful description of the benefits (e.g., payments or free treatment) to the subject from participation in the study; and

4. the location of the research and the person to contact for further information.

No claims should be made, either explicitly or implicitly, that the drug or device is safe or effective for the purposes under investigation, or that the drug or device is in any way equivalent or superior to any other drug or device. Such representation would not only be misleading to subjects but would also be a violation of the FDA's regulations concerning the promotion of investigational drugs (21 CFR 312.7 (a)) and of investigational devices (21 CFR 812.7 (d)).

FIG. 4.10. Letter from the FDA with information relevant for patient recruitment in trials regarding advertising for patients.

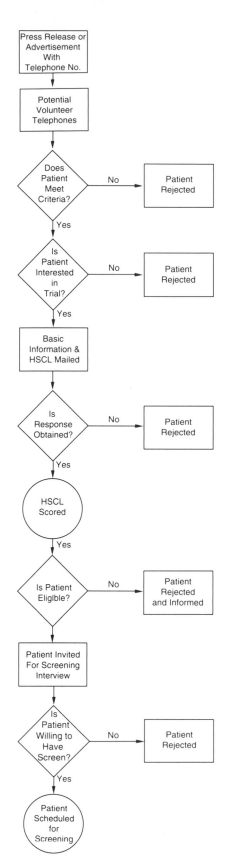

FIG. 4.11. Flow diagram of patient responses to newspaper advertisements or stories based on press releases. HSCL, Hopkins Symptom Checklist. Modified from Covi et al. (1979).

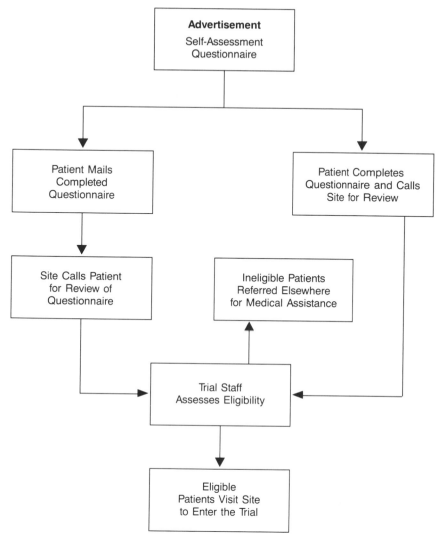

FIG. 4.12. Flow diagram of the recruitment of symptomatic volunteers. Modified from Covi et al. (1979).

Lung, and Blood Institute (NHLBI) frequently provide pamphlets to interested callers. Other examples of brochures or flyers designed for patients are shown later in this chapter.

Telephone Screening in Response to Advertising

Only a small amount of information about a trial is usually included in an advertisement but the suggestion is almost always made for interested persons to call for more details. The initial screening for eligibility is made during the telephone call. The simplest system is to have calls directed to the investigator or recruitment coordinator who can describe the trial and judge whether the caller is potentially eligible before making an appointment for further evaluation. Large clinical trials and those conducted over extensive geographic areas often establish a toll-free (800 number in the United States) line that directs inquiries to a central location. This method can simply be used to ask for the caller's name, address, telephone number, and other pertinent information as needed. The trial site nearest the prospective patient may be given the information to contact the patient, and the prospective patient is given the name of the nearest investigator and local recruitment coordinator who will make contact with them. In a more refined method, trained operators answer all calls and conduct preliminary screening for qualifying demographic and clinical criteria. If the caller meets the initial criteria, the operator reads a script describing the trial. Operators should be trained to answer some questions beyond the script and to refer special questions to staff monitors or clinical trial managers. The Parkinson Study Group (1989) advertised a national toll-free telephone number to recruit patients. Information about the trial was provided and patients were referred to one of the 28 sites in the United States and Canada. The central telephone group performed 2,424 patient telephone interviews totaling 39% of total inquiries.

The Computerized Patient Accrual System (CPAS) developed by Premier Research (Westchester, IL) is a computer-based telephone system using toll-free telephone numbers for rapid acquisition of patients for clinical trials. CPAS manages recruitment for numerous clinical trials using a centralized, trained staff. Scripts are designed for each trial and backup for unusual questions are referred to staff for the individual trial. The Pediatric Oncology Group developed a fully automated system that receives telephone calls and creates a dialogue without human intervention (Krischer et al., 1991). The microcomputer-based technology accepts dial tone pulses and creates spoken sound from text files using a Texas Instruments Speech System. Calls can be monitored on an external speaker. The advantage of the automated system is its ability to answer calls 24 hours a day, 7 days a week. The potential disadvantage is patient confusion or dislike of the computer-generated interview. Both systems can be designed to perform other tasks including making appointments, calling patients who miss appointments, tracking all eligible callers to determine whether they enroll, as well as tabulate the sources of publicity that led to calls.

Community Screening

Large scale, preventive trials usually require screening of a wide population to inform potential patients of their risk to develop a particular disease. These include the possible detection of (1) high cholesterol during lipid screening, (2) hypertension during blood pressure screening, and (3) breast cancer during mammography screening. Routine mass population screening is not intended for individuals whose personal medical care includes screening for those disorders. The purpose of community screening is to alert the remaining public to their potential risks. The clinical trial staff provide free or low-cost testing and return results to the individuals tested or to their physicians. Thus, no obligation to enter a trial is made when the person presents for a screening test. At this time, trial staff have an opportunity to describe the purpose of the trial and initiate contact with people who might be eligible. Thereafter, follow-up with patients for trial recruitment is made through standard medical channels.

Contacting appropriate areas of a community for screening can be accomplished through mail, telephone, or door-to-door interviewing using randomized or total sorting based on mail postal code, telephone area code, or regional demographics. Another method of preselection is to approach industrial sites and companies where workers are (or may be) stratified into occupational groups and age blocks. Unselected screening can be accomplished by solicitation in shopping malls in downtown areas or using mobile vans. News media stories and advertising will heighten the response to community screening by informing the general public of the purpose of the screening and the potential personal benefits to be gained from it.

Examples of Community Screening

Recruitment through community screening was reviewed by Melish (1982). He defined community screening as "mass screening linked to any event, location or organization," and described recruitment strategies used for the Coronary Primary Prevention Trial. Their method involved utilizing clinical trial staff and volunteers to attend health fairs, sporting events, exhibitions, and conventions and to establish temporary screening sites at shopping centers, parks, and other locations where large numbers of people congregate. Mobile vans were used in this trial to attract the target population and maintain a standardized office/laboratory area for cholesterol screening. Other trials have used simple tables and banners at appropriate locations to attract attention, collect names of potential participants, and perform a preliminary screening with a questionnaire. Schrott and Merideth (1982) described the development of media messages to remind people of the importance of blood pressure and cholesterol checks. A program called "Cholesterol Check! 75" was widely advertised as a free testing for cholesterol. Their Table 7 describes the system used to develop media participation. Other sites used mass mailing strategies including voter registration lists, drivers' licensee lists, and group membership lists in addition to direct mail services by postal code (McDearmon and Bradford, 1982). One advantage to a broad-based mailing is that the volume of the letters mailed weekly or monthly may be adjusted based on the current screening activity resulting from the prior list. Levenkron and Farquhar (1982) described specific methods of mass media recruitment including television, radio, local magazines, newspapers, programs for local events, billboards, brochures, and printed messages on municipal bus passes.

Community screening using telephone contacts in specific census tracts complemented by personal recruitment at the home of the potential participants was a successful method for the Coronary Artery Disease Risk Development in Young Adults (CARDIA) trial (Hughes et al., 1987). The Chicago site used random digit dialing of computer-generated telephone numbers, followed by census tract telephoning to balance demographic factors. The disadvantage to this method was the inclusion of many business and unused telephone numbers, although unpublished numbers were included (an advantage of this method). The Oakland site prepared a demographically balanced list prior to initiating the telephone campaign. The Birmingham clinic used random selection of telephone numbers. Simultaneous with the telephone campaign, local media and endorsement of community leaders were used to publicize the trial. In addition, the trial was able to reimburse participants up to $25.00 for expenses related to screening examinations.

Patient Registries

Newcomb et al. (1990) describe the use of a population-based cancer registry to recruit for a placebo-controlled, double-blind trial of tamoxifen. They used the Wisconsin Cancer Reporting System to identify 3,585 women of the correct age, stage of disease, and previous therapy. They sent letters to these women's physicians requesting them to sign letters about the trial and mail them, with a brochure, to potentially eligible women. Of the women who received a letter, 38% contacted the trial office. The goal of 140 patients enrolled was achieved over an 18-month period.

This approach could also be used where professional or lay groups maintain registries. Registries are particularly important for identifying patients with rare diseases. It would be essential to maintain patient privacy until the patient decided to contact the trial site or allow the trial site to contact them. Various types of registries are indicated in Table 4.7.

Patient Registries for Future Clinical Trials

Patients with certain chronic diseases (e.g., cancer) or rare diseases may be listed in a registry (Herson, 1980). This practice enables recruitment activities to be much more efficient and rapid if and when a clinical trial is proposed for that group of patients. Registries could be maintained by a regional center (e.g., oncology coordinating center), by a lay organization focusing on a rare disease, by a professional society, or by any interested group. This group of patients serves as a pool that should expedite the recruitment process.

Journal Notices, Letters, and Editorials

The journal *Oncology* regularly describes ongoing clinical trial protocols under the heading "Clinical Trials: Referral Resource" (compiled by Bruce Cheson, MD, of the National Cancer Institute). Cheson presents a structured abstract of each trial which averages about one-third to one-half of a page per trial. The abstract indicates

1. Type of cancer in bold heading and large type
2. Disease status of patients
3. Protocol number
4. Title of protocol
5. Principal investigator
6. Background of the trial
7. Eligibility criteria

TABLE 4.7. *Types of registries to use for obtaining prospective names of patients*

1. Medical records in an office practice
2. Medical records in a hospital
3. Blood bank donor lists
4. Public health registries
5. Societies of patients with a special disease
6. Insurance records
7. Government registries of patients with a specific disease

8. Treatment
9. Expected total number of patients to be enrolled
10. Total accrual as of the latest date
11. Telephone number to call

A 6-page summary of previously described trials was presented in the January, 1991 issue. This approach could be adopted by various other journals for appropriate trials. A variation of this approach is to present a news story in a journal describing the need for recruitment (Anonymous, 1988).

Letters to the editor are published in many clinical journals and may be used to solicit patient referrals to clinical trials. A representative example describes an ongoing ophthalmological trial (Macular Photocoagulation Study, 1984a).

Editorials in clinical journals may be used as a vehicle to stimulate patient recruitment in a specific clinical trial (Fine, 1980; Beck, 1988). Editorials are also used as an attempt to increase patient recruitment in a large number of trials (Friedman, 1987; Wittes and Friedman, 1988). Editorials about a specific trial may also be detailed and discuss recruitment issues (Fine, 1984).

Card-Return System to Contact Patients

Some Ethics Committees/IRBs require that investigators use a card-return system to contact patients about enrolling in an epidemiologic study. In this method, the investigator contacts a physician and requests permission to contact one or more of his or her patients. If permission is granted the investigator writes to the patient explaining the study and encloses a card that the patient is requested to return by mail to the investigator. The Ethics Committee/IRB usually limits the investigator to following up with only those patients who return cards. Additional contact of patients who have not returned their cards is considered unethical. Similarly, cards included in brochures or coupons in advertisements can be returned by patients interested in obtaining information about a trial. This method may obviate the need for mass mailing or telephoning.

One criticism of this method is that if the percent of patients who return a card is low, it then may indicate that they differ in some way from those who do not return their cards. This in turn would suggest that substantial bias may be inherent in the study. McTiernan et al.(1986) examined this issue in a case-controlled study of thyroid cancer in western Washington State women. They compared demographics and clinical characteristics of 124 women who returned a card and 35 women who did not but were subsequently interviewed. The authors observed differences between the groups. Risk factors also differed between the groups. These data suggest that serious limitations may exist with this method.

Use of Pharmacies

The Upjohn Company conducted a postmarketing surveillance study of prescription acne medications (Facklam et al., 1990) and enrolled 58 pharmacies using methodology described by Borden and Lee (1982). The pharmacists were "nominally reimbursed for their participation." The pharmacists described the study to all patients who presented a prescription for an acne medication and 13,465 of these patients were registered. Of these, 10,282 (76%) signed an informed consent agreeing to further follow-up and access to their medical records. The study consisted of two computer-assisted telephone interviews. Patients were not paid for their participation. Complete data were obtained from 6,453 patients. This method would seem to be an excellent means of assessing adverse reactions and other health events related to use of specific medications as part of a postmarketing surveillance study. Some of the limitations to this method identified by the authors are:

1. Invitation to participate in the study is probably not complete nor random. Pharmacists may invite patients when they are not busy and have time to discuss the study. Pharmacists also may invite primarily friendly patients.
2. All prescriptions for the medicine usually are not audited to assess the percent approached and enrolled, or to determine whether patients on all medicines used were approached at an equal rate.
3. Data are not collected on first time versus repeat use, duration of prior use, dose, and regimen.

Random Telephone Dialing to Obtain Controls

Numerous case-controlled trials have obtained controls using random-digit telephone dialing. Controls may be matched to cases for (1) sex, (2) race, (3) age, and (4) geographic location (Grufferman et al.,1984). In the approach described by Grufferman et al.(1984), age could be within 3 years, except for patients less than 5 years old whose controls, had to be within 1 year. Geographic area control was assured by using the same three-digit telephone number and area code as for the patient identified as the case.

Various procedures (too detailed to describe here) may be used to minimize the number of telephone calls to nonworking and nonresidential numbers (e.g., the computer randomly generates only the last two numbers of the telephone number, that number is dialed up to 15 times, including days, evenings, and weekends). Readers are referred to an article by Waksberg (1978) for additional details.

If there is a response, the person making the screening calls should state his or her university affiliation and ask for basic demographic data on family members to determine if any qualify as a control. If so, their interest in participating in the trial is discussed. A consent form is obtained by the center, and a telephone interview is scheduled.

CHANCE AND LUCK

There are numerous types of clinical trials where everything is planned perfectly and a perfect recruitment strategy is developed, but the trial still fails because of patient recruitment problems. Several examples are:

1. *Trials that depend on seasonal factors.* Most seasonal factors are out of anyone's control (e.g., for trials that evaluate treatments for seasonal allergies). Some years are better or worse than others for allergy sufferers depending on rain, temperature, and other factors. In some cases, a backup clinical trial could be initiated in another region or country where seasonal allergies are either worse or not im-

proved that particular year. The study of colds or influenza symptoms also fits this pattern because the number of patients affected vary greatly from year to year.

2. *Trials that depend on acute problems that have not yet occurred.* The incidence of many acute problems cannot be accurately predicted for any particular site. Wide variation in prevalence may occur, particularly when problems are based on chance or unknown factors (e.g., back sprains, burns, drownings, tennis elbow).

3. *Trials that depend on weather conditions.* Trials to study effects of medicines in skiers (e.g., for herpes labialis) or scuba divers (e.g., for baropressure problems) can be markedly affected by weather conditions that prevent people from doing these activities.

Countering these problems is not always possible, and sometimes the only options are to proceed despite the limitations, delay the trial, or cancel the trial. Other approaches are to modify the protocol so that more patients are eligible to enroll, intensify recruitment efforts, or initiate more sites (or a separate trial) at geographically different locations.

CHOOSING METHOD(S) FOR PATIENT RECRUITMENT

In choosing methods, it is better to consider the overall recruitment strategy and the advantages and disadvantages of each major method that could be used rather than apply a single formula. Some authors suggest using referring physicians only when referring physicians have no concerns about losing patients and there is no recognized form of therapy. However, there are numerous exceptions to all of these and other principles. The investigator who understands the pros and cons of most recruitment methods can do much better in choosing the most appropriate one(s) for a specific trial than can someone who sticks to a series of rules.

Choice of method(s) for recruitment is based on the overall assessment of several factors. These include (1) number of patients required; (2) type and availability of patients required for the trial; and (3) special requirements of patients that might be difficult, unpleasant, or onerous to many. For example, the Aspirin Myocardial Infarction Study (AMIS) sought patients within the first two months after a myocardial infarction. Thus, a search of hospital records was chosen as the most effective method to use. This method accrued 40% of all enrollees. The next largest group came from self-referral after media announcements (35%) (Schoenberger, 1987). Even though almost all patients were inpatients and in a hospital at the time when screening could have taken place, these investigators found that physicians were not a reliable or steady source of patient referrals. This finding in a trial of medically ill patients reinforces the problem of relying on medical staff for recruitment referrals. Schoenberger (1987) indicated that physicians require constant reminders to recall a trial and its need for enrollments when they are seeing patients. In contrast, the Thrombolysis in Myocardial Infarction (TIMI) trial fulfilled recruitment needs using patients identified in an emergency room or coronary care unit (Knatterud and Foreman, 1987). The availability of special cardiac care teams probably resulted in more careful screening of all patients, especially when team members were interested in studying tissue plasminogen activator therapy, which was a novel medicine and only available at that time to randomized patients within the trial.

Both small and large clinical trials would benefit from the advice given by Hunninghake et al. (1987) about choosing methods for patient recruitment: maintain several recruitment methods at all times. Not depending on a single method is prudent; realizing that no one method is optimum to reach all potential patients is wise; and acknowledging that no one can predict how well a method will function in your trial is conservative. On the other hand, there are numerous trials (e.g., pharmacokinetic, Phase I safety, Phase II pilot) where a single method is sufficient to enroll the usually small number of patients required. A final factor to consider are the regulatory guidelines of each particular country. These guidelines may preclude using methods that are highly successful in other countries. A letter describing FDA policies that would influence recruitment is shown in Fig 4.10.

COMPARISON OF RECRUITMENT METHODS

Albanes et al. (1986) compared three methods of direct patient recruitment in a lung cancer trial. The first method of direct invitation utilized mailing a brochure describing the trial along with a letter of invitation to prospective participants. The second method added a brief questionnaire inquiring about smoking habits and past history of cancer along with the brochure describing the trial. Patients deemed eligible based on questionnaire information were then invited to participate. The third method of self-determined eligibility structured the questionnaire so that if the person met the eligibility criteria, he or she was asked to visit the trial clinic at a scheduled time. Noneligible patients were asked only to return their questionnaires. The overall enrollment rate was 40%, with the highest rates coming from the group of self-determined eligibility. The direct invitation method yielded 38%, eligibility screening by mail 33%, and self-determined eligibility 49%. However, the authors mentioned that patients recruited by the second method required fewer initial screening visits than those from the other two groups. A similar chemoprevention trial for smokers planned two recruitment strategies for initial use: referral from other physicians and media promotion. The organizers planned additional recruitment strategies that would be held in abeyance pending the recruitment experience of the first year. The second set of options included occupational screening and addition of a second site (Arnold et al., 1989). The initial press release was developed for the investigators by the university public relations department for announcements on television, radio, and in newspapers. Thereafter, the investigators maintained contact with local media for follow-up stories, provided posters for local distribution, and paid for several advertisements. This trial anticipated increased contacts from the public after the press release and they hired extra staff and installed additional phone lines to facilitate the recruitment process. Newspaper advertising resulted in 65% of all participants who entered the trial. Overall, media publicity accounted for 93% of patient randomizations (i.e., entry). However, the efficiency of these methods was approximately 10%, meaning that one patient was randomized for every ten contacts. Mitchell et al. (1991) compared two strategies to recruit older women for cervical cancer screening. They compared (1) personal letters of invitation, (2) a community-based campaign, and (3) a combined strategy, finding the latter to be most effective. However, the letter alone was most cost-effective in terms of yield of eligible women.

Brauzer and Goldstein (1973) used a direct appeal to recruit symptomatic volunteers. The method (Fig. 4.9) consisted of a quarter-page newspaper advertisement that described the trial and included a 35-item, self-rating symptom checklist. The checklist was a short form of a standardized checklist that allowed readers to assess their level of anxiety and depression factors as self-determinants for eligibility. In addition, a general description of the program and eligibility criteria were provided. Symptomatic volunteers were asked to reply by mail, enclosing the checklist for eligibility review by the research team. The advertisement was used repeatedly, obtaining 100–175 replies from a newspaper that had a circulation of 400,000 copies. Most replies were received within 4 days of the advertisement, demonstrating the effectiveness of this method.

Covi et al. (1979) also used this method with an alternate system of telephone response in addition to mail replies (Fig. 4.11). Their system included a media release or advertisement describing the trial briefly and inviting potential symptomatic volunteers to telephone the research unit for further information. When patients telephoned the site a checklist was reviewed with them over the telephone to assess their eligibility. Investigators compared mail and telephone responses to the advertisement and found that both processes resulted in the same proportion of respondents accepted for the trial. In the first method, a large newspaper advertisement included a short form of a standardized checklist that allowed readers to assess their level of anxiety and depression factors as self-determinants for eligibility. In addition, a general description of the program and eligibility criteria were described. Symptomatic volunteers were asked to reply by mail, enclosing the checklist for eligibility review by the research team. The alternate method included a media release or advertisement describing the trial briefly and inviting potential symptomatic volunteers to telephone the research unit for further information, at which time a checklist was reviewed over the telephone to assess their eligibility. The direct method of recruitment requires that appropriate information be provided to the self-referred symptomatic volunteers who do not qualify for the trial but who do need medical attention.

Recruitment methods were compared for letters sent to 100 general practitioners near a large city hospital and for newspaper advertisements (Tiller and Biddle, 1991). Four formats were used for the letters (i.e., short or detailed, with or without an offer to visit the practice) seeking patients with generalized anxiety disorders. All letters to physicians resulted in ten referrals, two of whom met DSM-III criteria for generalized anxiety disorder. The format used was not found to be important. The newspaper advertisement resulted in over 500 contacts, screening interviews were scheduled for 136 patients, and 56 of the 120 individuals who attended met the DSM-III criteria. This latter approach was much more economical in terms of time and effort than the letters to physicians.

A sequential approach to patient recruitment beginning with media publicity about the trial, followed by mass mailing and targeted telephoning was used effectively in the Systolic Hypertension in the Elderly (SHEP) trial (Petrovich et al., 1991).

PREPARING A BROCHURE DESCRIBING THE CLINICAL TRIAL TO MAIL TO PROSPECTIVE ENROLLEES

A wide variety of brochures are being used as adjuncts to other methods of enhancing patient enrollment in clinical trials. Brochures that are not trial-specific are prepared by and about individual clinics (Fig. 4.13). They encourage patients to visit the clinic and to consider enrolling in trials. Other brochures describe the nature of

Text continues on p. 147.

Today's Research

Tomorrow's Health ™

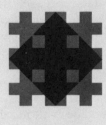

VOLUNTEERING

UPJOHN RESEARCH CLINICS

BCIU/JASPER

Today's Research

Tomorrow's Health ™

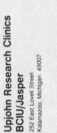

Upjohn Research Clinics
BCIU/Jasper
252 East Lovell Street
Kalamazoo, Michigan 49007

BCIU is located at 252 E. Lovell Street on the 5th floor of Bronson Methodist Hospital's Center Building.

The Jasper Clinic is located at 526 Jasper Street (*east of the hospital*).

Parking for both visitors and volunteers to the Upjohn Research Clinics is available at the south parking ramp located on the corner of Jasper and Walnut Streets. The entrance to the ramp is off Healthcare Plaza. (*Across from the helipad*). Parking is available in the reserved parking spaces marked BCIU/JASPER.

FIG. 4.13A–X. Brochures for patients. All are reprinted with permission. (4.13A and B are a single brochure.)

A

124

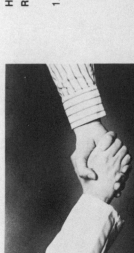

Only through a team

effort of scientists,

physicians, and YOU

can medicine advance

to conquer diseases.

HOW TO BECOME A MEDICAL RESEARCH VOLUNTEER

1. Call 384-9644 (long distance 1–800–458–6072) or visit the Recruitment Office in The Bronson Clinical Investigation Unit (BCIU) Monday through Friday 8:00 a.m. – 4:30 p.m. for an interview.

2. Attend an informed consent meeting. At this time the research staff will provide a detailed explanation of the study.

3. Sign a consent to participate.

4. Complete a medical history form and undergo a physical examination including laboratory studies.

5. Comply with all the study requirements, if you are selected as a participant.

HOW YOU BENEFIT

● Gain a sense of contributing to the advancement of medical science.

● Receive a free physical examination.

● Receive payment for study participation.

For further information please call 384-9644.

WE LOOK FORWARD TO HEARING FROM YOU!

B

FIG. 4.13. *Continued.*

Figure continues on next page.

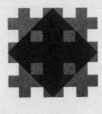

Today's Research

Tomorrow's Health ™

MEDICAL RESEARCH

UPJOHN RESEARCH CLINICS

BCIU/JASPER

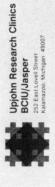

Upjohn Research Clinics
BCIU/Jasper
252 East Lovell Street
Kalamazoo, Michigan 49907

Parking

Parking for both visitors and volunteers to the Upjohn Research Clinics is available at the south parking ramp located on the corner of Jasper and Walnut Streets. The entrance to the ramp is off Healthcare Plaza. *(Across from the helipad).* Parking is available in the reserved parking spaces marked BCIU/JASPER.

Hours

Normal business hours are Monday through Friday, 8:00 a.m. to 4:30 p.m.

For Further Information

For further information concerning the Upjohn Research Clinics - BCIU/Jasper please call 385-7620. For information on current study activities, the Upjohn Research Clinics have established a 24 hour Hot Line 385-6861. For further information on volunteering for a study please call 384-9644.

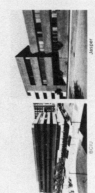

BCIU

Jasper

C

FIG. 4.13. *Continued. (4.13C and D are a single brochure.)*

126

Before permitting the marketing of a new medication, the Food and Drug Administration in Washington, D.C. requires proof that the medication is safe for human use and is effective in the prevention or treatment of disease.

For this reason the Upjohn Research Clinics were created in 1973 by Bronson Methodist Hospital and The Upjohn Company. The clinics are comprised of the Bronson Clinical Investigational Unit (BCIU) and the Jasper Clinic located in Kalamazoo, and the Victoria Clinic located in London, Ontario, Canada. The Kalamazoo facilities provide our community with the opportunity for education and experience in the clinical testing of new and existing medications, and studying their effect on various diseases.

The need for research volunteers is constantly growing. Within the first ten years, the Upjohn Research Clinic completed over five hundred studies, involving approximately ten thousand human volunteers. These volunteers range in age from 18 to 90 years, and include hospital and Upjohn employees, college students, business people, factory workers, self-employed individuals and many others.

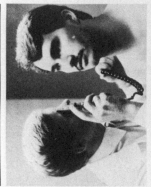

Volunteers are fully informed of the nature, risks and benefits of each study before they agree to participate

Some studies can be completed in a single day. Others require overnight stays in which the volunteers are comfortably housed in either BCIU or Jasper.

D

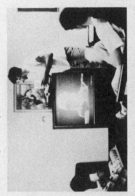

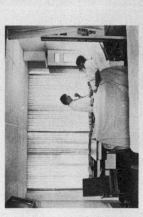

Most studies are preceded by a brief medical history, physical examination and laboratory studies.

Volunteers are encouraged to ask questions and are free to withdraw from a study at any time.

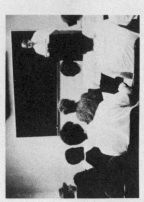

There are nicely decorated and furnished lounges, bedrooms and recreation areas. The facilities also include televisions, videogames, a pool table, quiet rooms for studying and even a sun deck.

Each study is reviewed by committees of experts in ethics, pharmacology, law, medicine, human rights, religion and social work to ensure the study is appropriate and scientifically sound. Each volunteer is protected according to the international code of ethics regarding volunteers in experimental studies.

Volunteers participate for various reasons. They receive compensation for their participation according to the time required, inconvenience incurred and study requirements. Most feel they are making significant contributions to the solution of human suffering. Others have an interest in how medical research is conducted, and some believe that their research involvement is a human responsibility.

General Comments of Volunteers:

"It was very much enjoyable. The staff explained every step that was taken and I felt very comfortable with them."

"I really don't see how my experience could be improved upon. I enjoyed it from the very beginning and look forward to the possibility of taking in another study."

"The importance of teamwork was clearly a good example in this program."

"I gained insight on how drugs are tested, their effectiveness and side effects. I felt I was really contributing something to the future. I hope that someone might benefit because of my involvement."

"Best treatment I've ever received at a medical facility, commendable staff!"

Only through a team effort of scientists, physicians, and YOU can medicine advance to conquer diseases.

FIG. 4.13. Continued.

Figure continues on next page.

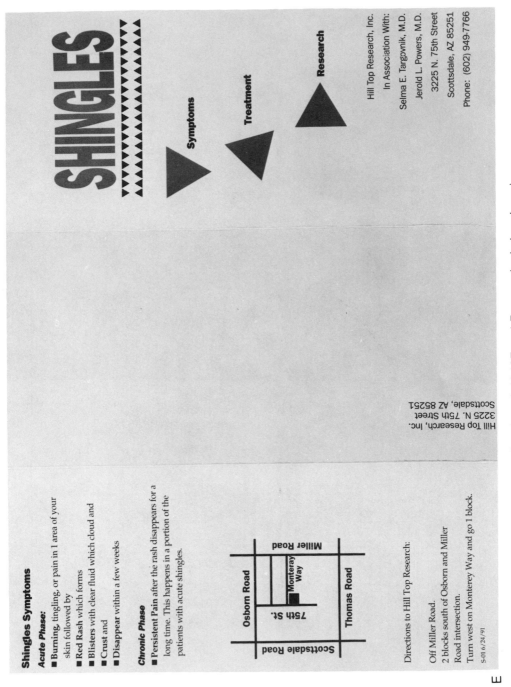

Shingles Symptoms

Acute Phase:

- Burning, tingling, or pain in 1 area of your skin followed by
- Red Rash which forms
- Blisters with clear fluid which cloud and
- Crust and
- Disappear within a few weeks

Chronic Phase

- Persistent Pain after the rash disappears for a long time. This happens in a portion of the patients with acute shingles.

Directions to Hill Top Research:

Off Miller Road.
2 blocks south of Osborn and Miller Road intersection.
Turn west on Monteray Way and go 1 block.

5-01 6/24/91

Hill Top Research, Inc.
3225 N. 75th Street
Scottsdale, AZ 85251

SHINGLES

Symptoms

Treatment

Research

Hill Top Research, Inc.

In Association With:

Selma E. Targovnik, M.D.
Jerold L. Powers, M.D.
3225 N. 75th Street
Scottsdale, AZ 85251
Phone: (602) 949-7766

E

FIG. 4.13. Continued. (4.13E and F are a single brochure.)

128

About Shingles

Perhaps you have known someone who has experienced the discomfort of shingles. About 20% (1 out of 5) of the population is affected at some time during their lives. Everyone who has had chicken pox has the potential to develop shingles. The chicken pox virus may hide dormant in the body for years until one day it reactivates, this time as shingles. No one knows why the virus becomes active a second time, but stress or a dip in immunity seems likely to be involved.

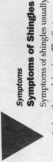

Symptoms
Symptoms of Shingles

Symptoms of shingles usually appear before the rash begins. The first symptom is burning, tingling, pain, or extreme sensitivity in one area of the skin. The trunk and the buttocks are the most often involved areas, but shingles can appear anywhere on the body, including the face. One to three days after the first symptoms, a red rash develops which becomes a group of blisters that cloud up and then crust, usually within 10 days.

People with shingles are often very uncomfortable. One of the complications of the condition is pain which may last for years. Research is ongoing to attempt to find a new effective treatment against shingles and the pain associated with it.

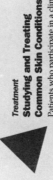

Treatment
Studying and Treating Common Skin Conditions

Patients who participate in a clinical research study can often make a difference in the lives of many others who have the same condition by helping test investigational drugs and treatments. At the same time, volunteer patients can be assured of participating in a study that has been carefully designed by physicians and researchers. Patients in a clinical research study are directly overseen by a medical staff that is personally concerned about its volunteers. We are in the process of recruiting patients for a study of shingles.

You may qualify for this study if:
- You are 18 or older
- Have a rash you think might be shingles
- Your rash is less than three days old

Research
The Current Study About Shingles

We are currently studying volunteer patients who are diagnosed with shingles in its earliest phase, hoping to find a drug that will both decrease the rash of shingles and minimize the pain that often follows it. The drug being studied is a new form of a drug that is available by prescription for the treatment of shingles. If you or a friend or family member develop a rash you think is shingles, please call us and you'll be seen promptly at no charge. If you do have shingles, the study will be explained to you in greater detail. If you have any questions regarding the study, please feel free to contact us at the number listed on the front of this pamphlet.

FIG. 4.13. *Continued.*

Figure continues on next page.

F

Finding New
And Better Ways
To Control
Cancer

*Getting Involved
In Clinical Trials*

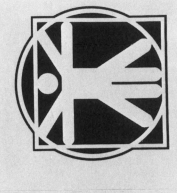

For More Information
On Clinical Trials

Your doctor may be able to give you more information about clinical trials. You can also get information about clinical trials, specific types of cancer, and cancer prevention, detection, and treatment, by calling the American Cancer Society's toll-free number at 1-800-ACS-2345.

*The American Cancer Society's
toll-free number is
1-800-ACS-2345.*

Testing Promising
Ideas About Cancer

Until all types of cancer can be cured, researchers are always looking for new ways to prevent, detect, or treat cancer. Studies done with cells and animals can only rule out some ideas and bring others to the point where they are safe enough to test in people.

That is where clinical trials come in. A clinical trial is a study to see if a new medical theory may actually help people. Although most clinical trials involve those who already have cancer, some trials test new ways of preventing cancer. Others look for ways to find cancer at an early stage when it can be cured more often.

*A clinical trial is a study to see
if a new medical theory may
actually help people.*

Most studies for cancer treatment are called Stage III clinical trials. This means the newer treatment has been tested first among animals and then among a small group of people to make sure it is safe.

If you are in a clinical trial to test a new cancer treatment, you will receive either the best standard treatment or a new one. You and your doctor will not be told if you are getting the standard treatment or the new one.

G

FIG. 4.13. *Continued. (4.13G and H are a single brochure.)*

130

Your Doctor Is Your Key to Clinical Trials

If you want to find out more about clinical trials, ask your doctor. Some people think that asking about a new type of medical care would insult the doctor, but it just shows you want the best for you and your family. Your doctor should feel the same way and want to tell you about other sources of good medical care. This includes new methods of preventing, detecting, and treating cancer—methods often tested in clinical trials.

Doctors who tell patients about clinical trials are leaders in medical care.

Doctors who tell patients about clinical trials are leaders in medical care. They are willing to take the time and effort to keep up-to-date about medical advances and how these can help their patients. Your doctor can refer you to a clinical trial, help you enroll, and follow your progress. Even after you enroll in a clinical trial, your doctor may continue to provide many important parts of your medical care.

Who Can Join Clinical Trials?

Everyone has the right to apply to a clinical trial. However, because each trial is planned to answer a specific research question, strict entrance rules must be followed. This will make sure that the results are due to the methods being compared, rather than to the type of cancer, how serious the disease is, or personal traits or habits.

Guidelines to decide who can participate in clinical trials make the results more reliable and protect you as well. There must be at least a good chance that you will be helped by the clinical trial. Even patients who receive the standard treatment seem to do better than patients who receive the same treatment but are not in clinical trials. This may be because patients in clinical trials are so closely watched.

Because each trial is planned to answer a specific research question, strict entrance rules must be followed.

People in cancer prevention trials must also meet entrance guidelines. Studies to test if certain foods could help prevent cancer would not include people with eating problems that could force them off the diet. Studies to find ways to detect certain cancers early are usually limited to those most at risk. It wouldn't be a wise use of research money to look for early lung cancers in people who never smoked or for prostate cancer in young boys.

Being Involved In a Clinical Trial

Before entering a clinical trial, you must know about the trial's purpose and methods and sign a consent form stating you do know. If you have any questions about the clinical trial, keep asking them until you get the answers you need.

The American Cancer Society and other groups are urging insurance companies to cover more of the costs of clinical trials.

You are free to leave any trial, at any time, for any reason. If it is found that the newer treatment is clearly not as good as the standard treatment, the trial will be stopped. If it is found that the new treatment is clearly better, the trial will also be stopped and the newer treatment offered to all who were in the trial.

Clinical trials take place at large cancer centers, community hospitals, and the offices of local doctors. Often, the costs of the treatment itself are paid by the sponsors of the trial. You or your insurance company will still have to pay for hospital stays and medical tests. To avoid unexpected bills, find out ahead of time what is covered and what is not. Your doctor, social workers at hospitals, and agencies such as the American Cancer Society can help you find out about insurance coverage and other forms of funding. The American Cancer Society and other groups are urging insurance companies to cover more of the costs of clinical trials.

Figure continues on next page.

FIG. 4.13. *Continued.*

TABLE OF CONTENTS

04/01/91

——————————— ♦ ———————————

The **DIRECTORY OF HIV CLINICAL RESEARCH IN THE BAY AREA** is published by the Community Consortium and is updated three times per year. The **DIRECTORY** is intended solely as an informational resource on clinical trials in the greater San Francisco Bay Area which are currently enrolling patients. No endorsement is made of any specific trial described herein.

The **DIRECTORY** is as comprehensive and up-to-date as possible. However, any listed trial may close to patient enrollment at any time. The Community Consortium solicits updated information about clinical trials available throughout the Bay Area; any trial which has been reviewed and approved by an Institutional Review Board may be included. Anyone with information appropriate for publication in this directory is asked to call Zach Weingart at the Community Consortium office at 415/ 476-9554.

A name and telephone number to contact for further information is provided for most of the clinical trials listed. *For those trials conducted by the Community Consortium, patients should contact their personal health care provider.* A listing of providers affiliated with the Consortium is printed on page 14. Providers not affiliated with the Consortium may call our office at 476-9554 for information about our Clinical Trials Program.

FIG. 4.13. *Continued. (4.13I, J, and K are the first three pages of the Directory of HIV Clinical Research in the Bay Area.)*

HOW TO USE THIS DIRECTORY

HOW THE DIRECTORY IS ORGANIZED

Eighty-four studies are listed in this research guide, arranged according to the type of study or the group of people for whom the study is intended. The **Table of Contents** lists thirteen groups of studies, most of which are treatment studies. This means that people are given an experimental drug under carefully controlled conditions to see if it helps them get better.

The first grouping deals with **Antiretrovirals**, drugs intended to fight HIV infection. Listed here are trials of drugs such as AZT, ddI and Compound Q.

The second grouping is of **Combination Therapies**. In these trials antiretrovirals are used in combination with immunomodulators, drugs intended to improve the function of the immune system. Immunomodulators include such drugs as interferon and thymopentin.

The next seven groups of studies deal with treatments for various kinds of opportunistic infections (secondary diseases which often accompany HIV infection), such as *Cytomegalovirus* (CMV) disease, *Pneumocystis carinii* Pneumonia (PCP) or thrush.

Treatments for HIV-Related Malignancies includes drugs intended to treat the cancers which sometimes accompany HIV infection, such as Kaposi's Sarcoma (KS) or lymphoma.

Miscellaneous Interventional Trials is a "catch-all" category which includes treatment studies that do not fit into any of the categories listed above.

Women sometimes think they are excluded from taking part in clinical drug trials. In most cases this is not true. Pregnant or nursing women <u>are</u> generally excluded, because it is not known whether taking an untested drug might cause damage to the baby. Therefore, women who have sex with men usually must agree to use birth control during the course of the study. Children are also frequently excluded because their bodies are undergoing rapid growth processes and might be harmed by taking an untested drug. **Studies Specifically for Women and Children** contains a limited number of studies for pregnant women and children, who have traditionally been excluded from experimental drug studies.

The last group of studies deals with **Observational / Epidemiologic Studies**. These are basically "data-collection" studies, which help to increase our knowledge about HIV disease in various ways. An observational database may, for example, collect information on people taking an approved medication to find out if long-term use of this medication has side-effects which were not apparent when it was first licensed. An epidemiologic study may look at the origins and spread of the HIV epidemic and how this affects different groups of people over a long period of time.

HOW TO FIND INFORMATION ABOUT A SPECIFIC TOPIC

The **Index**, found on page 16, may be the easiest way to look up specific information in the Directory. Drugs being studied, diseases these drugs are intended to treat and sites where the trials are being conducted are listed alphabetically for quick reference.

An example may help you understand how to use the Index. Let's assume you live in the South Bay and want to know about trials in your area dealing with prevention of *Mycobacterium avium* Complex. If you look up "*Mycobacterium avium* Complex" in the index, you will find that it is discussed on pages 4 and 5. Turning to page 5, you will find that a drug called rifabutin is being studied for the prevention of MAC, and that AIDS Community Research Consortium in Redwood City and Santa Clara Valley Medical Center in San Jose are two of the sites conducting trials with rifabutin. If you wanted more information, you could call the contact person(s) listed for either of these sites.

FIG. 4.13. *Continued.*

Figure continues on next page.

DRUG NAME	ELIGIBILITY	STUDY TITLE	SITE / CONTACT PERSON

ANTIRETROVIRALS

DRUG NAME	ELIGIBILITY	STUDY TITLE	SITE / CONTACT PERSON
D4T	HIV+ or AIDS, with fewer than 500 CD4 cells	A Dose-Ranging Safety, Pharmaco-kinetics and Preliminary Efficacy Study of BMY-27857 (D4T) Administered Three Times Daily to Symptomatic HIV-Infected Patients	Davies / Ann Conroy, RN 565-6649
AZT	Caucasians, African-Americans or Latinos, scheduled to begin AZT therapy at 500 mg / day. CD4 cell counts between 100 and 500. Prior use of AZT is not permitted	A Prospective Comparison of Zidovudine's Effects on CD4 Responses in HIV-Infected Caucasians, African-Americans and Latinos	SFGH / AIDS Research Group 821-5089
ddI plus AZT	HIV+ with fewer than 400 CD4 cells. Must also be p24 antigen positive. No progressive KS or active opportunistic infection	A Phase I Study to Evaluate the Pharmacokinetics, Safety and Antiviral Effects of Concurrent Administration of Zidovudine (AZT) and 2',3'-dideoxyinosine (ddI) in Patients with Human Immunodeficiency Virus (HIV)	SFGH / AIDS Research Group 821-5089
ddI	AIDS. Intolerant of AZT and ineligible for ACTG Phase II ddI trials	Videx™ (ddI) Treatment IND	Note: This is the ddI "expanded access" program. Any health care provider can enroll eligible patients into this study. Ask your provider for details.
ddI	AIDS, with disease progression despite AZT therapy. Ineligible for ACTG Phase II ddI trials	Videx™ (ddI) Open Label Study	(See Note: above)
ddI vs. ddC	HIV+ with CD4 cell counts less than 300 or AIDS. Unable to tolerate AZT or with disease progression despite AZT therapy	A Randomized Open-Label Comparative Trial of Dideoxyinosine (ddI) and Dideoxycytidine (ddC) in HIV-Infected Patients Who Are Intolerant Of Or Have Failed Zidovudine (ZDV) Therapy (CPCRA 002)	Community Consortium / Ask your health care provider (see page 14) Kaiser San Francisco / Allen Harris, RN 929-4848
ddC, AZT or both	Asymptomatic HIV+ with fewer than 200 CD4 cells, or symptomatic HIV+ with fewer than 300 CD4 cells. Patients must have taken at least 500 mg. of AZT per day for at least 24 weeks	A Randomized Double-Blind Comparative Study of Dideoxycytidine (ddC) Alone or ddC / ZDV Combination Versus Zidovudine (ZDV, AZT) Alone in Patients with HIV Infection Who Have Received Prior ZDV Therapy (ACTG 155)	Kaiser San Francisco / Gretchen Van Raalte, RN 929-4848 SFGH / AIDS Research Group 821-5089 Stanford ACTG / 723-6231

K

FIG. 4.13. *Continued.*

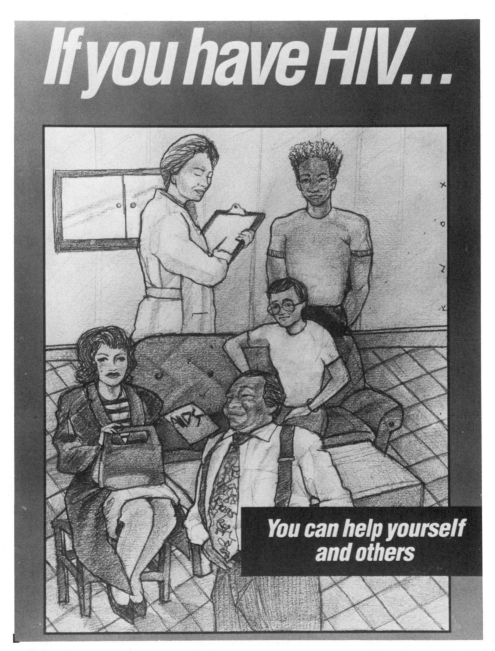

FIG. 4.13. *Continued. (4.13L through W are patient information sheets provided by the Community Consortium—An Association of Bay Area HIV Health Care Providers. 4.13L is the cover.)*

Figure continues on next page.

Join a Community Consortium clinical trial

The Community Consortium is a group of doctors and nurses in the Bay Area who take care of people with HIV. We believe that, together with our patients, we can help in the search to find better treatments for people with HIV. That's why we offer clinical trials that you can join right in the doctor's office or clinic where you go for your regular care.

What is a clinical trial?

A new drug goes through many tests in the lab before people take it. If the results are good, the drug is tested in small groups of people. When people take a new drug as a part of a study, it is called a clinical trial.

The results of a clinical trial are very important. They tell us about the safety of the drug when people take it. They also tell us if the new drug helps people get better.

Clinical trials in your doctor's office - A new idea

Most clinical trials take place in big hospitals. Many people do not take part in these trials. Some may not live near one of the hospitals, and others may not want to go to a special research clinic.

Now there are programs, like ours, in doctors' offices and clinics in the community. These "community-based" clinical trials are important because more people can take part in the testing of promising new drugs.

Some good reasons to join

■ You may be helped by the new drugs that are being tested.

■ The drugs that are being tested are free.

■ Any extra lab tests you need for the clinical trial are free.

■ You don't have to go to a big hospital or special clinic.

■ You can help speed the search to find better treatments for people with HIV.

M

FIG. 4.13. *Continued.*

Informed Consent

Researchers are required by law to give you all the facts about a study before you join. This information must be explained in a way that you can understand. Before you join a study, you will be asked to read and sign a consent form. This is called giving **Informed consent**. When you sign the consent form, it means that you have been given all the information about the study, and that you agree to join.

The consent form is <u>not</u> a contract. You do not give up any rights if you sign the consent form. You can leave the study at any time.

What should I know before I sign the consent form?

Before you sign the consent form, you should know:

☑ the reasons for using the experimental treatment

☑ the risks and benefits of taking part in the study

☑ any extra costs, doctor visits, lab tests, etc.

☑ what drugs you will have to take

Are there other questions I should ask before I sign the consent form?

Before you decide to join a trial, you may want to know:

☐ How will information about me be handled to protect my privacy?

☐ Can I take the drug after the trial is over? Will I have to pay for it?

☐ If I get sick or develop health problems while on the trial, will I be taken off the trial?

☐ How can I find out the results of the trial?

(over) ➡

N

FIG. 4.13. *Continued.*

Figure continues on next page.

☐   Are there other studies of this drug I should know about?

☐   (For women) Do I have to use birth control? If so, what
      kind? If I become pregnant will I have to leave the study?

What should I do if I don't understand something?

Do not sign the consent form until you understand everything in it. Keep asking questions. The staff should be able to answer most of them. However, there may not be enough information about certain drugs to answer some questions.

Are there other places to get information about clinical trials?

For free information about clinical trials, you can call:

☑ Community Consortium at **415/ 476-9554**. Ask for the
     Directory of HIV Clinical Research in the Bay Area

☑ AIDS Clinical Trials Information Service at **1-800-TRIALS-A**

☑ San Francisco AIDS Foundation at **415/ 863-AIDS**. Ask for
     BETA - (Bulletin of Experimental Treatments for AIDS)

☑ AIDS Treatment News at **1-800-TREAT-12**

☑ Project Inform at **1-800-334-7422**

☑ E.A.C.H. Program at **415/ 864-1214**. (Bilingual and culturally
     sensitive treatment advocates for gay men of
     color)

An Association of
Bay Area HIV
Health Care Providers

3180 - 18th Street
Suite 201
San Francisco, CA 94110
415/ 476-9554

FIG. 4.13. *Continued.*

Patients' Rights and Responsibilities

In a clinical trial, patients and health care providers work together. As a patient in a clinical trial, you need to know your rights. You also need to know what your health care provider has a right to expect from you.

What are my rights as a patient?

The people involved in your care must treat you with consideration and respect. You have the right to:

- ☑ be told all the important details about your care
- ☑ ask questions and have them answered
- ☑ say no to any test, procedure or medication
- ☑ go to another health care provider to get more information
- ☑ know the names of anyone you talk with
- ☑ read your medical records with your health care provider
- ☑ make your own decisions about your health care
- ☑ know that your medical records will be kept confidential.

What are my responsibilities as a patient?

The researchers have a right to expect certain things from you, too. As a patient, you have the responsibility to:

- ☑ be honest about your medical history and anything in your lifestyle which may affect your health
- ☑ follow health advice and instructions
- ☑ keep appointments or re-schedule them at least 24 hours in advance

P

(over) ➡

FIG. 4.13. *Continued.*

Figure continues on next page.

☑ report any changes in your health

☑ be sure you understand the facts before you make a complaint

What should I do if I think my rights are not being respected?

If you have problems with someone involved in your care, you can:

☐ talk to them and tell them how you feel

☐ ask questions so that you understand their reasons for doing things that make you uncomfortable

☐ act fairly and calmly (losing your temper may not help to solve the problem)

What if I've done all these things, and think my rights are still not being respected?

If you still think your rights are not being respected, you can:

☐ ask for an opinion from another staff person

☐ make an appointment to talk with the supervisor

☐ write your complaint down and bring it with you to the appointment. If it is hard for you to write, ask someone to help you.

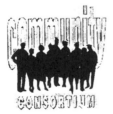

An Association of
Bay Area HIV
Q   Health Care Providers

3180 - 18th Street
Suite 201
San Francisco, CA 94110
415/ 476-9554

FIG. 4.13. *Continued.*

Women and Clinical Trials

Women with HIV can take part in clinical trials. Often, women don't get enough information about clinical trials and think they can't join. Some women think they must have an abortion if they become pregnant while in a study.

Some facts about women and clinical trials . . .

Every clinical trial has requirements about who can join. If a woman meets these requirements, she can join. A woman can't be excluded just because she is a woman.

In many studies, women must agree to use birth control if they have sex with men. Pregnant or nursing women usually can't join a trial of an untested drug because it is not known if the drug might harm the baby. However, there are now a few studies for pregnant women.

What happens if a woman becomes pregnant while in a trial?

A woman should know what the rules are about pregnancy before she joins a trial. Different trials have different rules about whether a woman can continue in the trial if she becomes pregnant. Every woman **always** has the right to make her own decisions about her pregnancy. No one can force her to have an abortion.

If you become pregnant, you may want to talk to the Bay Area Perinatal AIDS Center (BAPAC) at San Francisco General Hospital. They will be able to give you the most current information about pregnancy and HIV disease. **BAPAC (415) 821-8919**.

Talk to your health care provider about clinical trials. This will help you make the decisions that are best for you.

R

(over) ➝

FIG. 4.13. *Continued.*

Figure continues on next page.

Women with HIV may have special problems.

Women sometimes have problems in their female organs. For women with HIV, these may be related to their HIV disease. Here are some of the problems that you should know about:

☐ An infection (such as a yeast infection) in the vagina that doesn't go away after taking medicine for it. Or, the infection comes back after the medicine is finished

☐ Pain in your belly when you don't have your period

☐ Fluid coming from the vagina. This fluid may be thick or thin, white or green, and may smell

☐ Open sores or bumps in or outside the vagina or anus

☐ Pain during sex

☐ Diseases that you may get from having sex. These are called sexually transmitted diseases. They are also called S.T.D.'s. The names of some of these diseases are: herpes, chancroid, syphilis, genital warts, pelvic inflammatory disease (P.I.D.), human papilloma virus (H.P.V.), gonorrhea and chlamydia

☐ Women with HIV disease may have a higher risk for cancer. **It is important to have a pelvic exam (an exam of your female organs) and a Pap smear (a test for cancer) every 6 months.**

If you have any of these problems, talk to your health care provider. Also, be sure to get a pelvic exam and Pap smear every 6 months. Ask for a referral to a gynecologist (a doctor who treats women) if your health care provider can't do this exam.

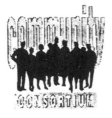

An Association of
Bay Area HIV
Health Care Providers

S

3180 - 18th Street
Suite 201
San Francisco, CA 94110
415/ 476-9554

FIG. 4.13. *Continued.*

The Observational Database Project

The purpose of this project is to gather information about the symptoms, treatments and illnesses affecting a large group of people with HIV. The information we collect will help us to better understand HIV disease and its treatments. It will also help us to know what new research is needed. We will be able to monitor changes in your health over time. You will not be required to take a drug as a part of this study. This project takes place in your doctor's office or your clinic.

Women, people of color, drug users and other groups of people who have not been in studies before are encouraged to enter.

How long will this study last?

You may be in this study indefinitely.

Who can join this study?

You can join this study if you:

☑ are HIV+ or have AIDS or ARC

☑ are at least 13 years old

What will I have to do if I join this study?

Your doctor or nurse will ask you some questions about your health. This will happen during your regular visit. You will not need to make extra visits or have any extra lab work. The results of some of your regular lab tests will be part of the information collected. All the information is confidential.

T

(over) ➡

FIG. 4.13. *Continued.*

Figure continues on next page.

Some of the questions you will be asked include: "How have you been feeling? . . . What are your symptoms? . . . What drugs do you take for your illness?" There will be other questions as well. It will only take a few minutes to answer the questions.

How do I join this study?

You must be under the care of a doctor to join. Talk to your doctor if you are interested. You may be able to join during a regular visit. If you have questions, call the Community Consortium at 415/ 476-9554.

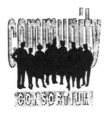

An Association of

Bay Area HIV

U   Health Care Providers

3180 - 18th Street
Suite 201
San Francisco, CA 94110
415/ 476-9554

FIG. 4.13. *Continued.*

Toxo Information Sheet

A very common parasite or "bug" called ***Toxoplasma gondii*** causes a disease called Toxoplasmosis ("Toxo" for short). Many healthy people have been exposed to the bug which causes Toxo. It can sometimes live in our bodies for many years without making us sick.

Why should people with HIV disease know about Toxo?

Because people with HIV disease may have weak immune systems, they can have problems with the Toxo bug. It can cause a dangerous brain disease called toxoplasmic encephalitis (TE). TE can cause headaches, vision problems, seizures, numbness in the arms and legs, and difficulty with balance, body control and thinking processes.

How do people get Toxo?

Most people get Toxo by eating raw or undercooked meat or fish. It is also possible to get it from dirty cat litter.

Can Toxo be treated?

There are drugs that can be used to treat Toxo. Most people get better with these drugs. But, the Toxo bug is still in their bodies and may cause problems again.

Therefore, people with HIV must take medicine for the rest of their lives so they don't get TE (the brain disease) again.

How can I find out if I have the Toxo bug?

Your doctor or health care provider can perform a simple blood test to find out if you have the Toxo bug. A positive test result means that you have the Toxo bug in your body. You are "Toxo positive." It does not mean that you have TE.

V

(over) ➡

FIG. 4.13. *Continued.*

Figure continues on next page.

How can I help protect myself from Toxo?

It is important that you take care of your general health. Here are some other things you can do to lessen your chances of catching the Toxo bug:

- ☑ do not eat raw or undercooked meat or fish
- ☑ wash your hands after touching animals
- ☑ wear a mask and gloves when cleaning a litter box
- ☑ keep the litter box away from places where you eat
- ☑ talk to your doctor to learn the facts about toxo

Information about Toxo can be confusing. Ask questions about anything you don't understand.

Are there Toxo studies?

The Community Consortium is conducting a study at certain doctors' offices and clinics. This study will find out if there are drugs that can stop people who are Toxo positive from getting TE.

How do I join the Toxo Study?

Read the fact sheet in this brochure about **The Toxoplasmosis Prophylaxis Study**. You must be under the care of a doctor to join. Talk to your doctor if you are interested. You may be able to join during a regular visit. If your doctor is not doing the study, you or your doctor can find out where else you can go by calling the Community Consortium at 415/ 476-9554.

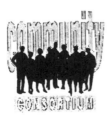

An Association of
Bay Area HIV
Health Care Providers

W

3180 - 18th Street
Suite 201
San Francisco, CA 94110
415/ 476-9554

FIG. 4.13. *Continued.*

HERPES ZOSTER CLINICAL STUDY

—Oral medication and daily clinical evaluations will be provided.

—Patients <50 years of age receive active treatment vs. placebo.

—Patients ≥ 50 years of age receive active treatment.

—The following criteria must be met.

1. ENROLLMENT MUST BE WITHIN 72 HOURS OF RASH ONSET.
2. Patient must not have received antiviral meds or immunomodulating meds or Zostrix (capsaicin) within the past four weeks.
3. Patient must not be immune compromised, HIV positive, or receiving cytotoxic or immunosuppressive drugs.
4. Female patient of child bearing potential must not be pregnant or nursing and must be using appropriate means of birth control.
5. Patient must not be intolerant or hypersensitive to acyclovir.
6. Patient must not be receiving tricyclic antidepressants or probenecid.
7. Patient must have no impairment of hepatic or renal function.
8. Patient must have no gastrointestinal dysfunction that might interfere with absorption.
9. Patient must be available for 6 month follow-up.

** Patients with Zoster Ophthalmicus will only be admitted in study of patients ≥ 50 years of age.

X

RG-C456

FIG. 4.13. *Continued.*

a clinical trial. These have been prepared by pharmaceutical company clinics (Fig. 4.13A–D), disease societies (Fig. 4.13G,H), government agencies (Table 4.9), investigators (Fig. 4.13E,F,X), and consumer-community group alliances. Another approach is to prepare a video presentation that describes a specific trial or type of trial and encourages patients to enroll. For example, the American Cancer Society prepared an excellent 15-minute video that encourages patients to enroll in clinical trials by allaying their fears of what may be involved (G. Murphy, *personal communication*). Brief videos suitable for showing on television could be prepared as spot advertisements or to complement news stories. Slide shows with accompanying sound could be prepared for patients as a less expensive visual alternative to videos.

Before developing a brochure for a clinical trial, look at examples used in other trials and evaluate their good and poor features. A most convenient approach to prepare a brochure to mail to prospective enrollees (e.g., Fig. 4.13E,F) is as follows:

1. Take a standard full-size sheet of paper.
2. Fold into thirds (as for a letter) suitable to be placed in an envelope or taped (or stapled) and mailed as is.
3. Complete each of the six panels. For convenience these are referred to with the letters A to F.
4. Panel A (Front) should contain the name of the trial and a photo, logo, drawing, or design as appropriate.

5. Panel B is on the left after the brochure is opened, and is the back of Panel A. This panel should describe the purpose of the trial, its design, name of the principal investigator, his or her affiliation, any sponsoring group (if desired), treatments, and any special requirements expected of patients. General inclusion criteria should also be listed. This amount of information will often require the use of a second panel.

6. Panel C is in the center of the opened brochure next to B. The remainder of information from Panel B should be placed on Panel C. Alternatively, Panels B and C may be used as a large double-sized panel. One or more of the panels could contain a fact list about the medicine, disease, or trial.

7. Panel D is on the right side of the opened brochure next to C. It should contain information for the patients to complete and return to the site. This information must include the prospective patient's name, address, telephone number (where he or she can be reached during the day), and whether he or she desires more information, wishes to be screened, or is responding to another request that is being made.

8. Panel E (on the reverse of Panel C) is on the left when the brochure is opened with Panel A on the far right. This should contain the address of the site and investigator's name for returning Panel D. A stamp may be placed on panel E or a prepaid mailing identifier may be printed. Panel E should be tucked inside when the brochure is folded.

9. Panel F is the mailing address panel which should contain the return address of the site in the upper left-hand corner and space for a label with the mailing address or for the patient's name and address to be written.

10. The number of colors (if any), photographs, type, and weight of paper used should be discussed with the printer.

Examples of the patient brochures used by The Upjohn Research Clinics are shown in Fig. 4.13A–D.

TABLE 4.8. *Contents of a recruitment guide for individual trial sites*

A. Administration
   1. Total number of patients required, and number required per time period
   2. Any subclass suggestions of groups where high (or low) representation is desired
   3. Method(s) to be used to monitor recruitment
   4. Method(s) to be used to provide feedback on recruitment to each site
   5. Consequences for failure to meet recruitment quotas
   6. Policy on providing medical follow-up to referring physicians
   7. Who to contact at the central site or sponsor for assistance

B. Recruitment strategy of the trial
   1. Outline and description of the trial's strategy
   2. Explanation of the sequence of methods to be used by all sites as well as flexibility allowed at individual sites

C. Methods of recruitment
   1. Acceptable and unacceptable methods of recruitment for the trial
   2. Acceptable and unacceptable sources of patients for the trial
   3. Advice on interactions with patients prior to screening, requesting an informed consent, conducting an exit interview
   4. Use of thank you (or other) letters to patients and referring physicians
   5. Pointers to assist staff in the recruitment process

TABLE 4.9. *Table of contents to the booklet "What are Clinical Trials All About"*[a]

A. Introduction
   1. What is a clinical trial?
   2. Why are clinical trials important?
   3. Why would a patient be interested in a clinical trial?
   4. Are there risks of side effects in clinical trials?
   5. Why does cancer treatment have side effects?
   6. What is being done to lessen side effects of treatment?

B. If you are thinking of entering a clinical trial. . .
   1. Are you eligible for a clinical trial?
   2. What trials are available for your type of cancer?
   3. What is best for you?
   4. What are important questions to ask about a clinical trial?
   5. What is informed consent?
   6. What is it like to be a patient in a clinical trial?
   7. Can you leave a trial at any time?
   8. What protection do you have as a patient in a clinical trial?
   9. What can help you learn if a trial is sound and well run?
  10. What kinds of clinical trials are there?
  11. How are trials divided into phases?
  12. How are clinical trials conducted?

C. The National Cancer Program and clinical trials
   1. Glossary
   2. Cancer Information Service (CIS)
   3. Notes

[a] This 23-page booklet is by Eleanor Nealon and is a production of the National Cancer Institute (NIH publication no. 90-2706) reprinted in 1989. Numbers of sections and part A added. This booklet is available free of charge by calling the NCI's Cancer Information Service (1–800–4–CANCER).

Another type of brochure is a guide for each site in a multicenter trial that describes the recruitment methods to be used. This should contain all relevant information from the list in Table 4.8. The table of contents to the booklet "What are Clinical Trials All About" is shown in Table 4.9. Information on obtaining this booklet is given in a footnote to this table.

5

Ethical Issues in Patient Recruitment

This chapter focuses on a number of ethical issues that arise during the recruitment of patients into clinical trials. The discussion is somewhat restricted in that it does not cover (1) the ethical background, history, or current thinking about protecting participants in trials from unnecessary risk; (2) the ethical responsibilities of investigators in clinical research; or (3) the functioning of Ethics Committees and IRBs. Numerous monographs (e.g., Levine, 1986) present these and many other related topics in great detail. This chapter considers a few of the practical ethical issues related to recruitment that are widely discussed today.

The term volunteers is sometimes used to denote either healthy normal individuals or patients who volunteer for a trial (Macrae et al., 1989). Most commonly (and in this book) the term volunteer is only used in the former capacity.

OFFERING PAYMENTS TO RECRUIT VOLUNTEERS OR PATIENTS

Offering Money to Recruit Volunteers into a Phase I Trial

Because volunteers receive no medical benefit from participation in a clinical trial, and are often at risk to suffer adverse effects (usually transient), it is reasonable to pay them for their participation. This is standard practice by many academicians and at almost all pharmaceutical companies and is accepted as both ethical and appropriate. Money should not be given only to those volunteers who complete an entire trial because this places undue pressure on volunteers to remain in a trial from which they might rather withdraw (e.g., because of moderate or severe adverse reactions). Money given to volunteers should be prorated based on the extent of their participation unless there are legal requirements to give all volunteers the entire sum, even for partial participation. The amount of money offered cannot be so excessive that volunteers would feel strong pressure to remain in a clinical trial from which they would rather withdraw.

Offering Money to Recruit Patients into a Phase I Trial

In a clinical trial in which patients are not expected to receive significant medical benefit (e.g., a pharmacokinetic trial), it is both appropriate and acceptable to pay them for their participation. The same two caveats that were presented above (i.e., not paying only those subjects who complete a trial, and not offering an excessive amount of money for participation) also apply to patients who are paid. If it is necessary to recruit severely ill patients because of the medicines' known or potential toxicity, then the possibility of paying them must be discussed among the various groups (e.g., investigators, Ethics Committees, sponsors) involved in the trial. It would be valuable to include a bioethicist in these discussions, or to invite one to chair a discussion.

Offering Money to Recruit Patients into a Phase II or Phase III Trial

Participation in Phase II or Phase III trials usually offers some medical benefit to patients. Thus, the consensus of most academicians and pharmaceutical companies, is that it is inappropriate and sometimes unethical to offer patients more money than that required to reimburse them for transportation, meals, and out-of-pocket expenses, possibly including child care. The rationale is that payment introduces an element of coercion and makes it unclear whether patients are sometimes remaining in a clinical trial for the money they will receive, when it is in their best interests to drop out. Patients may also distort their true feelings in answering questions and report fewer adverse events if they fear being discontinued from a clinical trial that provides an otherwise unavailable investigational medicine. These events could affect the type of data obtained and the interpretation of results. One means of addressing this issue is to offer all patients the same amount of money regardless of their length of participation.

Some pharmaceutical companies do offer money to patients for Phase II trials, particularly if little or no benefit is expected to accrue to the patient. This practice would be acceptable to most Ethics Committees/IRBs if patients were asked to exert themselves significantly or to participate in a test for which it was otherwise extremely difficult to find patients who would volunteer. Another category of Phase II or III clinical trials where payment might be considered is where patients are offered a redundant form of a standard medicine and do not see any reason to enroll in the trial except for the money. Whether patients should receive additional money above their costs for participating in a clinical trial depends on the country, the Ethics Committee/IRB, and the particular investigator, as well as the practical issues concerning the difficulty of finding patients to enroll and the influence that the money would have on their behavior. Offering patients excessive sums is again considered unethical. The issue of compensating people who volunteer to enroll in clinical trials is discussed by Ackerman (1989).

Basing Payments on Reasons for Leaving a Trial

When patients or volunteers decide that the adverse reactions to a medicine or treatment they experience are unacceptable, they are technically considered *discontinued* from the clinical trial by the investigator. Such patients represent treatment failures even if they initiate discussions about withdrawing before information about adverse reactions is disclosed, or if patients state they will definitely leave the trial for medical reasons. When the reason for leaving the trial before its conclusion is based solely on personal preference (e.g., moving, cannot continue to take time away from work to attend clinic, disinterest, failure to improve), that situation is defined as patient *drop out*. Patients and volunteers often are unable to state their specific reason for withdrawal, or simply fail to return for follow-up. It is important for the investigator to determine if and to what degree the treatment contributed to the dropout. If any link, however remote, is found with the treatment, the situation should be categorized as medicine- or therapy-related. Such instances would require full payment to the patient or volunteer who provided important data on adverse effects leading to discontinuation of treatment. Not only should the patient or volunteer not feel that he or she disappointed the investigator by stopping the protocol, but each person should be encouraged to report their reasons for leaving the trial as fully as possible. Patients who feel vaguely uncomfortable should be encouraged to express this effect rather than deny any problem when asking to withdraw.

Although a volunteer or patient may not have completed a trial for personal reasons, he or she should be given partial payment based on the proportion of the protocol fulfilled. It would be unfair not to provide compensation for activities that might have taken time and effort even if the data cannot be used in clinical trial outcome analyses.

OFFERING PAYMENTS TO REFERRING PHYSICIANS

The practice of providing a monetary payment to physicians who refer patients for clinical trials has recently been strongly debated (Lind, 1990; Higby, 1990; Hsia, 1990) and is generally considered inappropriate. Lind (1990) describes the process in detail and eloquently offers several strong arguments against the practice. Lind asks, for example "What would patients think if they suspected that their physician's enthusiasm might result from the prospect of a finder's fee, particularly one that is not just tied to a referral but contingent on enrollment?" If one accepts all of Lind's arguments, then the logical conclusion or extension of the argument is that clinical investigators also should not gain personally by conducting a clinical trial. The fact that many, but not all, clinical investigators do gain personally (e.g., prestige as well as funding for staff, equipment, travel) also may influence their decision about whether to seek to enroll specific patients in their own trial or refer patients to a competing trial. Also, the degree to which an investigator attempts to convince a patient to enter a clinical trial may be influenced by these motives. It is not always possible for an investigator who has to decide whether to refer a patient to one of several available trials to objectively and fully consider the patient's interests. While inclusion criteria theoretically prevent investigators from enrolling nonqualified patients, enrollment of ineligible patients is in fact a common practice in many clinical trials.

The above discussion is not primarily presented to disagree with the conclusions of Lind, but to suggest that the funds received by investigators for clinical trials, above expenses, may ethically be used to support other research they are conducting, purchase and maintain medical or scientific equipment, and help support their department or university. Awards from grants and contracts routinely go to the institution or department that manages the use of funds for allowable purchases, salaries, or travel. Moreover, a physician who refers a patient to a clinical trial may not charge that patient for an office visit, and thus may feel that it is appropriate under the circumstances to accept a finder's fee as alternative payment based on time spent performing a preliminary screening and discussing the trial.

USING COERCIVE TACTICS TO RECRUIT PATIENTS

Any time there is a superior–subservient relationship between two individuals, it is impossible to ensure that coercion was not felt by the person in the subservient position, even if coercion was not overtly used in the recruitment process. Three examples of this relationship in clinical research are (1) an investigator recruiting his or her staff or students, (2) a professor recruiting his or her students, and (3) a pharmaceutical company conducting a clinical trial and recruiting its junior level employees. The second example describes what commonly happens when psychology professors recruit students to participate in their clinical trials.

It is the responsibility of the Ethics Committee/IRB to be aware of this issue and to protect those volunteers (or patients) in a subservient relationship. Unfortunately, this is rarely done for several reasons.

1. The specific recruitment plans for a trial are not always presented to the Ethics Committee/IRB.
2. Any changes in recruitment methods are not generally presented by the investigator, but are implemented when he or she desires.
3. If the investigator states that patients will be recruited from specific sources using specifically named methods, but does not state in the recruitment plan what groups of individuals will *not* be contacted, the investigator may change the plan unbeknownst to the Ethics Committee/IRB. The same principle applies to identifying methods that will *not* be used, or stating that *only* certain methods will be used.

The best means of ensuring the protection of each major group of patients or volunteers that requires some protection is to increase the publicity about them. This was done for prisoners in the 1970s and led to their exclusion from clinical trials because they were unable to provide a true informed consent. Similarly, the groups discussed above cannot provide a true informed consent if the volunteers believe that refusal to enroll may result in being fired, may affect their career prospects, or influence their course grades.

The patient–physician relationship is sometimes similar to that described above

TABLE 5.1. *Selected groups of vulnerable patients for whom special recruitment considerations exist*

1. Patients on welfare
2. Ethnic and racial minorities
3. Patients with limited capacity to consent
4. Patients confined to institutions (e.g., prisoners)
5. Patients who are mentally retarded
6. Patients who are mentally psychotic
7. Patients who are under legal age (i.e., children and adolescents)
8. Patients who are unable to provide an assent (i.e., children who are less than 6 or 7 years of age)
9. Patients who have a strong dependency relationship with the person or group attempting to enroll them in the trial

in that a simple, low-keyed request by a physician for the patient to consider enrollment in a trial may make some patients feel as if they have no choice but to enroll. For some patients, the statement that they are under absolutely no obligation to enroll does not help. The mere request to consider enrolling, even by the physician's nurse, will be interpreted by some patients as either a command or a request that cannot be refused. There may not be an easy way to protect these patients from feeling coerced. It is hoped that this group represents a minority of patients. Nonetheless, this phenomenon is real. The same principle applies even when the physician is not the trial's investigator and asks a patient to consider joining another investigator's trial (i.e, the physician is referring the patient). Many patients are becoming involved in their own medical treatment, and this tends to minimize the coercion they might feel. Nonetheless, this is an important issue for physicians to consider before discussing a clinical trial with patients. Giving patients a copy of the informed consent early in the discussion phase is another means of minimizing this coercion. Additional steps (e.g., discussions with family and friends) could be taken if desired. In addition to patients, employees, students, or staff, there are other groups of potential trial participants who are vulnerable and whose rights must be protected (Table 5.1). These patients' rights are discussed in detail by Levine (1986) and by Spilker (1991, Chapter 27).

ETHICAL GUIDELINES FOR RECRUITMENT OF HEALTHY VOLUNTEERS

Macrae et al. (1989) discuss several of the ethical issues concerning normal volunteers. These include:

1. Use of an informed consent that includes standard elements [see Chapter 27 of *Guide to Clinical Trials* (Spilker, 1991) for the accepted list of United States elements]. The most important element that differs between the vast majority of volunteers and most patients involves the statement that the research is unlikely to be of any direct personal benefit to the volunteer. Similarly, some patients (e.g., severely ill patients in Phase I trials) are unlikely to benefit from their participation in a trial.

2. Normal volunteers should not be enrolled in clinical trials where there is perceptible risk. The definition and application of the term risk raises numerous other issues (e.g., how is perceptible risk measured and how much risk is excessive). The balance should be determined by considering the benefits to be gained by society

as a whole versus the risks to the individual (i.e., considering issues of collective ethics versus individual ethics).

3. Volunteers should not be sought where a dependency relationship exists. For example, it is unethical to seek trial volunteers in the following superior–subservient relationships (1) researcher and student, (2) parent and child, or (3) employer and employee. Elements of coercion, duress, or a desire to please may mitigate against the possibility of the "volunteer" being able to provide a voluntary consent. This issue was previously addressed.

4. Volunteers sought from any organized group (e.g., firemen or students at a specific school) should only be contacted after officials of that organization have been informed and have fully discussed the issues with those who will conduct the trial.

5. Self-experimentation or experimentation on colleagues or friends of the investigator should be subjected to the same professional and ethical reviews as for other more conventional clinical trials.

6. Issues of liability for injury should be considered and discussed for both negligent as well as nonnegligent causes. It should be determined who is responsible for payment and how payment would be determined. Numerous options and proposals exist in this area (e.g., see Macrae et al., 1989).

INFORMED CONSENT ISSUES

Is the Informed Consent a Form of Bias in Patient Recruitment?

There is little doubt that the informed consent procedure introduces bias into the patient recruitment process. The patient population that meets all inclusion criteria and has passed all screening tests must provide informed consent to be officially enrolled in a trial. Signing the informed consent is often considered the final step of the patient's recruitment process. (Alternative descriptions are given in Chapter 1.) Patients who refuse to give their informed consent may or may not represent a cross section of the population of patients screened. If they are, then no bias would be introduced into the trial by their refusal. However, data from a number of trials demonstrate that there are sometimes important differences between patients who provide informed consent and those who do not (Edlund et al., 1985). Unfortunately, extremely few publications describe the characteristics of patient refusers (Edlund et al., 1985). Any clinical differences that exist between patients who sign and those who do not sign informed consents means that bias has entered the clinical trial that would not otherwise be present. The bias created by using an informed consent may cause either false-positive or false-negative results. Several authors have indicated that the mere use of an informed consent has a substantial impact on patient enrollment into some clinical trials (Jack et al., 1990).

An informed consent written in a negative emotional tone, or which describes all potential risks to patients in a dramatic way, will have a more negative effect on patient recruitment than would a form that contained more balanced statements.

Reasons for Problems in Obtaining Informed Consent

Many trials are unable to achieve their recruitment goals because the investigators fail to obtain informed consent from patients who pass (or would pass) screening examinations. This failure may occur for the following reasons.

1. Culture and tradition of the country, or the investigator's own background, make it emotionally difficult for the investigator to ask patients for their informed consent. The easiest way to resolve this problem is to have someone else ask the patients. This person should be more comfortable with the process and could be another investigator, a nurse, the trial coordinator, or a special resource person (e.g., a translator).

2. The investigator who asks for informed consent may be rather stiff or brusque in describing the trial and in asking for the patient's informed consent. In this case, the investigator should spend more time with each patient and not rush the process. For example, he or she could describe the status of treatments for the patient's disease and then indicate that the best approach is currently uncertain. At that point the investigator could state briefly (a) that there is a clinical trial that the investigator is participating in, (b) the reason(s) why the investigator is participating in the trial (e.g., to scientifically determine the optimum treatment), and (c) the possible reasons why the patient should consider enrolling. It would then be appropriate to discuss the patient's level of interest. If the patient expresses interest, the physician should describe (a) what an informed consent is; (b) the reasons why an informed consent helps protect the patient; (c) the fact that the form may be shown to and discussed with friends, relatives, or others; and (d) the types of information it contains. At that point the patient should be shown the informed consent and given ample time to read and digest its contents. This may involve the patient taking it home and discussing the trial with the investigator or other professional at another time. Only after inquiring whether the patient has questions, and answering them, should the investigator ask the patient for his or her agreement to enter the trial and signature on the informed consent. A study on the amount of information to present to patients found that physicians underestimated the amount of information and discussion desired by patients (Strull et al., 1984). Interestingly, the same study found that clinicians overestimated the patients' desire to make medical decisions.

Is the Use of Deception Acceptable in Obtaining an Informed Consent ?

"Deception" is defined as providing only partial information so that important details of the clinical trial are not fully revealed to the patient, either in advance or not at all. Deception also includes providing misinformation to the patient. Planned use of deception to obtain patients' informed consent and participation in trials or other clinical research is inappropriate. Unfortunately, this practice remains in common use today, primarily in research in psychology, sociology, and other humanities that recruit normal volunteers.

Typically, deception is justified on the basis that if the volunteers were informed about the nature of the trial or study conducted, their knowledge would prevent the study from being conducted. For example, a placebo lead-in trial cannot reveal the fact that all patients will receive placebo for a period of time before receiving active medicine. In this circumstance, patients can be informed that they will receive a placebo at some point during the trial without specifying when. Similarly, volunteers may not be told that they are drinking a low alcohol content beverage when in fact it contains no alcohol. The issue is that people who believe they are drinking alcohol, but are not, behave differently than people who believe they are drinking alcohol and really are. Many trials like this could not take place without deceiving some volunteers into believing they really were drinking alcohol when they were not, and vice versa. Ethics Committees/IRBs often have allowed this type of research when there are no alternative means of testing a hypothesis and they consider the proposed research scientifically important enough that some deception is acceptable. Provisions must be made in those cases to inform patients about the deception after their participation has been completed. It is also necessary for the investigator to provide any counseling or help required by patients after the trial as a result of the deception. Deception in clinical trials is discussed in more detail by the American Psychological Association (1982) and by Spilker (1991). The former group provides guidelines of when deception may be justified and how it may be handled ethically.

A common pattern of deception is when patients are recruited by telling them that the data are being collected for their treating physician or for their medical records (and thus does not require informed consent). In many cases the investigators believe that they are doing no harm because they justify to themselves or to an Ethics Committee/IRB that the research is really part of patient care. There is a gray area between collecting medical data for the patients' medical benefit and for conducting clinical research. Ethics Committees/IRBs must be extremely careful about this practice and ensure that patient rights are protected. At a recent Institute of Medicine meeting on Quality of Life studies, several academic investigators who claimed their research was performed for the patients' benefit were soundly chastised by the large majority of professionals present. As one person stated " If it walks like a duck, sounds like a duck, and looks like a duck—it is a duck." In other words, clinical research should not be disguised as part of the patient's medical care to avoid obtaining an informed consent. If an Ethics Committee/IRB has questions about this topic, they should ask the investigator what he or she will do with the data and then evaluate the response.

The teacher–student relationship deserves an additional comment because this approach is commonly used in psychological research, an area with an extremely high rate of deception [see Chapter 64 in Spilker (1991) for references]. Another coercive practice in this area involves giving student volunteers classroom credit for participating in research studies (Royce and Arkowitz, 1977).

Kaufman (1983) reported that "physicians tended to withhold information from patients; and that the tendency to withhold information varied directly with the degree of the status differences between physicians and patients. Middle-class patients were more likely to receive answers to their questions than were patients of lower socio-economic status." This interesting observation raises another caution for investigators to keep in mind as they conduct discussions relating to informed consents.

Should Patients Be Informed If the Investigator is Receiving Payment for the Patient's Participation in a Clinical Trial?

This question undoubtedly sounds like heresy to many, if not most, clinical investigators, although there is clear logic and an important issue underlying the question. If the informed consent requires information on issues pertinent to the patient's decision to enroll in a clinical trial and people's behavior is motivated in part by receiving money, then patients should be told this information. If an investigator informs a patient that the institution receives money for a trial, the patient's thinking about reimbursement for out-of-pocket expenses or about receiving additional payment for their participation could be influenced. Trial enrollment could be affected if patients learn that the investigator (instead of the institution) receives money for the trial. This topic was recently discussed in the literature (Shimm and Spence, 1991). Those authors state that it is ethically necessary for patients to be informed about payments to the institution or to an investigator prior to the patient's signing an informed consent. Future trends in the informed consent process may include debates on this controversial issue.

INTERACTING WITH ETHICS COMMITTEES AND IRBs ON DIFFICULT ISSUES

Ethics Committees/IRBs may change a protocol in a way that affects recruitment into a clinical trial (e.g., adding more restrictive inclusion criteria). The investigator should discuss these changes with the committee. In some cases, an Ethics Committee/IRB may impose draconian rules on how to recruit patients under the guise of protecting patient rights. For example, recruitment may be limited to patients who already have failed three types of therapy, have extremely severe disease, or have more than three episodes per month. Another type of restriction could be the requirement to use inpatients or to offer permanent follow-up therapy to responders. The investigator should do everything possible to ensure that unreasonable restrictions are not imposed, or if they are, he or she should be prepared to debate the issues with the Ethics Committee/IRB.

One consideration for physicians who anticipate problems with the Ethics Committee/IRB that would affect patient recruitment or other aspects of the research is to consult the hospital's attorney about national laws and guidelines prior to the Ethics Committee/IRB meeting. A written statement on these points may be submitted with the protocol, presented when the protocol is discussed, or presented after the Ethics Committee/IRB makes a statement that the investigator wishes to discuss further.

Because recruitment methods and even sources may vary among different sites of a multicenter trial it does not generally pose problems for the entire trial if one or more Ethics Committees/IRBs make recruitment more restrictive. But if the committee attempts to influence recruitment by modifying inclusion criteria or the protocol itself, major problems generally result. Such a change often requires compromises, or one (or more) sites may have to drop out of a multicenter trial, unless the investigator is able to convince the Ethics Committee/IRB to revise its decision.

6

Economic Issues in Patient Recruitment

COSTS OF RECRUITMENT

Why Measure the Costs of Recruitment?

Investigators usually have choices to make regarding both sources and methods of recruitment. Economic issues are a major influence on the decision of which sources and methods to use. Whether costs of various types of sources and methods are known from previous trials, pilot work, or careful estimates, or are merely guesses based on general impressions, the clinical trial budget must be sufficient to cover the anticipated costs of conducting the trial, including recruiting participants. The more accurate the economic data used by the investigator, the more confidence can be placed in the recruitment strategy developed.

What Are the Costs of Patient Recruitment?

Costs of patient recruitment vary from nil (when the investigator performs all recruitment tasks), to providing the salary necessary to obtain a minimum of staff time devoted to screening patients and obtaining informed consent, to providing large sums of money to support major national trials where publicity campaigns are used to spur recruitment. These latter trials often include a full-time recruiting staff. Recruitment costs include some, but rarely all, of the items listed in Table 6.1.

How to Estimate and Measure Recruitment Costs

The first step to estimating or measuring patient recruitment costs is to identify each of the separate elements involved (Table 6.1). Because some decisions may be based on costs (e.g., how much advertising should we do?), it is desirable to obtain multiple cost estimates for relevant factors and success rates (i.e., yields) of different sources and methods.

A minimum of three success rates (e.g., average yield expected for patient enrollment, better than average, or worse than average) should be measured. For example, the average expected success rate could be 25% of patients contacted by method A (e.g., chart review) will eventually enroll, and 5% of patients contacted by method B (e.g., advertisements) will eventually enroll. Better rates then can be calculated by using increments of 10%, 20%, or another percent. Lower rates also may be chosen to cover a broad range of possibilities.

Cost estimates for advertising should involve several options. For example, if a short radio advertisement is planned, it may be useful to obtain cost estimates for several different stations. Estimates of the potential audience to be reached by each station should include the number of people who might qualify for the trial. The cost also should be obtained for 2, 10, and 25, or other numbers of times the advertisement will be run.

Data on the cost of professional and other staff should be calculated and presented in terms of hours or months of time, or as the number of full and part-time staff. These data should also be subdivided by the level of staff and whether they are

---

TABLE 6.1. *Representative items that constitute recruitment costs*

A. Personnel
  1. Staff time in planning recruitment
  2. Staff time in contacting referrals and implementing other recruitment methods
  3. Staff time in conducting initial interviews with patients—on the telephone, as written responses, or face-to-face
  4. Staff time in conducting the entire screening process
  5. Staff time in obtaining informed consent
  6. Staff time to meet to solve problems or address issues
B. Direct expenses
  1. Printing costs for brochures, notices, advertisements, letters
  2. Mailing costs (e.g., to referral physicians, to investigators)
  3. Advertising costs for newspapers, radio, television, magazines
  4. Telephone costs
C. Travel expenses
  1. Costs to hold meetings to discuss recruitment plans, progress, problems
  2. Costs for trial coordinators to visit various sites
  3. Costs for trial staff to travel to outlying screening sites
  4. Costs for potential enrollees for visits to clinic for screening
D. Other expenses
  1. Interactions with a central recruitment group
  2. Interactions with an Ethics Committee/IRB

presently employed or must be hired. Hired personnel may also be evaluated as either temporary (e.g., telephone operators hired for 2 months) or permanent staff.

An alternative approach is to ask one or more contract research organizations to provide an estimate of recruitment costs. Depending on the nature and size of the trial, it may be reasonable to consider contracting the recruitment aspects to such a group. If recruitment depends on methods using direct patient interviews in shopping malls or contacts by telephone, then it is sensible to consider using an outside group with special expertise in the method(s) to be used.

USES OF COST DATA

How Should Recruitment Cost Data Be Used?

Two opposite approaches may be used. It is possible to start with the available budget and then to determine what it can purchase in terms of patient recruitment. The opposite approach is to generate a budget for patient recruitment by calculating the ideal patient recruitment costs and then to determine how far the resources will go. The latter approach is generally preferable, because if the costs of the desired recruitment approach are not matched by resources, increased resources should be sought. If additional resources cannot be found (as is often the case), it then becomes necessary to pare down either the extent to which each method will be used, or to decrease one or more of the more expensive recruiting methods.

It is important to evaluate yield when financial resources for patient recruitment are an issue. Yield is defined as the percent of contacted or screened patients who enroll. Once yield is determined, the cost per enrolled patient can be calculated for each proposed recruitment method. The cost of each method is then compared. Prior to a trial, it is usually necessary to use a series of cost estimates rather than actual cost data because the data will not have been generated on which to calculate actual costs and actual yields per method. Using data from previous trials conducted by the same investigators, plus data from colleagues and the literature, it may be possible to derive reasonable estimates for both the cost and yield data for each recruitment method planned. Actual data are shown in Tables 6.2 to 6.4.

Why Costs Are Not the Sole Factor in Choice of Recruitment Methods

It is important to estimate the cost per enrolled patient for a variety of recruitment methods. These data coupled with the available budget will help planners choose the most appropriate recruitment methods to use in the trial.

There are a number of reasons why it is not appropriate to choose recruitment methods solely on the basis of cost. First, it is important not to disturb the time frame of the trial. Less expensive methods may take longer to implement, resulting in prolongation of the trial beyond the planned or required time. Even if time is considered in all of the calculations (e.g., compare only those methods that are expected to lead to successful recruitment within the required period), there are still other factors to consider.

1. Are all of the methods expected to enroll patients who are similar in terms of:

a. disease characteristics,
b. social and economic status,

TABLE 6.2. *Recruitment costs*

Step exclusion and no. of conditions	Number entering step	Relative cost	Cost per person entering step[a]	Total cost for step	Percent of total cost
Brochure mailing					
0 NA	223,815	0.12	$ 0.35	$ 77,500	9.7
Telephone interview					
1 Age, medications, etc.	11,810	1	2.97	35,076	4.4
BL 1					
2 No-show	8,662	10	29.70	37,422	4.7
3 Outside weight limit	7,402	5	14.85	109,920	13.8
4 Outside 1st DBP limits	7,059	10	29.70	209,652	26.3
5 Miscellaneous	3,262	5	14.85	48,441	6.1
BL 2					
6 No-show	2,993	20	59.40	36,115	4.5
7 Outside 2nd DBP limits	2,385	10	29.70	70,834	8.9
8 Miscellaneous	1,074	33.6	99.83	107,213	13.4
BL 3					
9 No-show	960	10	29.70	2,911	0.4
10 Miscellaneous	862	24.4	72.57	62,557	7.8
Total	841		$948	$797,641	100.0

From Borhani et al. (1989) with permission.
[a] Cost per person for steps 2, 6, and 9 are based on number of no-shows. Laboratory costs are included in steps 8 (serum) and 10 (urine).
BL, blood level; NA, not applicable; DBP, diastolic blood pressure.

c. expected drop-out rate,
d. expected rate of discontinuation,
e. expected reliability in keeping appointments and cooperating with staff during clinic visits, and
f. expected compliance with taking medicine and following protocol directions outside clinic visits?

2. Will the efforts and stress level of trial staff be similar with all methods of patient recruitment? A less expensive method that places more stress on the staff may prove to be far more "expensive" in the long term and from the perspective of the trial's ultimate successful completion and overall quality.

TABLE 6.3. *Costs of strategies to locate patients for clinical trials*

	Total direct costs $	Persons assessed n	Cost per person assessed $	Persons confirmed for COAD n	Cost per confirmed case $	Confirmed cases not previously diagnosed n	Cost per case not previously diagnosed $
Hospital records	1,887	75	25.20	63	30.00	NA[b]	NA
Physician referral	4,209	352	12.00	247	17.00	94	44.80
Advertising campaign	12,499	475	26.30	204	61.30	104	120.20
Mailed questionnaire	37,260	932	40.00	409	91.10	198	188.20

Reprinted from Barlow et al. (1984) with permission.
COAD, chronic obstructive airway disease; NA, not applicable.

TABLE 6.4. *Recruitment costs in the HDFP trial*

Site	Percent of screenees enrolled	$ Cost per enrollee
Housing project	6.4	235
Census tract	15.8	250
Door-to-door	12.6	470
Random sample	4.5	836

Reprinted from Ford (1987) with permission.
HDFP, Hypertension Detection Follow-up Program.

3. Some methods will not yield any patients. This could arise if patients are unaware of a problem and it is uncommon. Alternatively, the methods used may not reach the patients of interest.

RECRUITMENT BUDGETS

What Percent of a Clinical Trial Budget Should Be Spent on Patient Recruitment?

The proportion of a total clinical trial budget devoted to recruitment varies enormously among trials. The Utah Hypertension Trial (Williams et al., 1987) spent $59 for each patient recruited, totaling 10% of the $1.5 million overall budget. In contrast, the Hypertension Prevention Trial spent $948 per person randomized, totaling $798,000 in recruitment costs (Borhani et al., 1989). A stress incontinence trial spent an average of $83 per randomized patient, with various recruitment method costs (see Table 6.5) ranging from $3 to $338 per entry (Burns et al., 1990). Cost per patient entered into the Hypertension Detection and Follow-up Program ranged from $235 to $836 at four sites (Ford et al., 1987). Newcomb et al.(1990) utilized a cancer registry to recruit patients for a clinical trial. They calculated recruitment costs of $8 per potential enrollee or $135 per actual enrollee. These costs included mailing and computer costs, but not additional screening costs. They stated that their recruitment costs compared favorably to a "similar study," the Hypertension Detection and Follow-up Study. The costs for creating and maintaining the registry are not included in these calculations. Unfortunately, few trials have reported recruitment costs, or the relative efficiency of one method over another. Thus, at this time,

TABLE 6.5. *Cost/retention of recruitment methods*

Recruitment method	Cost ($)			Per subject randomized		Total respondents	Retention/entry ratio
	Printing	Personnel[a]	Total				
Posters	1,321	3,388	4,709	196	(24)	313	13:1
Newspaper	1,690	2,278	3,969	45	(87)	521	6:1
Suburban papers	917	308	1,225	122	(10)	61	6:1
Brochures	538	139	677	338	(2)	29	15:1
Media presentation	No charge	222	222	28	(8)	89	11:1
Doctor	No charge	250	250	0	(0)	15	None
Other referrals	No charge	124	124	3	(4)	14	4:1
Total	4,443	6,711	11,154	732	(135)	1,042	8:1

Reprinted from Burns et al. (1990) with permission.
[a] Includes time expended to implement the method and screen the responses.

the data are insufficient to address the question, What percent of a clinical trial budget should be spent on recruitment? The number will vary widely depending on protocol requirements, inclusion criteria, availability of patients, and other factors.

Effect of Limited Financial Resources on Clinical Trial Planning

Lack of sufficient funds for a small multicenter trial leads to many trials being undertaken by a solitary investigator. Limited funds may also lead to clinical trials being initiated as pilot trials instead of larger single site or multicenter trials.

Source of funding may determine the way that funds can be utilized (e.g., grants that can share resources as needed versus contracts that stipulate various constraints). It is possible to apply for small grants that fund specific aspects of an overall project, allowing the investigator to undertake a clinical trial. Although the initial request for funding is based on an itemized budget, grants usually provide an overall sum that can be reallocated as needed. This fiscal freedom is particularly helpful for support of peripheral subprojects, pilot studies for future trials, or follow-up of prior trials. In contrast, contracts usually stipulate payment only for specific tasks as accomplished.

Financial requirements of a trial are markedly influenced by sample size. Sample size in turn is based on the magnitude of the expected effect. Knowing that a desired endpoint would require 500 patients might lead investigators to alter the hypothetical magnitude of difference considered important so that only 200 patients would be necessary. This can be easily justified because during the development of a protocol for a new investigational medicine, it is often difficult to know what is a clinically meaningful effect. But, the entire cost of a clinical trial may be wasted if the number of patients enrolled is too small to answer the question of interest.

Budgeting Recruitment Costs

Trial budgets should be estimated based on the number of patients who must be found, screened, and sign the informed consent, to obtain the requisite number to enter the trial (McDearmon and Bradford, 1982). If patient deaths, dropouts, or discontinuers are to be replaced by new patients, then an estimate of these two categories also must be made.

A recruitment budget could be created as a total sum, or separate budgets could be created for:

1. *Finding patients.* Costs for advertising, printing, contacting patients and physicians about a clinical trial. These administrative costs can be quite expensive (Table 6.5).
2. *Screening patients.* All costs for initial telephone contacts and questionnaires, through to the advanced testing of patient prerandomization. If these data also are used as baseline values, then a case could be made for apportioning part of these costs to another category.
3. *Enrolling patients.* Time spent by staff in discussing the trial, answering questions, and obtaining informed consent.
4. *Administrative costs.* Time spent by staff completing all administrative activities required to recruit patients into the trial.

5. *Other costs.* Depending on the nature of the trial, additional costs are incurred to hold special meetings to address problems, or to adopt new recruitment methods.

Effect of Protocol Changes on the Recruitment Budget

The determination of funding required for a trial is based on the items listed in the protocol, ranging from the number of staff to the cost for special tests. Once funds are appropriated for academic and government sponsored trials, it is cumbersome, if not impossible, to attempt to increase the budget allocation. In such cases, a late decision to add another site, establish a central laboratory, or include expensive radiographic tests would cause a major drain on the budget, unless other items can be reduced. The Program on Surgical Treatment of the Hyperlipidemias (POSCH) (Buchwald et al., 1987) suffered delays in recruitment because of restrictions in transferring funds to open replacement sites. Changing the inclusion criteria to enlarge the potential pool of patients allows a fixed recruitment budget to be more effective.

Conversely, the decision to discontinue a special test or reduce staff can create a cash flow bonus that may be used for an underfunded aspect of the trial. For example, moving the salary for a recruitment coordinator from one site to another could increase productivity at the expanded site without necessarily having an impact on the reduced site if other staff could take on the recruiter role or recruitment is so slow that lack of a coordinator will not alter enrollment rates. Alternatively, the coordinator could serve two or more sites. In single-site studies, the ability to juggle funds within a program allows the investigator to meet unexpected demands as well as to add extra features as desired. For example, the salary saved when clinical staff assist with the trial can be allocated for newly incorporated laboratory tests that were not anticipated when the protocol was prepared.

In industry sponsored trials, additional costs are more readily budgeted so long as the company remains committed to the development of the medicine or device.

Amortizing the Cost of a Central Recruitment Coordinator

Multicenter trials often are coordinated by a central group that provides efficient services for all the sites. One role that can be undertaken by a coordinating center is the centralization of recruitment efforts. In particular, a recruitment coordinator can efficiently assist sites in developing strategies that work locally, can spread information among sites about recruitment practices that work well at one or another site, and can generally manage the overall recruitment effort. This role can be established at each site in large trials, as was done in the Lipid Research Clinics Trial (1983).

Although the hiring or designation of a specific person as recruitment coordinator is costly, the expense is shared by all sites when the position is centrally located. Energies and efforts are expended where needed (e.g., spending the time necessary to assess why a slow site is not increasing screening, or determining why a site has a low yield of enrollees despite an active screening program). Because it is rare that a clinical trial has no recruitment problems, the hiring of a central (or site) recruitment coordinator is usually a wise allocation of funds that should be considered during the trial's planning stage.

COLLECTING COST DATA

Tracking Costs of Patient Recruitment

Data should be collected on various aspects of recruitment to compare actual costs with projected or estimated costs. These data will be invaluable if problems arise and choices must be made about allocation of more (or less) money among methods. Data are, therefore, required on the amount of staff time spent contacting various recruitment sources by different level individuals (e.g., physicians, research assistants). Data tracking the amount of money paid for printing, postage, radio and television promotions, newspaper advertisements, and other direct expenses are also useful, as are data on screening activities in terms of time, and costs for laboratory or other tests.

Screening costs are part of the cost for conducting the clinical trial, in addition to recruitment costs. They may be divided or allocated entirely to either category when calculating total recruitment costs. The approach taken should be based on the use of the data. For example, if a comparison of the costs of using different recruitment sources is desired, all screening costs should be included as part of recruitment. This enables different yields of enrollees (i.e., number of patients screened to yield one enrollee) to affect the conclusion as to which sources are most cost-effective.

The data for total time expended may be converted to number of staff per year at the level required to conduct the specific activity. Data also may be expressed as the number of staff hours spent to enroll one patient into the trial. Depending on the size and importance of the trial, these data may be calculated separately for each site and then compared.

Actual data on patient yield are also important to collect both by source of patients and methods of recruitment for each. Recruitment costs are presented in detail for the Hypertension Prevention Trial by Borhani et al. (1989). Table 6.2 presents a summary of their data. These authors discuss the issues in deriving an optimal cost strategy and indicate seven of the numerous factors that affect this determination. Table 6.5 describes specific costs incurred for each recruitment method used by Burns et al. (1990). The entry ratio demonstrates the efficiency of each method based on patient enrollment. Definitions of how costs for time and staff labor were calculated are provided by Silagi et al. (1991).

Costs of Clinical Trials Borne by Patients

Insurance companies have increasingly been unwilling to pay for investigational therapy in clinical trials (American Medical Association Council on Scientific Affairs, 1991). These costs must be paid for by patients, the principal investigator's grant or contract, the department sponsor, or the institution in which the trial is conducted. Occasionally, other sources of funds may be found. Some tests required by the protocol may be interpreted by an insurance company as unnecessary for the patient's well-being and appropriate medical care and, therefore, will not be covered. Ancillary costs in a clinical trial (e.g., special tests, extra days of hospitalization related to the trial) that are above those of usual care also must be paid for. In some trials these costs are passed on to the patient. Other costs, such as travel, meals, and lodging (particularly for accompanying family members) are often paid by patients. In many trials and for many patients, these costs may be substantial and may be a barrier to enrollment. The nature and amount of costs covered by patients should be discussed with them before and during the informed consent process when details are outlined about who will pay for the various parts of the trial.

Cost Per Screenee Versus Cost Per Enrollee

Not every recruitment plan is efficient. Some recruitment strategies are able to gather large numbers of screenees, but few patients are found to be eligible for entry. Because the number of patient entries, rather than the number screened, is more important, trial staff must keep their attention focused on enrollment into the trial. Typically, referrals from physicians will have a relatively high yield of trial enrollment whereas community screenings have a relatively low yield (see Chapter 3). Thus, the staff cost to use various types of recruitment sources and methods should be calculated before, during, and after the process is initiated. For example, waiting for appropriate referrals from medical colleagues may provide high quality trial candidates, but the rate of referrals may be too slow to keep staff active full-time. In contrast, placing an advertisement in the newspaper might bring a flurry of phone calls requiring extensive evaluation by trial staff and medical personnel, but may ultimately provide a low yield. Not only is much time involved but extra staff might have to be hired temporarily and trained. Thus, the screening of large numbers of potential enrollees in a major community might be found to be no more cost-effective than screening in a small community, which may achieve a lower recruitment rate but is accomplished with fewer staff.

SELECTION OF A RECRUITMENT METHOD BASED ON COSTS

Various recruitment methods are generally evaluated prior to a clinical trial, and one or more are chosen. Ford (1987) described the experiences of four sites participating in the Hypertension Detection Follow-up Program. Each site used a different recruitment method and the costs varied, but not in proportion to the patient yield. The New York site approached people in a housing project; Atlanta focused on households in census tracts; Jackson, MS used door-to-door canvassing in specific districts; and Davis, CA used a stratified random sample.

Table 6.4 demonstrates that although the census tract system yielded the highest number of randomizations from the screening pool, it was not more cost-effective than the housing project approach. Staff using census tract and door-to-door methods reached more eligible people but not more economically. The stratified random sample method was not only costly, but resulted only in a small proportion of screenees who were actually randomized. Unfortunately, these data cannot be extrapolated to other trials because of the many site-specific factors that must be considered (e.g., personnel costs in different cities, transportation and logistics in urban versus suburban areas).

TABLE 6.6. *A comparison of recruitment costs using personalized letters plus phone calls or letters alone*

	Letters and phone calls	Letters only
Goal	1,700 appointments	1,700 appointments
Letters sent	8,500 letters	22,000 letters
Listing names	$ 1,080	$ 2,797
Supervision	$ 486	—
Finding phone numbers	$ 610	—
Phoning	$ 3,894	—
Stamps required	$ 2,720	$ 7,040
Letterhead	$ 595	$ 1,537
Envelopes	$ 340	$ 878
Copying	$ 160	$ 414
Secretary	$ 1,008	$ 2,606
Total	$10,893	$15,272

From Baines (1984) with permission.

Economic Comparison of Recruitment Methods

A comparison between two methods was made by Baines et al. (1984) for the National Breast Screening Study (NBSS). Table 6.6 shows the cost of letters followed by telephone calls or letters alone to reach prospective patients. The letter alone gave a 7.6% yield. When a letter was followed by a phone call, a 20.3% yield was obtained. The investigators concluded that it was more economical to use the dual technique with a smaller list in order to recruit the requisite number of patients.

A detailed description of the initial process of finding patients is presented by Burns et al. (1990), and is shown in Table 6.5. They found that newspaper advertisements were the most efficient method and yielded the highest retention of respondents. Less expensive methods were generally less efficient. Burns and co-workers calculated the overall study recruitment costs as $11,154, and the average cost per patient as $83. An advantage of the more expensive poster method they used is that the smaller (but constant) number of patient contacts made led to less stress among the staff in processing patients. Newspaper advertisements created a

TABLE 6.7. *Cost-effectiveness of recruitment approaches*

Recruitment approach	Preparation time hr	Screening visits hr	Baseline visits hr	Total time hr	Nurse cost $	Doctor cost $	Mail cost $	Total cost[a] $
Electoral roll	64	124	52	240	3,360	1,620	957	5,937
Community-based	27	49	57	133	1,862	2,100	29[b]	4,254
General practice	56	69	56	181	2,534	2,000	302	4,836

Adapted from Silagy et al. (1991) and reprinted with permission.
[a] The total cost per person randomized is calculated by dividing the total cost by 100. All costs are in Australian dollars.
[b] Includes cost of distributing posters and leaflets.
[c] Costs for the general practice approach was also calculated excluding one inefficient site, resulting in a total cost of $4,372.

great number of responses over a short period, but also led to many logistical problems that created more stress.

The cost of each aspect of approaching elderly patients using three different sources is detailed by Silagy et al. (1991) (Table 6.7). They calculated preparation time, screening and baseline visit time, mailing costs, as well as nurse and doctor time costs. A community-based approach required the least amount of hours and the lowest salary and mailing expenses, whereas the use of electoral rolls was least efficient in both respects. General practice referrals were of intermediate cost, but varied by site because of inefficiencies in retrieval of names of potentially eligible patients. The average total cost for each enrollee ranged from $42.54 to $59.37 (Australian dollars) in this trial conducted in the Australian health care system.

THE COST OF PROLONGING THE RECRUITMENT PERIOD OR USING AN ALTERNATIVE APPROACH

Prolonging any aspect of a clinical trial increases costs (Schoenberger, 1979). Because salaries are a major portion of the cost of maintaining a trial, an extension of time to complete a trial greatly increases the budget. Gaston et al. (1987) stated that lengthening the recruitment period in their trial from 24 months to 27 months primarily increased personnel costs. The economic impacts of the major ways of altering patient recruitment are discussed below.

Additional Time for Recruitment

If a trial protocol is maintained with a fixed duration of follow-up for all patients, extension of the accrual period by a number of months or years may be needed to enter an adequate number of patients. The cost overrun of extension depends mainly on staff salary, tests used for screening, and site administrative expenses including rental of space or equipment. Extension of the trial has a redeeming value in that if the trial is not completed properly (i.e., with an adequate number of patients), then the entire initial investment by the sponsor may be wasted. The cost overrun to extend the accession period generally can be calculated because the slope of the patient accession curve is known well in advance of the end of the designated period for completing recruitment. Various other aspects of the trial can be modified so that additional costs are minimized. For example, trial staff could be reduced to a part-time basis near the end of the trial when the number of clinic visits are reduced. Screening tests or other tests conducted during the trial sometimes may be reduced or accomplished using a less expensive method. These modifications must be discussed at length with statisticians and others to ensure the trial's integrity is not compromised. It may be possible to centralize some functions to save cost and duplication at each site (e.g., selected data or blood samples can be sent to a central laboratory for analysis).

Even if extra funds are allocated to extend recruitment, one problem that occurs is staff fatigue. Staff become exhausted and upset if there is continuous goading to meet quotas. They may feel like Sisyphus eternally striving uphill trying to reach an elusive goal. Although the end of a long trial may mean the termination of employment for some staff, both they (and the investigators) usually are relieved to see the end in sight. Not only is the pace of activities altered when recruitment ends, but the desire to hear the results of the trial also leads to a desire to reach the conclusion of the follow-up period.

On the other hand, the announcement of additional funding to support extended recruitment often serves as a stimulus for the team to persevere toward the goal within the brief extension period. Everyone affiliated with a trial is likely to feel encouraged as the overall enrollment climbs and approaches the total number of patients needed. There is also a feeling of pride knowing the trial is considered worth an extra investment by the sponsor.

Reducing the Duration of the Follow-up Period

One strategy to maintain the overall cost of a clinical trial as planned without shortening the entire duration of the trial, is to reduce the length of patient observation during a follow-up period. Careful thought must preface this plan to be sure it does not compromise the trial's results. Trial planners must decide if the trial's design can provide adequate answers to the major hypothesis with a shorter observation period. Biostatisticians must be involved in this decision to assess the effect on the data if the sample size or duration of follow-up are altered.

Reducing Patient Drop-out Rates to Shorten the Recruitment Period

An alternative to changing the recruitment period is the possibility of taking measures so the patient drop-out rates will be lower than anticipated, thereby reducing total sample size requirements. The VA Epilepsy Cooperative Studies (Cramer et al., 1988) specifically targeted patient retention as a major factor combined with steady recruitment, to meet revised sample size requirements. Using demographic data available at screening, investigators identified the types of patients most likely to drop out of an epilepsy clinical trial and targeted those patients for special attention (e.g., extra education about the diagnosis and need for medication, referral for other support services). The specific efforts needed to retain patients in different trials are likely to differ and should be discussed by those responsible for recruitment activities.

Changing the Number of Clinical Trial Sites During a Multicenter Trial

As discussed in issues of altering a trial protocol, the decision of whether to change the number or size of clinical sites during a multicenter trial sponsored by academicians or government agencies is based largely on cost because of the difficulty in obtaining extra funds to expand a trial once it is underway. The situation is often quite different if the sponsor is a pharmaceutical company. A company's decisions about recruitment are made primarily on the basis of minimizing the time required to recruit patients and to conduct the trial. Money is usually available to spend on recruitment activities considered important. The following are options that may affect recruitment costs.

1. Eliminate a Site. Removal of a site that does not provide a reasonable number of patients (i.e., meet quotas) saves money but also eliminates even the few patients being entered at that site. Some trials start with an excess number of sites and have the intention to eliminate weak performers after one year or a predetermined review point. This approach was suggested by the Lipid Research Clinics Program (Lipid Research Clinics Program, 1983). This apparent inefficiency is based on the principle that it is not possible to know in advance which teams (i.e., sites) will be good recruiters. Previous history of a site's performance is not necessarily a good predictor of how it will perform in the planned trial. Many factors may differ and significantly affect the ability of a particular site to recruit patients in the current trial.

2. Replace a Site. It is possible to tentatively enlist one or more sites that are prepared to take over the funding and initiate a trial as soon as a weak site is eliminated. Although the net cost superficially appears to be the same, the time lost during the transition and startup of the new site reduces the cost-effectiveness of this plan. In addition, Collins et al. (1980) caution that: "there is no certainty that the replacement facility will perform better than the one replaced."

3. Add One or More Additional Sites. The possibility of adding an extra site to a trial depends on whether additional funds can be obtained. Extra sites should be selected as early as possible. Time required for planning and startup reduce the total efficiency of this plan, but it often represents a sound approach. This approach is often used by pharmaceutical companies when they are faced with major recruitment problems.

4. Expand Recruitment at Existing Sites. If a site with high recruitment rates can be expanded with existing or additional staff for screening, or an auxiliary office, this approach could be more cost-effective than adding or replacing an entirely new site. The proven capacity of a smooth functioning team is often a better approach to increase recruitment than depending on the unknown performance of a new site. Funding can sometimes come from elimination of an existing site, reduction of the enrollment quotas of one or more sites, or reallocation of the trial budget (e.g., reduce salary funding for selected sites, or provide less advertising funds to slow recruiting sites).

5. Reduce Recruitment Activities at Existing Sites. If a site has consistently recruited fewer patients than planned into a trial, it may nonetheless be functioning at its optimum pace. However, this pace may not require as much support as is needed at sites with both higher screening and recruitment rates. In this case, reduction of support (e.g., fewer staff, part-time instead of full-time staff, less money for advertising) at that clinical site may not affect the site's productivity. It might be more cost-effective to retain a slow site that maintains a low but steady pace of patient recruitment and to continue patient follow-up than to close the site. Cost savings can be distributed as described above.

PART II

Putting the Elements of Recruitment Together

Initially, we planned an analysis of successful and unsuccessful approaches. This analysis was, however, of little relevance since it emphasized that unsuccessful approaches are determined by a combination of local conditions and the skills, talents, and focus of the individual clinic recruitment staffs. For example, churches were an effective focus of recruiting only in Birmingham; mass mailings were most successful in Portland; senior housing screenings were particularly successful in Chicago, and so on. Yield rates from the group of persons invited to screening after medical record reviews were much higher than from unselected groups, but the effort that was required to obtain the review made the approach less than ideal. Mass cover mailings, on the other hand, had low yields but required comparatively less personnel time per person contacted, and [were] successful approaches to recruitment.

—Vogt et al. (1986)

7

Developing a Recruitment Strategy

Although many trials are initiated with a general plan of where and how to seek patients (i.e., sources and methods), the protocols of few trials include detailed plans for a recruitment strategy. Even when addressed, the strategy usually does not go beyond questions of "where" and "what," to address questions such as: When should each method be used? Who should be involved with each step? How much will it cost? How much can I afford? Are there quotas? Are there special issues to consider? Unfortunately, lack of foresight and planning added to overoptimism frequently lead to a shortage of enrolled patients. Any single factor or any combination of factors may be responsible for poor (i.e., undesirably low) rates of patient recruitment. To minimize the likelihood of poor recruitment, investigators should develop a recruitment strategy prior to initiating a trial, and should develop, as well, multiple contingency plans. This chapter describes the basic elements that make up a recruitment strategy, how to create this strategy, and the types of choices that

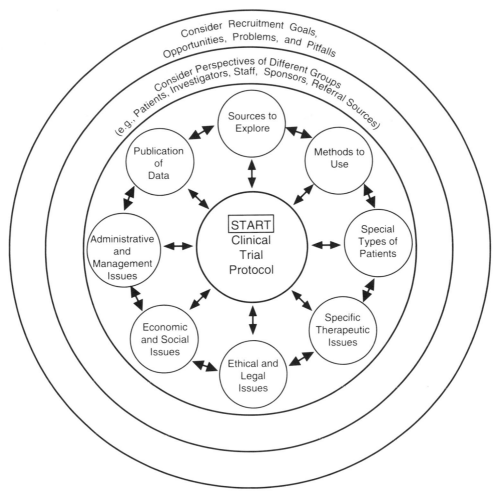

FIG. 7.1. Development of a patient recruitment strategy. Beginning with the clinical trial protocol, one next considers the elements listed in separate circles, all of which may interact. These are considered in the context of different perspectives in the outer circle and finally in relation to goals, opportunities, problems, and pitfalls shown in the outermost circle.

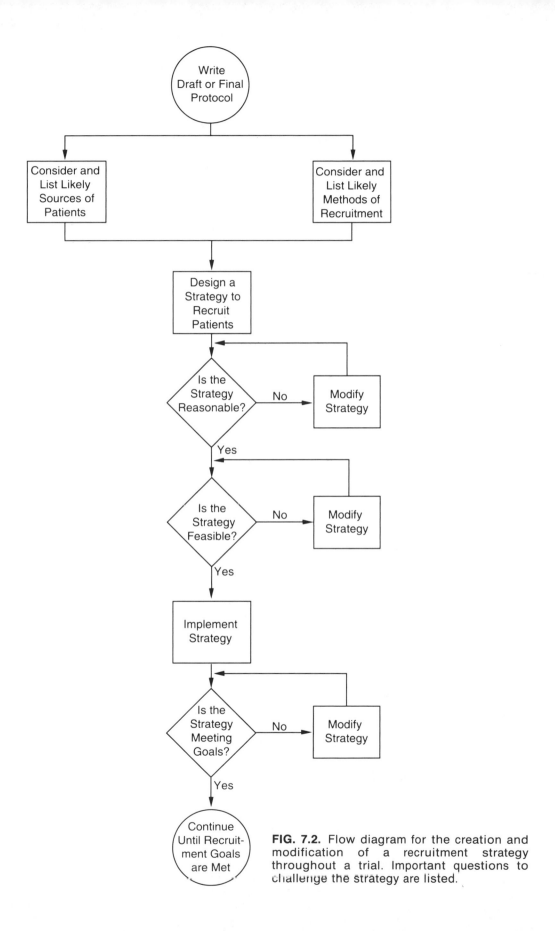

FIG. 7.2. Flow diagram for the creation and modification of a recruitment strategy throughout a trial. Important questions to challenge the strategy are listed.

usually must be made. The next chapter discusses various contingency plans that can be implemented if the strategy does not work perfectly.

WHAT IS A RECRUITMENT STRATEGY?

A recruitment strategy is a plan that encompasses the basic elements of recruitment in a clinical trial (e.g., patients, sources, methods, time, and resources) (Fig. 7.1). The strategy includes a decision on whether and when to use multiple plans. The strategy should encompass all aspects of recruitment, from the initiation of the trial through to the signing of informed consent by individual patients or patient random-

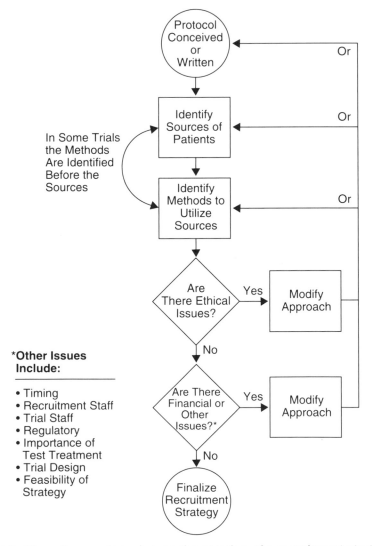

FIG. 7.3. Flow diagram focusing on the creation of a recruitment strategy.

ization (see Chapter 1). The general process is shown in Fig. 7.2 and Fig. 7.3 is a more detailed diagram focusing on the creation of the recruitment strategy.

Patient retention in a clinical trial is extremely important because patients who drop out or are discontinued often must be replaced. Even if replacement is not required, the successful completion of a clinical trial successfully depends on many, if not most, patients completing the trial. Problems with retention, rather than recruitment, of patients in a trial may suggest that there are problems with the requirements of the trial, the conduct of the trial, or almost any other aspect (e.g., staff). Thus, patient retention is not a subpart of patient recruitment and is not discussed at length in this book.

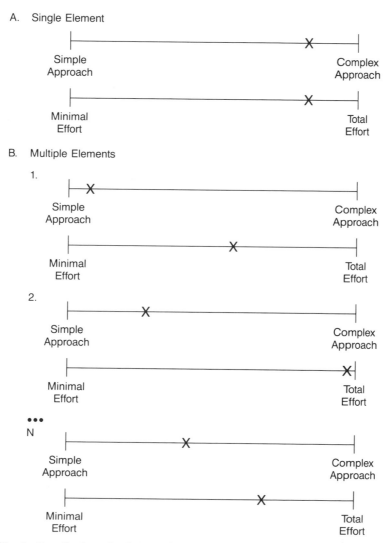

FIG. 7.4. Illustrating that each element in the recruitment strategy may be viewed along two spectra: from simple to complex in approach, and from minimal effort to maximal effort. In A, the strategy consists of a single element. In B multiple elements are used to create the recruitment strategy. The three dots represent any number of intervening elements between 2 and N.

The Need for a Systematic Recruitment Strategy

A systematic recruitment strategy is required because most clinical trial investigators (even experienced ones) markedly overestimate the projected rate of patient recruitment. This has been referred to as both Lasagna's Law (Spilker, 1991) and Muench's Third Law (Bearman et al., 1974; Ederer, 1975). The former states that the number of patients available for entering a clinical trial falls markedly when the trial is initiated and rises markedly after the trial is complete. Muench's Third Law states that the number of patients estimated to be entered is more than ten times the amount available. Willford et al. (1987) reported that eight of nine trials completed at VA medical centers overestimated the rate of patient recruitment.

ELEMENTS OF A PATIENT RECRUITMENT STRATEGY

The following are descriptions of the essential elements that should be included in a recruitment strategy planned in advance of the trial or during the course of a trial that is not meeting recruitment goals. Each element may be viewed along two axes—one representing complexity of approach, the other representing the amount of effort expended (Fig. 7.4).

Element One: Description of Patients or Volunteers

The primary element in a recruiting strategy is the patient to be enrolled. The most essential points that must be considered are:

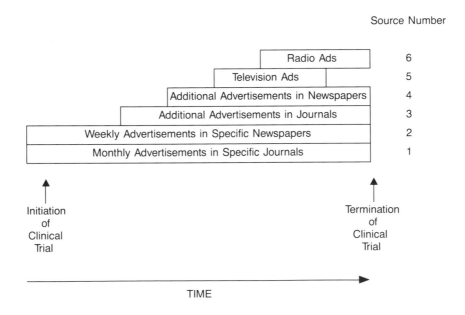

Note: Sources 3 to 6 would be initiated if patient recruitment did not achieve prespecified goals.

FIG. 7.5. Illustrating how a single recruitment method (i.e., advertising) can utilize various sources in a stepwise manner over the course of the trial. Sources 3 to 6 usually would only be initiated if patient recruitment did not achieve pre-specified goals. Nonetheless, the entire plan shown could be used regardless of actual recruitment.

1. The number of patients needed.
2. The type of patients needed in terms of demographics, classification of disease, severity of disease, prognostic characteristics of disease, and the other inclusion criteria.

Element Two: Selection of Sources

Potential sources for patient recruitment should be carefully considered prior to starting the trial, and a choice should be made of the one(s) to be used. This decision is often not made in a systematic way until the trial is underway and poor enrollment rates are noticed. The probability that the sources chosen can provide a sufficient number of appropriate patients within the necessary time frame must be assessed as carefully as possible. The two major aspects of sources to consider are (1) the various types that can be used, and (2) the number of each type that will be necessary.

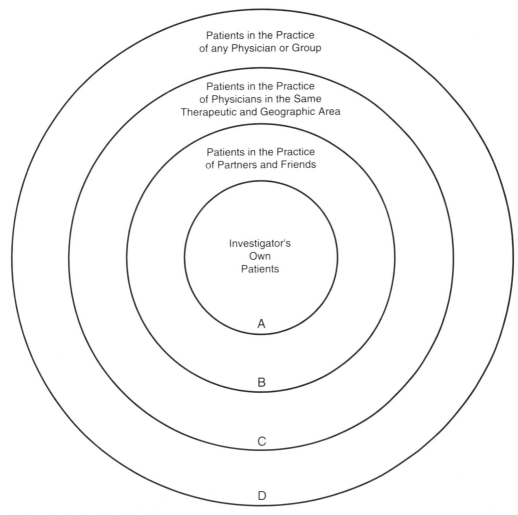

FIG. 7.6. Patient referral spectrum visualized as a series of four concentric circles including progressively more and more referrals from groups and areas that are progressively distant from the investigator.

Possible sources to consider are identified in Chapter 3. Sources may be added in a trial in a stepwise (i.e., cumulative) manner (Fig. 7.5). The sources used may also be viewed as progressive levels starting from the investigator's own practice (Fig. 7.6).

Element Three: Selection of Methods

Recruitment methods also should be evaluated and one or more chosen prior to the trial. The overall recruitment strategy should choose to use (1) a single method, (2) multiple methods simultaneously, or (3) multiple methods sequentially. The more different the recruitment methods used are from each other, the more questions will be raised about whether data obtained may be combined and how well the data may be extrapolated to other patients. Methods may be added in a trial in a stepwise (i.e., cumulative) manner (Fig. 7.7). Methods may also be viewed as progressive levels (Fig. 7.8). Flow diagrams may be made for using any method. Fig. 7.9 shows a flow diagram for using medical records.

Element Four: Length of Time for Recruitment

Several factors influence the allocation of time to patient recruitment. First is the pattern of patient enrollment (see Fig. 7.10): Will all patients be enrolled simultaneously or will they be enrolled sequentially over a period of time? In many short-term trials and in some long-term trials, all patients begin the trial on the same day;

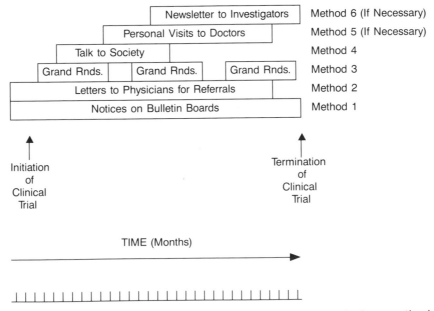

FIG. 7.7. Stepwise model of a recruiting strategy. In this example four methods have been chosen for use, and two others will be used if necessary. Grand Rnds. presentation at grand rounds. Stepwise refers to adding new methods onto the existing strategy. If recruitment was too successful (e.g., temporarily overloading staff), then methods could be terminated or the efforts on them reduced.

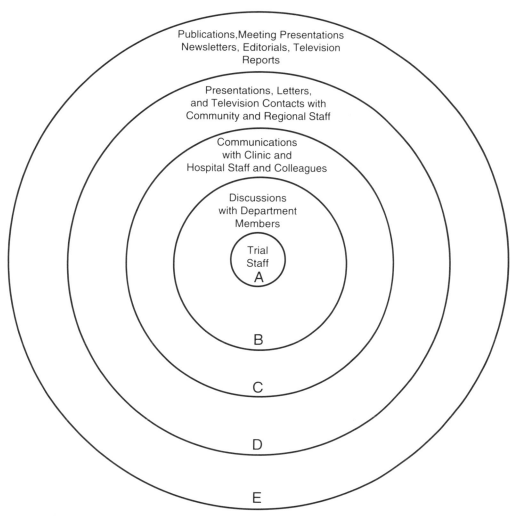

FIG. 7.8. Five concentric circles illustrating how publicity can be spread progressively to professionals stepwise from the trial staff.

but in the most common type of clinical trial patients enter and complete the trial at various times. The second factor is the duration of treatment. In general, the longer the treatment period for each patient, the longer is the recruitment period. However, even if the trial lasts only a single day for a patient, it could take years to enroll all patients necessary. This could occur if (1) the disease is rare, (2) the selection process excludes most patients, (3) the treatment effect is unpleasant and patients drop out, or (4) if an extremely large number of patients must be enrolled.

Element Five: Resources to Support Recruitment

Trial organizers should determine the resources needed to achieve the recruitment goals. Resources include money, sites, staff, facilities, experience, personal contacts, and investigator time. Financial resources include costs of screening and en-

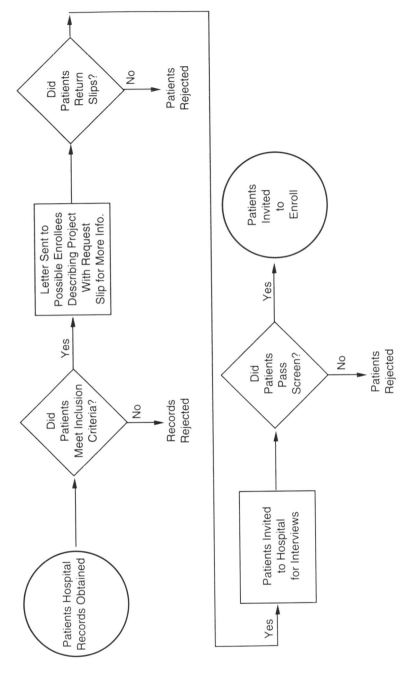

FIG. 7.9. Flow diagram illustrating one means of recruiting patients as a result of chart review. The term clinic or office could be substituted for hospital.

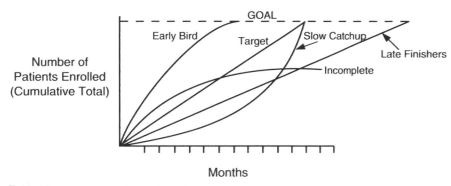

FIG. 7.10. Common enrollment patterns observed by plotting the number of patients enrolled in a clinical trial versus time. Although the target is shown as a constant rate, any other pattern could be used as a target rate of patient enrollment. *Early bird* sites reach their recruitment goals ahead of time, *slow catchup* sites increase their recruitment rate toward the end of the trial, but finish on time or nearly so. *Incomplete* sites never achieve their goals and *late finishers* reach the goal later than intended (or scheduled).

rolling patients. It is a quite obvious but often overlooked fact that having a higher percent of successfully screened patients enter a trial makes it less expensive. If a large number of patients must be screened and only a few are expected to pass and enter the trial, then other groups (e.g., coinvestigators, colleagues) may be asked to help with the screening process in terms of contributing or loaning staff, rooms, and equipment.

DEVELOPING A RECRUITMENT STRATEGY IN TEN STEPS

Step One: Identify the Number of Patients To Be Recruited

The number of patients to be recruited in a clinical trial is always greater than the number to be enrolled. Even if 100% of the patients enrolled are expected to complete the clinical trial, as in some pharmacokinetic and other Phase I trials, the number who must be screened and the number who will sign the informed consent are invariably larger. This reduction from the number of patients recruited to those entered mandates that a larger number of patients be recruited than the number needed for a clinical trial.

Using the Funnel Effect

The "funnel effect" describes the rate of attrition at each stage of the recruitment chain. The person responsible for identifying the number of patients to be recruited should start with the number of patients the investigators want to complete the trial and work backward through each step of the recruitment chain to estimate the total number to be used as the initial goal for recruitment. It is usually best to assume that a certain percent of patients will drop out after enrollment (i.e., *after* the recruitment period is complete). These will have to be included in the estimate of the total number to recruit.

Use of estimates commonly known as "fudge factors" (i.e., allowances for problems that may or may not be specifically known or anticipated in advance) is a means of providing a comfort level to those responsible for the trial. On the other hand, the calculated number of patients may be unrealistically high in terms of availability of patients, or of one's resources. In most clinical trials, the use of other probability factors on top of realistic probability estimates of drop-outs at each step of the recruitment chain is unnecessary.

Most investigators find it extremely difficult, if not impossible to accurately estimate, let alone calculate, the number of patients who will proceed from one stage of the recruitment chain to the next. These investigators prefer the pure guess approach. That approach uses a single guess and states that if X number of patients are needed to complete (or to enter) a clinical trial, then Y number of patients should be recruited. This approach may or may not turn out to be as accurate as determining individual probabilities for each stage of the recruitment chain.

Ignoring the Funnel Effect

A third approach to identifying the total number of patients to recruit is to basically ignore the funnel effect and merely state that patients will be recruited until there are a sufficient number to complete a clinical trial. In moderate and large size trials, particularly those in which recruitment is conducted over a long period (e.g., 6 months or longer) it is possible to use this approach. A drawback of ignoring the funnel effect is that the rest of the recruitment strategy developed may be inadequate to recruit a sufficient number of patients to complete the trial within the desired period. If that occurs, then a change in recruitment strategy may be necessary. Peer review groups are usually reluctant to fund open-ended recruitment strategies.

Step Two: Identify Source(s) of Potential Patients

This step may be extremely easy or difficult to conduct. In some cases, requirements in the protocol obviate the need to consider options. For example, a trial may be designed to evaluate patients within one or more particular wards, clinics, hospitals, or medical practices. Alternatively, two specific groups may be compared (e.g., patients in a Veterans Administration hospital and community hospital).

When choices exist, the possibilities should be listed and discussed among the pertinent members of the team designing and conducting the clinical trial. If the trial is sponsored it is essential that this step be conducted with the investigators who will conduct the trial. What may seem to be the "obvious" sources to the sponsors who have prepared the protocol may be totally unrealistic or inappropriate to the investigators. The investigators usually have a far better understanding of the true possibilities of recruiting patients from different sources.

A critical element in the decision is whether to use a single source or multiple sources of patients. A single patient source should be used whenever possible in Phase I and II trials and specialized Phase III trials (e.g., liver failure patients), because this allows for better characterization of the patients and better extrapolation of the results. Broad patient population trials conducted in Phases III and IV usually should involve multiple sources to enable better extrapolation of the results.

Three different private practices that are used as a source of patients by three separate physicians should be considered a single type of source if the patients are generally comparable. If the patients have different social, economic, and disease characteristics, however, then each practice may be considered a separate type of source. A single physician with separate practices in a poor clinic, a wealthy suburb, and a community hospital should be considered to have three different sources unless the patients are shown to be similar. If not, then that investigator may be requested by the sponsor to use only one or two of the sources, to be consistent with the other sites in the trial. It makes little difference how the term *source* is specifically defined, except insofar as whether differences between the sources used to recruit patient are considered important.

Two major reasons for using multiple sources in a recruitment strategy are (1) to obtain patients more rapidly and easily, and (2) to enhance the ability to extrapolate the results of the clinical trial to a broader variety of patients, to ensure that other, similar patients from the sources will respond similarly to those who were enrolled in the trial.

Step Three: Determine Method(s) for Approaching Each Source

After deciding on what types of medical recruitment sources will be used, it is then necessary to identify which specific physician groups, hospitals, clinics, or other referral centers will be requested to participate, if any. The number of clinical centers of each source to be used should also be planned. If nonmedical recruitment sources will be used, the same considerations apply.

At that point it is relevant to determine whether contact with referral centers or groups will be made by telephone, letter, visit, or another approach. Individuals assigned the responsibility for conducting each step of the referral process, including follow-through, should have demonstrated relevant skills. To increase the chances of successful recruiting it is sometimes desirable to identify individuals who have a special relationship to people at the referral source and can make initial or follow-up contact with those sites. List all relevant details on paper (or in a computer), including a system for follow-up to ensure each contact has been made and that appropriate actions are being taken. Individuals who are unsuccessful in this activity should be replaced.

Step Four: Determine Methods for Processing Patients

The procedures to move prospective enrollees through the stages of recruitment may be extremely simple or complex. For a large or a complicated small clinical trial, it is usually necessary to prepare special forms for assisting staff personnel with:

1. Initial screening on the telephone,
2. More detailed screening at the clinical trial site,
3. Explaining the nature and specific aspects of informed consent.

A form for initial screening on the telephone should include columns for (1) name (or initials), (2) date of contact, (3) critical demographic information, (4) telephone number, (5) answers to critical inclusion criteria, and (6) interest in the trial. (This presupposes that data from multiple patients can be put on a single page; in many cases each patient's responses and data will have to be put on separate pages.) Forms should be easy to complete while conducting the interview on the telephone. A test run should be made with real or staged patients via telephone calls before this form is finalized. A sheet of instructions for telephone interviewers should be prepared that addresses such issues as (1) tone of voice to use, (2) how to describe the trial, (3) exactly what patients would be asked to do, (4) benefits and risks for patients, (5) how to assess whether the patient meets inclusion criteria, (6) what is the next step, and (7) how to obtain more information from patients.

The same considerations apply to forms for more detailed screening at the clinical trial site. The contents of the form depend primarily on the protocol. Forms for describing the informed consent are primarily instruction forms for the staff to use.

A pamphlet describing the clinical trial is a useful mechanism to boost enrollment in large trials. In addition to printing or photocopying forms, it is important to ensure the availability of a sufficient number of appropriate staff to interview patients and answer their questions. Having staff available to answer questions during a trial ensures that fewer patients will drop out because they could not reach someone at the clinical trial site when they tried to do so. This practice has major implications for recruitment because it may decrease the need for replacement patients. Another mechanism to retain compliant patients in a clinical trial is to prepare a manual of instructions for patients. Details of information that could be included in such a manual have been described (Spilker, 1991).

Identify each of the impediments to a successful recruitment plan, then identify a means of addressing each point raised. It is important to assess and discuss among the group responsible for recruitment the motivation of each group of people involved. Determine how to motivate physicians to refer patients and also consider whether to allow patients to self-refer themselves for a trial. Using a devil's advocate approach to challenge the proposed view is a valuable means of checking a strategy for major flaws.

Ensuring the smooth progression of patients through the recruitment chain requires discussions with colleagues, staff, sponsors, and other groups. These discussions should include consideration of unusual circumstances and situations that may arise, in addition to the more common possibilities. Rare events are not usually pertinent to consider, except if and when they occur.

Step Five: Plan the Informed Consent Process

A recruitment strategy includes an informed consent strategy (i.e., a predetermined plan of how to approach patients to seek an informed consent). Careful consideration should be given to all staff using a consistent style when explaining the scope and purpose of a trial to patients. Preparation of a staff training manual often improves consistency that could enhance enrollment rates. A large body of medical literature exists on this topic and may be searched if problems develop.

For large clinical trials involving many sites, or for treatment-IND trials, consider using a single national Ethics Committee/IRB. This procedure saves time. Moreover, some Ethics Committees/IRBs delay a trial's initiation by requesting changes in the protocol that may be inappropriate or cannot be made without compromising the integrity of the trial. It may be valuable to submit to each committee a synopsis of current scientific thinking underlying the trial.

Because Ethics Committees/IRBs often meet at infrequent or irregular intervals, it is important to check their schedule ahead of time and submit the protocol in a timely manner. Not to do so risks significant delays.

Step Six: Itemize Alternative Methods and Approaches for Successful Recruitment

The spectrum for this step ranges from doing almost nothing (because of little perceived need), to creating elaborate backup recruitment systems. A possible backup system would be to identify those mechanisms that will be used to enhance recruitment if targeted rates are not achieved. A stepwise plan should be developed (Figs. 7.6 and 7.7) describing how to increase the number or intensity of recruiting efforts at specified points during the trial. Resources available for recruitment will greatly influence the choice of methods used.

Step Seven: Document the Recruitment Strategy and Periodically Review It—Both Prior to and During the Clinical Trial

Numerous advantages exist for writing the strategy and periodically reviewing it, in addition to discussing it prior to the clinical trial. These advantages include those that accrue from focusing appropriate attention on various recruitment issues. Re-

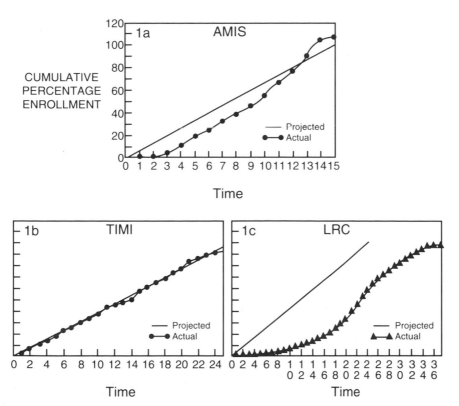

FIG. 7.11. Recruitment performances of AMIS, TIMI, and LRC–CPPT, respectively. These are plotted on graphs with the same dimensions and serve to illustrate the enrollment pattern as a percent of projected cumulative sample size versus time. The three studies required 15 months, 25 weeks, and 37 months, respectively, to recruit their final cohorts. Also depicted by the straight line in each figure is the projected constant rate accrual for each study using the planned recruitment time for each of the clinical trials. Reprinted from Probstfield et al. (1987) with permission.

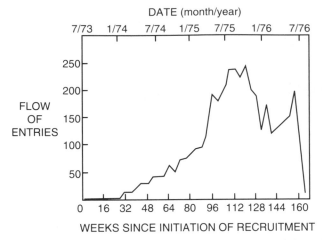

FIG. 7.12. Flow of patient entries per 4-week interval. Reprinted from Marshall (1982) with permission.

viewing the strategy provides opportunities to discuss various points and to fine-tune or modify the original plans and intentions. Recording decisions and outcomes of discussions at recruitment group meetings may be used to confirm points raised during future discussions. Finally, a written document provides a useful basis for publishing recruitment practices and experiences, if the trial results warrant.

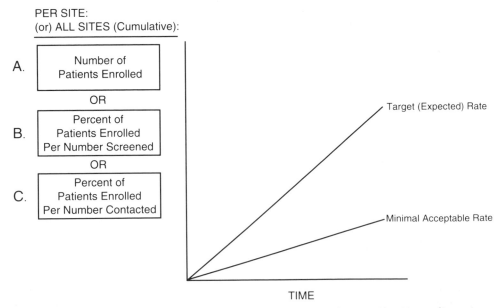

FIG. 7.13. Three possible ordinates that could be used to show patient recruitment over time for either individual or all sites. Two curves show the minimal acceptable rate (i.e., a quota) and the target (i.e., expected) rate.

A. Each Center Drawn Separately (cumulative data illustrated)

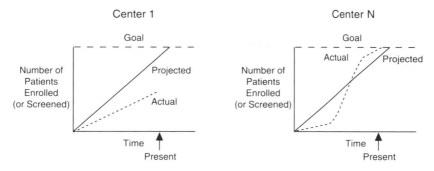

B. Each Center Drawn Separately (monthly data illustrated)

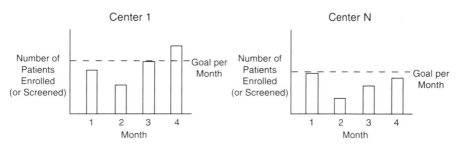

C. All Center's Data Combined (cumulative data illustrated)
D. All Center's Data Combined (monthly data illustrated)

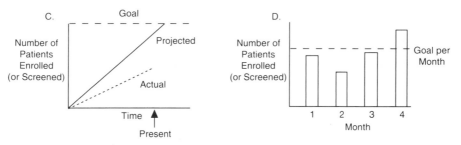

FIG. 7.14. Different means of showing patient recruitment over time for either individual centers (i.e., A, B) or combining data from all centers (i.e., C, D). Time periods may show discrete segments (e.g., months, quarters) using histograms or continuous plots (i.e., A, C). Goals may be shown.

Step Eight: Determine How the Strategy Will Be Critiqued Prior to the Clinical Trial

Once a strategy has been created and written down it must be further critiqued and assessed. All recruitment strategies must be feasible and realistic. There are numerous other criteria that may be used to assess the likelihood that the chosen strategy is the most appropriate one for the clinical trial. One approach is to assemble a group of internal trial staff plus external ''experts'' or consultants to debate the strategy. Various ''what-if'' scenarios may be considered at that meeting.

Step Nine: Determine How the Strategy Will Be Reviewed During the Clinical Trial

Once the strategy is in place and the trial is underway, there should be a formalized system for reviewing and evaluating the degree of success of the strategy. This may involve use of goals and quotas as described in Chapter 9, or merely assessing the stage of patient recruitment and determining whether or not it is acceptable.

Whether the review stage will involve assessment of recruitment data submitted by each site should be determined prior to the initiation of the trial. That would enable the appropriate forms to be designed and discussed with each site. Implementation of additional paperwork during a trial is rarely received in a positive way.

Figure 7.10 illustrates the most common way to demonstrate recruitment progress and status (i.e., to plot the cumulative number of patients enrolled on the ordinate versus time on the abscissa). The planned (projected) rate is shown (i.e., target) as well as the actual data. Different hypothetical recruitment patterns are shown in Fig. 7.10 plus simple interpretations that describe them. Figures 7.11 and 7.12 show similar graphs for four actual trials, although the ordinate plots cumulative percentage enrollment in Fig. 7.11 and flow of entries per period in Fig. 7.12. Other examples are shown in Fig. 7.13 that also illustrates a second plot of quotas (i.e., minimal acceptable rate). Varieties of ways to illustrate patient recruitment over time per site or cumulatively, particularly through the use of histograms to show recruitment per period, are shown in Fig. 7.14. Interpretations of various histograms are given in Fig. 7.15.

1. Early Enthusiasm But Poor Finish

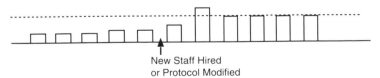

2. Investigator Who Needs Prodding

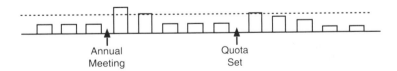

3. Investigator With a Specific Site or Protocol Problem

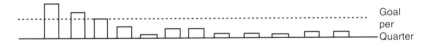

FIG. 7.15. Three patterns of quarterly recruitment rates and interpretation of the results.

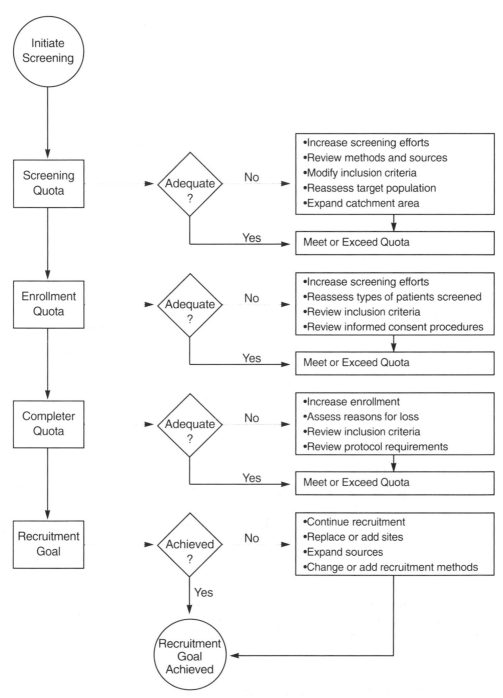

FIG. 7.16. Illustrating how the different types of recruitment quotas are related to each other and the recruitment goal of the trial. Methods to improve problem situations are also shown.

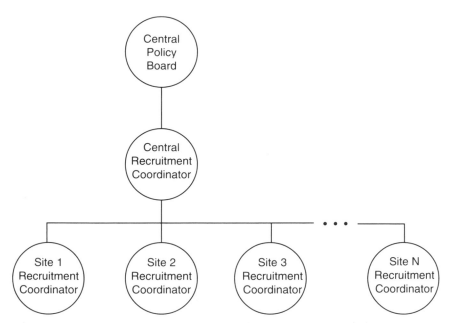

FIG. 7.17. An organizational structure for a trial with a recruitment coordinator at each site. An alternative for multinational trials is to appoint a national recruitment coordinator for each country involved in the trial.

The group of individuals who review data presented in one or more of these ways (Figs. 7.10 to 7.15) should address the questions shown in Fig. 7.16. This flow diagram should guide their thinking about how to deal with various issues.

Step Ten: Determine How the Process Will Be Administered

After a strategy is proposed, refined, and approved, its administration still must be determined. While the strategy's implementation and follow-through may correctly be viewed as part of the strategy itself (e.g., Will there be full-time recruitment coordinators?), it is convenient for the purposes of this chapter to consider it as a separate topic.

Figure 7.17 illustrates probably the most formal and comprehensive recruitment system for a multicenter trial. The recruitment coordinator could have other positions as well as being in charge of patient recruitment.

RECRUITMENT STRATEGIES OF SELECTED CLINICAL TRIALS

A few specific recruitment strategies are presented as examples. It is not considered worthwhile to present strategies used by a large number of specific trials. The interested reader can find discussions of many more recruitment strategies by referring to the references listed in Table 1.5.

A Pediatric Study

The Bogalusa Heart Study (Croft et al., 1984) was a 10-year study of cardiovascular risk factor examinations in children. This study's recruitment strategy involved (1) maintaining high visibility in the community, (2) employing a local field staff, (3) using community volunteers, and (4) emphasizing that the study belongs to the community. Each of these and other aspects of their strategy are described in detail in their publication.

A VA Multicenter Study

The VA Epilepsy Cooperative Study (Mattson et al., 1985) used a strategy of engaging all the neurology residents at each site as referral sources for newly di-

TABLE 7.1. *Mass media recruitment strategies*

Source	Example
A. Television	
1. News coverage	On-site coverage by local correspondent and film crew
2. Talk-show interview	Trial director appears on follow-up segment to special coronary heart disease related broadcast
3. Taped public service announcement	"Mr. Cholesterol" designed to educate and solicit self-referrals
B. Radio	
1. News coverage	Press release coverage of CPPT[a]
2. On-the-air interviews	Physician/patient interviews, accepting questions from callers
3. Recruitment messages	Periodic announcements by broadcast hosts during their regularly scheduled shows
4. Taped public service announcement	Repeat broadcasts during time-limited recruitment campaign
C. Newspapers	
1. Feature articles	Description of the CPPT and local LRC[a] follow-up
2. Brief news articles	Description of on-site occupational screening by LRC
3. Photo layout display	Coverage of LRC staff at work
4. Announcements/advertisements	Listing of screening locations or coupon insert for free cholesterol checks
D. Limited subscriber publications	
1. Magazines	Advertisements placed in local circulation magazines
2. Special audience newsletters and bulletins	Information appearing in publications for members of educational, professional, corporate, and religious organizations
3. Special event printed programs	Advertisements appearing in printed programs for recreational and cultural events
E. Other media	
1. Posters/billboards	Strategically placed in heavy traffic areas
2. Brochures	Distributed to selected groups
3. Bus cards	Printed message on monthly passes
4. Telephone messages	Announcement as preface to telephone weather report

Reprinted from Levenkron and Farquhar (1982) with permission.
[a] CPPT, Coronary Primary Prevention Trial; LRC, Lipid Research Clinics.

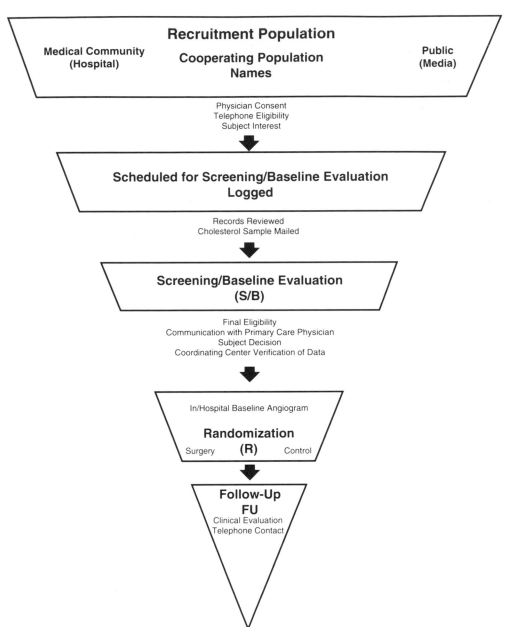

FIG. 7.18. A model clinic flow diagram. Reprinted from Buchwald et al. (1987) with permission.

agnosed patients. Strategies included (1) frequent emphasis on the importance of the trial hypotheses in talking to referral physicians, (2) high visibility of the coordinator and investigator in the medical center, and (3) continuous education of residents and other referring physicians and staff about inclusion criteria.

An Epidemiological Study

An epidemiological study conducted in Leningrad (Katrusenko and Sestov, 1981) used the following system.

1. Up to three written invitations mailed to each person identified within a given sample, born in a certain period.
2. Each person was contacted by telephone if no response was obtained.
3. Each person who could not be contacted was visited.

The authors presented the time required (in days) to achieve various levels of patient response for the best, average, and worst subpopulations contacted.

A Surgical Study

A surgical follow-up study of patients with congenital heart defects was conducted by O'Fallon et al. (1987). The investigators sent a packet to each patient who was

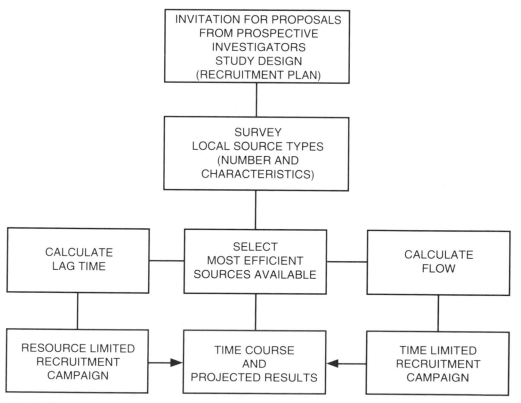

FIG. 7.19. Sequence of steps in local level planning of a recruitment strategy. Reprinted from Agras et al. (1982) with permission.

in the original trial using the following instructions:

1. Mail a packet to each patient. The packet includes:
   a. A letter informing the patient that he or she participated in NHS-1 and informing him or her of the present study.
   b. A questionnaire on status of health, history of medical events, and general life-style.
   c. A medical records release form.
   d. A return card on which the patient or parents can indicate agreement or refusal to participate or can request more information.
   e. A stamped, addressed envelope for the return of reply to the clinical center.
2. In 2 weeks, unless card indicating refusal to participate is received, send a thank-you/reminder note to the same address.
3. In 2 weeks if no response, call and/or mail another packet as described in item 1.
4. In 3 weeks if no response and no telephone contact, send packet as described in item 1 by certified mail (OFallon et al., 1987).

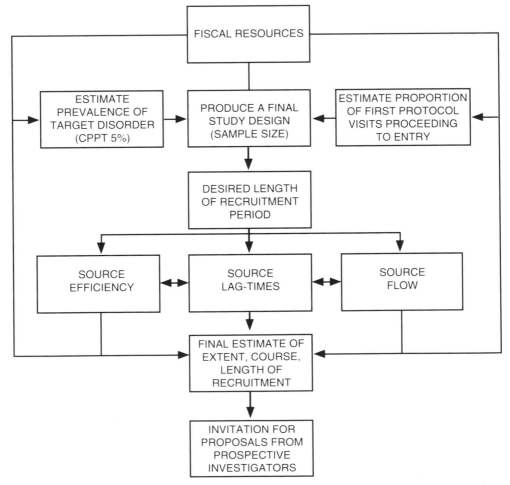

FIG. 7.20. Sequence of key steps in national level planning of a recruitment campaign. Reprinted from Agras et al. (1982) with permission.

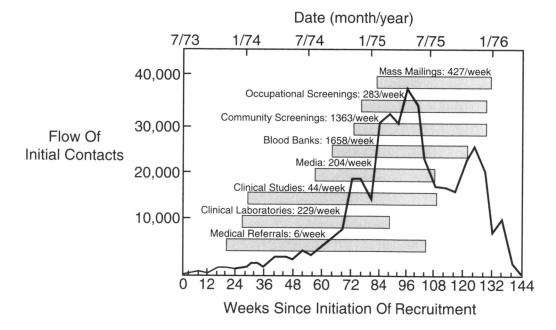

FIG. 7.21. Flow (number per 4-week interval) of initial contacts, over time, and period of major yield for each major recruitment source category. The data presented here included those who did not meet the age and sex eligibility criteria and reflect the temporal data that were available for 96% of the sample. The period of major yield depicted for each source excludes the time to acquire the first and last 10% of the total from the source, thereby minimizing both the initiation and termination phases. Temporal data were available for at least 90% of those from each source except clinical studies (88%), media (64%), and medical referrals (55%). Reprinted from The Lipid Research Clinics Program (1983) with permission.

TABLE 7.2. *Subject participation in pilot study by method of invitation*

| | Invitation method[a] | | | |
	Direct invitation no. and (%)	Eligibility screening by mail no. and (%)	Self-determined eligibility no. and (%)	Total no. and (%)
Category				
Invited	199	196	195	590
Non-response	11 (6)	28 (14)	9 (5)	48 (8)
Ineligibles based on smoking history[b]	80 (40)	66 (34)	52 (27)	198 (34)
Other ineligibles	7 (4)	6 (3)	8 (4)	21 (4)
Refusals	26 (13)	31 (16)	31 (16)	88 (15)
Randomized	75 (38)	65 (33)	95 (49)	235 (40)

Reprinted from Albanes et al. (1986) with permission.
[a] Column percentages exceeding 100% are due to rounding.
[b] Includes 47 smokers of self-rolled cigarettes (23, 13, and 11, respectively).

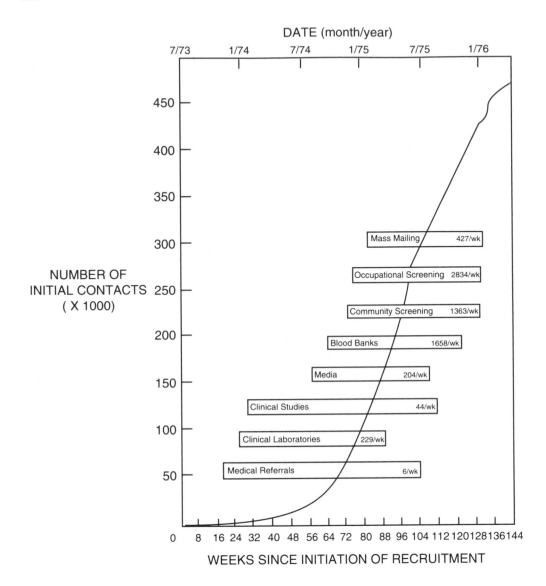

FIG. 7.22. Cumulative initial contacts over time and period of prime yield for each source category. The data include those who did not meet the age and sex eligibility criteria and reflect temporal data available for 96% of the sample. The period of prime yield depicted for each source excludes the time to acquire the first and last 10% of the total from the source, minimizing both the initiation and termination phases. Temporal data were available for at least 90% of those from each source except clinical studies (88%), media (64%), and medical referrals (55%). Reprinted from Marshall (1982) with permission.

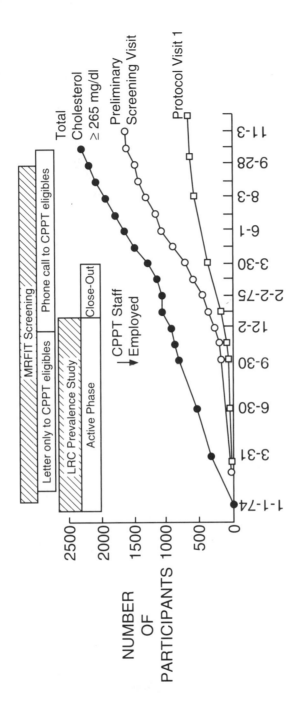

FIG. 7.23. Cumulative number of eligible plasma cholesterol levels, preliminary screening visits, and first protocol visits of MRFIT referrals to the Minneapolis LRC over time. This center conducted a preliminary screening visit for referrals before the first protocol visit. Reprinted from Hunninghake et al. (1982) with permission.

Use of Mass Media

The Coronary Primary Prevention Trial (CPPT) developed a sophisticated mass media strategy to use in their trial. This strategy is illustrated in Table 7.1.

Recruitment Strategies in Other Trials

Figures 7.18 to 7.23 illustrate recruitment strategies used in a number of additional trials. The trials are identified in figure legends. Note that although these examples represent large multicenter trials, the same strategies can be used in small single-site trials. The essential concepts are extrapolatable to almost all trials because multicenter trials depend on the same recruitment methods as those used in single-site trials (Table 7.2).

ISSUES IN DEVELOPING AND IMPLEMENTING A RECRUITMENT STRATEGY

Implementing a Recruitment Strategy

Depending on the magnitude of the clinical trial, it can be helpful to implement the recruitment strategy in a number of separate stages. The individual stages may be initiated such that Stage 2 (see Chapter 1) is scheduled to begin at a certain calendar date after the trial is initiated. Alternatively, Stage 2 may be scheduled to begin after a certain number of patients or a certain percent of the total have been enrolled (Table 7.3).

A better approach is to develop contingency plans to initiate Stage 2 if recruitment rates fall below the expected rates for a defined period of time (e.g., 3 months) or by a defined amount (e.g., 30% below projection after a minimum of X months from the initiation date), or by a combination (e.g., 30% below projection for any three consecutive months).

Most clinical trials do not require complex recruitment strategies to enroll a sufficient number of patients. In fact, most trials do not even involve a strategy for alerting the hospital staff, let alone those in the community, region, or nation about the trial. The golden rule about creating interest about a clinical trial is to choose one's method(s) carefully and then to adjust the intensity of efforts accordingly at the level of the specific hospital(s), community(ies), region(s), nation, or internationally.

A unified approach is required among those involved with a trial when approaching hospital staff. To build goodwill about an important trial in which staff involvement is important, it is usually appropriate to make announcements at major meetings to

TABLE 7.3. *Triggers that cause strategies to move to the next stage*

1. Specific number of weeks, months, or years
2. Specific number or percent of patients enrolled (per site or per trial)
3. Specific number or percent of patients not enrolled (per site or per trial)
4. Specific number or percent of patients not enrolled over a specific time period (per site or per trial)

the faculty and staff, to present information in newsletters, and to mail letters to each member of the hospital staff. Multiple exposures of the faculty to the existence of the trial is usually necessary to have it register in a manner that it is not easily forgotten. Nursing, laboratory, and other pertinent staff groups as well as interns and residents should also be made aware of the clinical trial. Patient recruitment may be solicited at the same time. The efforts expended presenting information should be commensurate with the importance of the trial and availability of resources.

Appointing a Recruitment Coordinator

It is desirable for most large clinical trials to have a recruitment coordinator who advises trial sites of their progress toward the goal(s), and recommends approaches they could take to enhance enrollment when recruitment problems develop. Expecting busy investigators and staff to solve often complex recruiting problems is not only unrealistic, but may be counterproductive as well. For example, steps taken by inexperienced investigators to improve patient recruitment could lead to (1) enrolling inappropriate types of patients, (2) spending time nonproductively attempting to boost enrollment, or (3) incorrectly diagnosing the recruitment problem. A recruiting coordinator was hired in the Coronary Prevention Trial and the specific roles of this individual were described by Prout (1981) as: (1) informing the public about the trial, (2) establishing a screening program, (3) equipping screening laboratories, and (4) developing a method for discussing informed consent with patients.

Strategy to Develop Medical Interest About a Clinical Trial Within a Community or Region

Appropriate staff should initiate contacts with local hospitals where referrals might be expected. Visit the chiefs of medical services and request permission to present synopses of the trial at staff conferences. Attend meetings of local medical societies after permission has been received to informally publicize the trial, present formal talks about the trial, or possibly display an exhibit. Mail information to, or telephone, those physicians who might be expected to refer patients to the trial. Write articles about the trial for local medical newsletters and regional medical journals.

Should a Strict Recruitment Period Be Established and Stated in a Protocol?

Deadlines usually tend to focus people's minds and thoughts. Being generous in a protocol and allowing investigators to "take all the time they need to enroll patients" may be sufficient to doom a clinical trial to failure. The opposite approach of placing undue pressure and stress on investigators to meet unrealistic recruitment goals is also unproductive. Finding the correct balance between these extremes is the challenge faced by everyone who writes protocols and plans trials, even if the author of a protocol is also the principal investigator who must apply the pressure on himself or herself. It is believed that a reasonable date should be established as part of the recruitment strategy (see Chapter 9, Goals and Quotas).

Calculating Patient Drop-out and Discontinuation Rates

Patients who do not complete the trial, either drop out on their own or are discontinued by the investigator. If either some or all patient drop-outs or discontinuers must be replaced in a trial, then additional patients must be recruited to achieve this state. Collins et al. (1984) list the drop-out rates for ten different multicenter trials managed by the same coordinating center. These rates vary from 1 to 50%. The authors mention four major factors that influenced these rates.

1. The outcome measure being used (e.g., mortality rates are easier to obtain than measures requiring patients to return to hospital).
2. The length of follow-up. Longer duration follow-up trials tend to have lower patient retention.
3. The type of study intervention (e.g., the more complicated, painful, or intrusive the intervention, the more likely it is that patients will drop out).
4. The trial population itself (e.g., the seriousness of the consequences of not receiving treatment and the mortality of the trial population).

Drop-out and discontinuation rates that are greater than anticipated threaten the successful completion of any clinical trial, particularly if a sufficient number of suitable replacement patients cannot be located and enrolled. The anticipated drop-out and discontinuation rates must be incorporated in sample size projections to determine the number of patients to be recruited. The obvious exception is if drop-outs and/or discontinuers are not to be replaced, according to the protocol.

Creating a Perfect Recruitment Strategy

One of the main reasons why a perfect recruitment strategy for a trial cannot be expected to be perfectly executed is that many unanticipated problems can arise that have a major negative impact on recruitment. Assume that an extremely well-considered recruitment strategy is developed. Assume further that a well-developed contingency plan is created. What could go wrong? The answer is "many things," and a few examples are listed.

1. The protocol design and requirements must be conducive with the patients' desire to join the trial. What if:

The chance of receiving placebo was considered unacceptably high to patients.
The length of the trial is considered excessive.
The cost of the trial to the patient is high and the costs are not reimbursed.
The number of uncomfortable measurements is considered high.
Too many baseline visits are required before the investigational therapy is initiated.

2. The personal relationships must be acceptable. What if:

Most patients do not care for the physician.
Patients see a different physician in the trial each week.
Patients have to wait an excessively long time in the waiting room.

3. The facilities must be acceptable. What if:

The building or parking lot is unsafe.
The facilities and waiting areas are unpleasant.

A mechanism must be established to obtain data on prospective patients. This may require 24-hour coverage 7 days a week . Beepers or answering services may be used to contact clinical trial staff whenever a patient is available for screening or entry.

Influence of Trial Size on Recruitment

Size may or may not influence the recruitment strategy developed. If two investigators each enroll ten patients in a two-site clinical trial, their recruitment activities will probably not differ greatly if they are part of a 50-site trial where each site enrolls ten patients. Of course, if the same two investigators are asked to enroll 50 patients each and not the ten they planned, it is certain that their original recruitment strategy will be reviewed and possibly altered. This example illustrates that the size of a trial *per se* does not necessarily influence recruitment activities. Numerous variations of this example could be described where, for example, the investigators' recruitment activities change drastically. Whether a trial is small, medium, or large in terms of patient recruitment has less to do with the success of recruitment than the nature of the protocol, the availability of patients, and the strategy developed to recruit them.

Assistance from Sponsors to Aid Patient Recruitment

There are few limitations on government, industrial (e.g., pharmaceutical companies), or other sponsors of clinical trials in assisting with patient recruitment. Apart from general discussions with investigators concerning the sources and methods to be used they may become directly involved in activities such as (1) designing and printing brochures about the trial, (2) preparation of posters, (3) preparation of press releases, (4) preparation of sample letters for investigators to send to colleagues and other referral sources, (5) contacting various potential sources to identify patient pools, or (6) most other activities discussed in this book.

It is essential that recruitment activities by sponsors are designed to assist the investigator and not to take over or control this function. This means that whatever is done is agreed to by the investigator(s). Because of the importance of recruitment and the difficulties often involved, it is unlikely that many investigators would object to most offers of assistance.

Pretrial Initiation Activities to Expedite Patient Recruitment

Most clinical trials do not begin with a "bang," charging ahead on a given date. Instead, they are gradually put into gear and progress to full-scale activity over time. As a result, there is usually a period of time for implementing recruitment that could even last for one or more years before the official start date of the trial (i.e., on or after the final approval by the Ethic Committee/IRB). During this time the investigator(s) may assess the potential of various sources, methods, and strategies of recruiting the patients needed to conduct their trial.

The activities to assess recruitment potential could be as simple as interviewing prospective patients to determine their interest in enrolling in a trial with specified

characteristics. Cautious or negative replies should be followed up to determine their causes and to identify what changes in the protocol would probably cause a large number of patients to change their mind. At the other extreme, a pilot clinical trial could be conducted solely to assess the ability of the proposed recruitment strategy to enroll enough patients, and to work out details of the strategy to be used in the full trial. A number of very large trials have used this approach (Croke, 1979) while also assessing the conduct of the trial and details of the protocol.

Another means of saving time for patient recruitment is to learn when the Ethics Committee/IRB meets and when protocols must be received to be considered at their next meeting. Because some groups meet relatively infrequently, it is important to have the protocol completed and most aspects of recruitment considered before the deadline. This consideration also concerns protocol modifications (e.g., changing inclusion criteria to expedite recruitment). The same considerations apply for any other group (e.g., clinical unit committee) that also has to review and approve a protocol and any changes.

Monitoring Recruitment in a Multicenter Trial

If a separate recruitment coordinator exists at each site and frequent status reports are sent to a central coordinating group, it may be unnecessary for that group to conduct monitoring visits to evaluate recruitment status on site. On the other hand, this desirable situation is uncommon and on-site inspections should be conducted to evaluate recruitment in almost all large multicenter trials. These recruitment assessment visits should be combined (if possible) with monitoring visits that evaluate data collection, data accuracy, and the clinical trial's conduct. Monitoring visits of any type should evaluate actual or potential problems and seek methods of correcting or preventing them.

Certification of Each Site's Recruitment Strategy by a Central Organizing Group

In a large multicenter trial it is relevant to review each site's recruitment plan and their expected ability to implement their plan prior to approving it. If the plan is a standard one developed by the clinical trial's organizers, it is still essential to ensure that (1) the plan is reasonable to apply at each particular site, (2) the subtleties of the plan are understood thoroughly at each site, (3) those who will implement the plan at each site are thoroughly trained, and (4) each site has the resources to implement the plan successfully.

If each site in a multicenter trial develops its own recruitment plan, the same four points listed above still apply. In addition, it must be determined that there is no potential or actual conflict among the methods to be used and that the patients recruited are not expected to differ systematically in any characteristics that are deemed important or that would affect the pooling of data and the extrapolatability of results.

Strategic Tips to Encourage Patient Recruitment

Identify the aspects of the protocol and treatment that may be of most interest to patients. These could include comments to the effect that:

1. This new medicine was recently discussed in a magazine or newspaper. Copies of appropriate articles may be given to patients.
2. For your transportation and other expenses we will reimburse you ($10 or $25) for each clinic visit.
3. We will offer free laboratory tests to follow your disease throughout the duration of the trial.

Details can be listed in a brochure or handout so that patients may literally bring the message home.

Establishing a Team to Handle Patient Recruitment for Multiple Clinical Trials

Any institution that conducts or sponsors many clinical trials may desire to hire one or more people to serve as full-time recruitment coordinators. The types of groups that should consider this approach are independent or academic groups that conduct multiple trials themselves (e.g., a pharmaceutical company that has its own clinic, an academic institution or department that maintains a clinic for conducting in-house trials).

One group that follows this practice is the Upjohn Company. Their clinics have three licensed practical nurses who recruit for all Upjohn trials conducted at their clinics. Half of the trials are Phase I trials and the balance are in Phases II and III. The company maintains a registry of over 10,000 volunteers in their pool of normal and diseased patients who live within a 50-mile radius (DeVries, *personal communication*). Their company's activities are described in brochures handed out to prospective enrollees (Fig. 4.13).

Providing Feedback to Referring Physicians

When patient recruitment has utilized referrals from other physicians, there are a number of additional issues that must be considered. Investigators should provide relevant clinical trial data and information about patients to the physicians who referred them to the trial. This can be done on one or more occasions, depending on the length and nature of the trial, and usually takes the form of letters or, possibly, telephone calls. This practice should be followed as a matter of courtesy as well as part of the ethical responsibility of temporarily caring for another physician's patient. Moreover, it will act as a stimulus for the physician to remember the trial and possibly refer additional patients. If the trial has a clinically significant effect on the disease for which the patient was being treated by the referring physician, then a detailed account of all clinically relevant events and data should be communicated to the original physician.

Thus, the recruitment strategy should be an integral part of the protocol. Every major aspect of recruitment that can be anticipated should be considered and planned prior to initiating the trial. The details will provide a stimulus for use of sources and methods throughout the trial. Nonetheless, despite the best of plans, nearly all trials will face problems that require revision, addition, or development of a new strategy as described in Chapter 8 on enhancing recruitment.

8

Strategies to Enhance (or Reduce) Patient Recruitment

One of the major reasons for insufficient patient recruitment in clinical trials is that investigators often rely on their personal assumptions about physician referrals and patient interest in a trial. Investigators who plan clinical trials often accept too many of the popular myths about recruitment as true and do not conduct pilot trials or interview a sufficient number of patients to assess how successful their recruiting efforts will be. In addition, many investigators depend on the goodwill of various groups to refer patients and have not accurately assessed the incentives for physicians or others to refer patients to their trial. This type of naivete can be observed in the medical literature that discusses patient recruitment and recruitment strategies. Moreover, the problems of recruitment that are published undoubtedly reflect the barest tip of the large iceberg of clinical trials that were never completed because of judgment errors in planning for patient recruitment.

This chapter explores how to improve recruitment after it is found to be insufficient—and thereby rescue a clinical trial. This is one of the most important aspects of patient recruitment. The initial approach to the problem is to identify the reason(s) for low recruitment and then to analyze the reasons and derive a remedy for the situation. The final step is to use the appropriate measures to increase the rate of enrollment.

Recruitment problems may occur at any point throughout a clinical trial. When they occur at the start of a trial, it may be because the appropriate population of patients was not found, was not approached correctly, or because of problems in the protocol. When recruitment problems are not evident during the early part of a trial but develop later in the trial, it is often an indication that the available pool of patients in the sources used has been nearly exhausted. The necessary steps to counter this problem are dependent on the potential to expand groups of patients from the sources used, or to approach new sources. Major recruitment problems that occur later in the trial also may indicate that the investigator is losing interest in the trial. Trial organizers should evaluate whether the same pattern or a totally different one occurs at each site in a multicenter trial.

IDENTIFYING REASONS FOR INSUFFICIENT PATIENT RECRUITMENT

There are several approaches to identifying the reasons for insufficient patient recruitment. The most common approach is for the investigator, or some other individual or group assessing another's trial, to pose a variety of direct questions. These questions are designed to identify the specific reason(s) for low patient recruitment. When asking these questions it is helpful to view recruitment in several discreet stages and to assess possible problems in each. Graphs of patients enrolled (or screened) over time are also a helpful tool (Figs. 8.1 and 8.2), as is the determination of the ratio of patients screened to patients entered (Fig. 8.3) for each site.

Seven major categories of recruitment problems are further subdivided into specific questions to pose when evaluating patient recruitment.

Evidence of a Problem

What is the evidence that patient recruitment is low at a specific time point in the recruitment period?

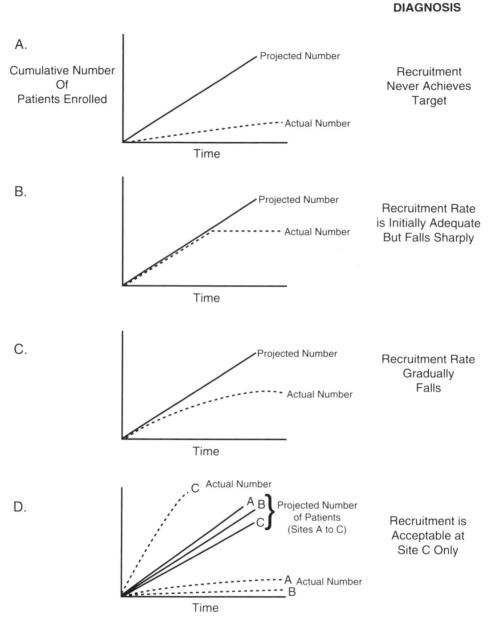

FIG. 8.1. Diagnosing common recruitment problems from the graph of cumulative number of patients enrolled over time.

Was patient recruitment ever satisfactory in the trial?
If so, for how long a period?
What is the specific magnitude of the problem in numbers and in percents?
How long has the problem existed?
Is it getting worse or is it generally stable?

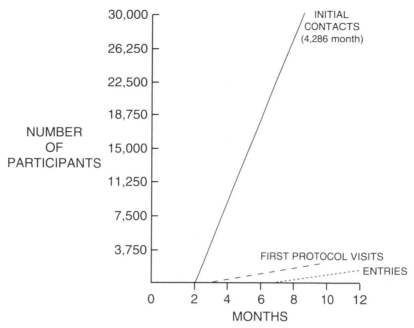

FIG. 8.2. Yield over time of initial contacts, first protocol visits, and entries. Reprinted from Agras et al. (1982) with permission.

Site-Specific Problems

How many sites (number and percent) in a multicenter trial have the problem?
Can one generalize about the types of sites that have the problem (e.g., are only community hospitals, hospital clinics, or veterans' hospitals affected)?
Are only certain types of investigators affected (e.g., less experienced investigators, investigators who have delegated part or all of the recruitment procedure)?

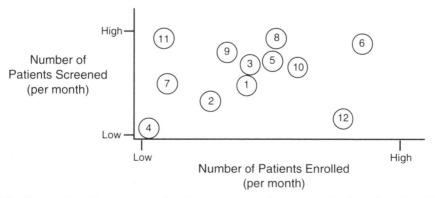

FIG. 8.3. Comparing the number of patients screened versus patients entered at 12 sites of a multicenter trial. Each circled number refers to a different site. Low enrollment despite high screening (site 11) suggests problems with their screening program. The high yield of recruited patients with few screenings (site 12) possibly suggests a unique source of patients, use of persuasive techniques, or a failure to record all patients screened.

Is the problem related to the size of the catchment area (e.g., large hospital in a small community, small hospital in a large city)?

Are the answers to questions listed below similar or different among sites?

Sources of Patients

Are all of the referral sources participating that agreed to do so?

Are there sufficient numbers of referral groups involved?

Are all of the sources of patients planned for in the recruitment strategy being used? If not, why?

Are problems primarily with one type of source? If so, which?

Are problems primarily with one specific source? If so, which one?

Are all physicians who could recruit patients aware of the trial?

Are all the physicians enlisted to recruit patients willing to do so?

Do these physicians have suitable patients to refer?

Why are physicians not referring patients in adequate numbers?

(Similar questions may be asked about the methods being used.)

Screening of Patients

Are the staff who screen the patients friendly and courteous?

Are there a sufficient number of staff?

What percent of patients are passing the initial screen?

What number and percent of patients are finding the tests difficult or too time consuming?

What number and percent of patients are returning for their second screen?

What complaints about the screen are most common? (e.g., too time-consuming, too long waiting, too arduous)?

Logistical and Administrative Problems

Is the screening site located in an area that is difficult to reach (e.g., no bus service)?

Is parking at the site inadequate? Parking fees are often expensive for patients attending screening visits.

Is the building where the clinical trial takes place confusing to find (e.g., a lack of signs to direct patients to the screening area)?

Do guards at the building entry appear to block access (e.g., ask for clinic appointment cards or other identification)?

Are telephone calls not answered because of lack of staff or are the telephone lines ''always'' busy because of an inadequate number of incoming lines?

Is there too much paperwork for either staff or patients to complete?

Is the paperwork too complex to understand and complete easily?

Is another trial siphoning patients away from the one of interest?

Personal, Nontrial-Related Problems of Patients

Numerous patients who might otherwise be willing to enter clinical trials may have personal nontrial-related problems. How many of each type of reason is given? The following are some types of reasons:

I am too busy
I live too far away
I can't afford the costs
I need to have babysitting
There are too many tests

Informed Consent Problems

Numerous informed consent issues are described in Chapter 5.

After asking the above questions, one will, it is hoped, know why enrollment is slow and whether the most important causes of poor recruitment are general, site-specific, or both. Numerous reasons for low patient enrollment are listed in Table 8.1 and other questions to pose and in Table 8.2.

Using a Questionnaire to Obtain Information from Patients

Prepare a simple questionnaire to determine how potential enrollees heard about the clinical trial. Information gained this way could indicate which are the most

TABLE 8.1. *Possible causes of low patient enrollment*

A. Disease related
   1. Incidence rate decreases
   2. Natural history of disease changes
B. Treatment related
   1. Better treatments become available
   2. More patients are receiving treatment
C. Patient related
   1. Perceived benefits of the trial are too small
   2. The trial is inconvenient
   3. Motivation is too low for many reasons
   4. Too few patients have the disease or problem being tested
D. Protocol related
   1. Inclusion criteria are too strict
   2. Requirements of the trial are too great
E. Investigator related
   1. Too little time to devote to recruitment activities
   2. Too much work to focus on the trial
   3. Too few funds to hire necessary staff
   4. Poor relationships and rapport with patients
F. Staff related
   1. Impolite or otherwise unfriendly staff induce negative feelings in patients
   2. Too few staff in a trial cause delays in taking care of patients
G. Practical issues
   1. Personal safety concerns exist at the facilities
   2. Too many visits are scheduled
   3. Each visit is too long or too arduous
   4. Too much money is required of the patients to pay for tests, transportation, baby-sitting, and other trial-related expenses
   5. Scheduling is inconvenient for working patients
   6. A period of hospitalization is required
   7. Parking is a major problem
   8. Public transportation is a major problem
H. Facilities related
   1. Buildings are old and run-down
   2. Buildings are large and intimidating
   3. The clinic is small and without privacy for interviews or examinations

TABLE 8.2. *Examples of questions to pose when patient recruitment does not meet the minimal threshold*

1. What is the gap between the minimal acceptable rate of patient enrollment and the history of patient enrollment at the site?
2. If the trial is a multicenter one, how many sites are having similar low rates of patient enrollment?
3. Are the reasons for low patient enrollment known? How have these reasons been established?
4. Are there sound reasons to believe the recruitment rate will increase without specific intervention?
5. Is a recruitment strategy in place to initiate the next stage of recruitment?
6. Have investigators, patients, and others (e.g., clinical trial staff, coordinating center staff) been questioned about reasons that could be responsible for the low patient enrollment rate?

productive sources of patients, particularly when multiple sources are being targeted. One also may ask why the potential enrollee contacted the center. For example, the patient may have wanted to learn more about his or her diagnosis, to obtain free screening and medical care, or to try a new medicine. Also, the influence of the potential enrollee's physician could be evaluated. In lieu of a questionnaire, one or more questions might be added to the initial telephone or written interview form to obtain the desired information.

Patients who qualify but decide not to participate in a clinical trial could be asked what changes in the trial would make them decide to enroll. Reasons might include more convenient scheduling, improving transportation, or less waiting time.

ADDRESSING THE CAUSES OF INSUFFICIENT RECRUITMENT: GENERAL APPROACHES

Collins et al. (1980) described five strategies used in Veterans Administration Cooperative Studies to improve inadequate recruitment. The problems of poor patient recruitment are described for seven different trials. Revised sample sizes were calculated for most trials. The five strategies used to enhance recruitment were:

1. Reevaluate the required sample size. Collins et al. (1980) described how the sample size for an aphasia trial was recalculated based on altered plans to test the hypothesis with all sites pooled instead of being tested individually (Fig. 8.6).
2. Add new hospitals (i.e., trial sites) to the trial.
3. Replace hospitals that had poor recruiting records.
4. Extend the patient recruitment period.
5. Modify the patient inclusion criteria.

These are probably the five most commonly used and important methods available to boost inadequate patient recruitment. In fact, the first and third methods do not directly help to boost recruitment, but lower the numbers of patients needed (method one) or free additional time to focus on productive centers (method three). Collins et al. (1980) show how appropriate use and balance of these approaches may improve poor enrollment. The critical factors are to diagnose the problem(s) accurately and to decide which of the above, or other antidotes, would be appropriate countermeasures to cure the problem.

Reevaluating and Modifying Inclusion Criteria

Screening logs should describe the major and minor reasons that patients fail to enter a protocol as originally designed. In some instances, the causes for rejection can be modified in a protocol's inclusion criteria so that more patients become eligible for the trial. If an eligibility criterion is altered, screening log data can be used to estimate how many additional patients become eligible for the trial based on the frequency of that item in the logs. Altering the trial's inclusion criteria must be done with extreme caution to avoid affecting the population's characteristics. A major change in inclusion criteria late in a trial could alter the population such that future patients enrolled late in the recruitment period are likely to differ significantly from the original group. An example of a change in inclusion criteria is the modification of a requirement for two episodes of the disease to allow entry for patients who have experienced only one episode but who have a family history of the disorder. This change could be limited to a maximum percentage of future entries to minimize the impact of the change on the trial cohort.

Modification of inclusion criteria does not always alter recruitment. One clinical trial that is noteworthy for the strictness of its inclusion criteria was described by LaRue et al. (1988). Only one of 192 patients screened was found eligible for enrollment. Moreover, 81% of patients were excluded by two or even more of the inclusion criteria. This trial protocol of acute stroke therapy underwent three revisions to boost patient recruitment. None of these revisions had any major effect on patient recruitment (Table 8.3). The enrollment of only one patient after nearly 2 years of screening 192 patients, plus the poor recruitment experiences of other sites involved in the trial, indicate that the protocol's inclusion criteria were too restrictive. The authors cite other stroke trials reported in the literature that enrolled 7.4%, 10.2%, and 32% of patients screened (LaRue et al., 1988).

The National Cooperative Gallstone Study (Croke, 1979) conducted a preliminary trial that included a biopsy prior to initiating a major trial. Figure 8.4 demonstrates a major improvement in both patient evaluations and enrollments (i.e., randomizations) in the major trial as compared with the pilot one. This change was attributed to three factors: (1) looser inclusion criteria, (2) the threat of nonrenewal of contracts with participating hospitals, and (3) deletion of the requirement for a biopsy. It is not possible to determine the influence of each factor individually on improved recruitment. The comparison of the priority score given to each site at the time of their selection with their ability to recruit patients is shown in Fig. 8.5. This indicates that the correlation is poor.

Modifying a Protocol to Enhance Recruitment

Most changes that are made to a protocol to enhance recruitment involve relaxation of the inclusion criteria. In addition, it is also important to consider whether patient recruitment would be enhanced by modifying another aspect of the protocol. It is critical to assess what aspect(s) of a protocol are responsible for the lower than desired recruitment rate. Apart from the inclusion criteria, it is possible that recruitment efforts are hampered by what patients perceive as:

1. An exceedingly long clinical trial.
2. Too many clinic visits.

TABLE 8.3. *Enrollment criteria for acute stroke multicenter clinical trial*[a]

	Initial (n = 94)		Revision 1 (n = 78)		Revision 2 (n = 20)		Final (n = 71)	
	Criterion	% Excluded	Criterion	% Excluded	Criterion	% Excluded	Criterion	% Excluded
Inclusion criteria								
Age (yr)	40–80	12	>35	3	>35	0	>35	0
Stroke type	Ischemic	12	Ischemic	17	Ischemic	0	Ischemic	0
Territory	MCA	18	MCA/ACA	26	MCA/ACA	15	MCA/ACA	20
Exclusion criteria								
Time of screening	>24 hr	24	>24 hr	23	>48 hr	25	>48 hr	27
Stroke	Unstable course	9	Unstable course	8	Unstable course	0	Unstable course	0
	Decreased level of consciousness	11	Decreased level of consciousness	14	Decreased level of consciousness	5	Decreased level of consciousness	4
	Lacunae/TIA	5	Lacunae/TIA	5	Lacunae/TIA	0	Lacunae/TIA	1
Severity	Plegia of one limb	14	Hemiplegia	12	Hemiplegia	20	Hemiplegia	11
Previous stroke	None allowed	31	Ipsilateral, contralateral with residual	18	Ipsilateral, contralateral with residual	15	Ipsilateral, contralateral with residual	14
Medical conditions	Hepatic or renal disease, alcohol or drug abuse	34	Significant hepatic or renal disease, alcohol or drug abuse	32	Significant hepatic or renal disease, alcohol or drug abuse	25	Significant hepatic or renal disease, alcohol or drug abuse[a]	18
Cardiac disease	Congestive heart failure, atrial fibrillation, valvular heart disease, clinically significant arrhythmias, cardiac surgery, and other[a]	28	Decompensated congestive heart failure, atrial fibrillation, valvular heart disease, clinically significant arrhythmias, cardiac surgery, and other[a]	13	Unstable atrial fibrillation, valvular heart disease, cardiac surgery <6 months, and other[a]	0	[a]	13
Gastrointestinal disease	Active peptic ulcer	4	Active peptic ulcer	4	Active peptic ulcer	5	Active peptic ulcer	0

216

Category	Item	Study 1	Study 2	Study 3	Study 4
Neurologic disease	Seizures	13	14	10	0 (Seizures nonexclusionary)
	All other neurologic diseases	9	21	25	0 (Severe movement disorder)
Psychiatric illness	Significant	2	4	0	— (Not specified)
Concomitant medications		30 [b]	15 [b]	0 (Nitroglycerine, β-blockers, anticoagulants, antiplatelet agents, and hypnotics allowed)	4 [c]
Laboratory tests	Clinically significant deviations from normal	19	8	5	0
Other	Untestable	10	17	15	0
	Intracranial surgery	3	3	0	0
	Questionable diagnosis	24	17	25	0
	Pregnant or lactating	0	0	0	0
	Nonneurologic deficit [d]	9	1	0	0

From LaRue et al. (1988) with permission.

MCA, middle cerebral artery; ACA, anterior cerebral artery; TIA, transient ischemic attack.

[a] Cardiac exclusions were myocardial infarction ≤4 months, acute or noncompensated heart failure, complete heart block, ventricular arrhythmia, unstable angina, cardiac, or carotid surgery ≤1 month, blood pressure of >190/110 or <90/60 mm Hg, or pulse of >110/min or <50/min.

[b] Exclusionary concomitant medications were vasodilators, barbiturates, naloxone, β-blockers, other calcium channel antagonists, dextrans including mannitol, anticoagulants, antiplatelet agents, corticosteroids, neuroleptics, antidepressants, and hypnotics.

[c] Disallowed concomitant medications were vasodilators, naloxone, other calcium channel antagonists, dextrans including mannitol, corticosteroids, and barbiturates other than short-acting; other medication allowed; 325 mg aspirin/day required in nonanticoagulated patients.

[d] Examples include amputations and other defects making assessment impossible.

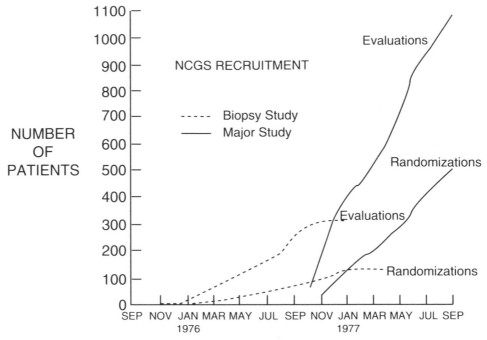

FIG. 8.4. NCGS recruitment in the biopsy study between November, 1975, and April, 1976, and for the major study from September, 1976, through August, 1977. Reprinted from Croke (1979) with permission.

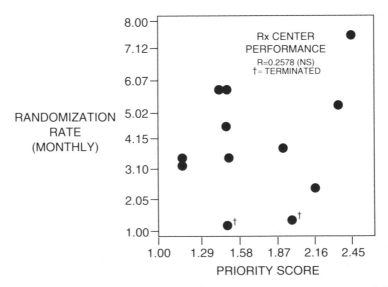

FIG. 8.5. Correlation of the priority scores given to the treatment centers at the time of their selection by the Steering Committee with the subsequent monthly randomization rate for each treatment center. Reprinted from Croke (1979) with permission.

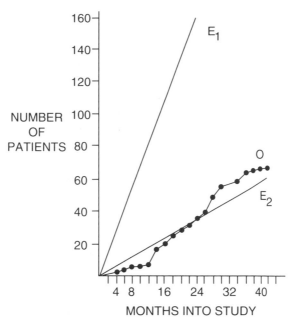

FIG. 8.6. Patient intake for Aphasia Study by month (E_1, original required sample intake; E_2, revised required sample intake; O, observed sample intake). Reprinted from Collins et al. (1980) with permission.

3. Too many tests conducted at each visit.
4. Clinic visits that are inconvenient in terms of the number of hours required.
5. Clinic visits that are inconvenient in terms of the time of day when they must be made.
6. Too many unreimbursed costs.
7. Too great a chance of receiving a placebo instead of an active medicine.

Most of these aspects may be modified through protocol changes. One must decide, however, whether the proposed protocol changes are justified and what effect they will have on the recruitment of patients. Major protocol changes may create major disruptions in the operation of the clinical trial so that it takes significant time to adjust and smooth operations again. In this regard, the experiences of the group that conducted the Macular Photocoagulation Study are valuable (Macular Photocoagulation Study Group, 1984b).

Improving the Quality of Interactions with Patients

All staff who interact with patients during the recruitment process should be evaluated for the appropriateness and professionalism of their contacts. This includes enthusiasm for the project, absence of feeling that staff are overworked, empathy for the patient, ability to discuss clearly benefits the patients will receive as well as ones they will not. Some patients who have completed a clinical trial can be asked if they are willing to share their experiences with other prospective patients on a one-to-one basis, or even using a group presentation. In some cases it may be desirable to produce a videotape to encourage new patients to enroll.

Staff should show genuine interest in the patient (e.g., in their family, hobbies, activities) and can note relevant details in a specific place in the patient's medical record or other place. For long-term trials, sending a birthday and holiday card is also a thoughtful idea that is usually well received.

Showing patients the facilities and equipment to be used prior to or at the time of screening may allay either general unfocused fears or highly specific fears. Describing the procedures to be followed in detail is another means of allaying fears that may not be addressed through a general presentation.

Address the concerns and questions of family or friends as well as those of the patient. The decision of whether or not a patient enrolls is often greatly influenced by the people the patient is close to. Moreover, the cooperation of family and friends may be needed during the course of the trial.

Developing a Plan

Before implementing specific methods to improve low patient recruitment, it is essential to develop a trial-specific plan of action. This involves ensuring that the person or people involved are convinced that the major reasons for inadequate recruitment are identified correctly. Do they make sense? In addition, it may be desirable to convene a meeting of investigators and staff to discuss these reasons, both individually (i.e., What steps will be taken to address each reason?) and collectively (e.g., What overall actions are possible within the resource constraints?). Also plan to discuss at that meeting how the decisions made will be implemented in time (e.g., deadlines). Assign responsibilities for each step of the plan. A Gantt chart (i.e., bar chart of activities over time as one axis) that summarizes the group's decisions would be a useful tool to help communicate and implement the group decision.

Monitoring a Change in Methods

The effectiveness of modifying a recruitment technique or initiating a new method can be monitored by observing changes in screening and enrollment rates after initiation of the new method. Evaluation of the demographic and prognostic characteristics of the screenees and enrollees will demonstrate whether a change in the recruitment strategy is reaching a new pool of candidates. Monitoring can assess whether use of the additional methods (or sources) is enhancing enrollment or recruitment from a different population.

EXAMPLES OF SPECIFIC METHODS TO IMPROVE RECRUITMENT

It is probably impossible to identify all of the potential causes for low patient recruitment. On the other hand, a relatively small number of reasons probably account for most experiences of low patient recruitment. Six of these are given below with approaches to enhance recruitment in those situations.

Inclusion Criteria are Too Restrictive

In considering a loosening of the inclusion criteria, a number of issues must be analyzed, including:

Should any inclusion criteria be loosened, as opposed to enhancing recruitment using other techniques?

Which criteria should be loosened?

To what degree should the criteria identified be loosened?

Will loosening the criteria tend to enroll patients with different characteristics that could affect the trial's outcomes?

Will loosening the criteria tend to alter the (statistically derived) number of patients that are necessary to be enrolled?

Boredom at Sites Leads to a Decline in Recruitment Rates

Sites that had been entering patients at an acceptable rate may experience a decline that can be attributed primarily to boredom. An entire series of activities should be planned to counter boredom (within the recruitment budget). Various steps that could be considered for stepwise implementation are:

1. Discuss with outside staff or those in a trial what action(s) will rekindle staff enthusiasm for the trial.
2. Determine what is motivating the affected investigator(s) to participate in the trial and then address that issue specifically.
3. Discuss the importance and implications of the trial outcome with staff, and the need to enroll patients.
4. Encourage the staff to explore the known and unknown clinical and scientific background of the trial therapies.
5. Create a newsletter and feature articles of special interest to the staff or on positive attributes of the investigators who appear least interested in the trial.
6. Offer the investigators opportunities to conduct other trials of interest to them or to initiate substudies within the current trial that would not adversely affect the trial.
7. Provide feedback to staff in terms of how close the recruitment or trial team is to achieving their recruitment goal.
8. Have all investigators meet to discuss recruitment problems and how the problems can be best addressed at each site and overall.
9. Bring selected staff to an investigators' meeting to stress their importance in helping the team reach the recruitment goals of the trial.

Another aspect of boredom may be administrative hassles of the investigator. Table 8.4 lists some of the reasons why physicians may be reluctant to enter patients into a trial.

The motivation of investigators and their staff must be carefully considered, as well as the motivation of physicians that an investigator counts on for referrals. For example, if the residents and other house staff have incentives (e.g., less work) to discharge patients as soon as possible, then enrolling their patients in the trial will slow the patient turnover for the house staff. Thus, the house staff would be reluctant to encourage their patients to enroll in a clinical trial. If it is possible for these patients to be transferred to a special ward, the house staff may develop an entirely different attitude about the clinical trial.

Inform investigators in a multicenter trial of how well they themselves are doing compared with other investigators. Encourage friendly competition among investi-

TABLE 8.4. *Selected reasons why some physicians are reluctant to enter patients in clinical trials*

A physician may have discomfort with the:
 1. Inclusion of placebo
 2. Size of the group given placebo
 3. Randomization process
 4. Informed consent procedures
 5. Restricted eligibility requirements
 6. Excessive time required to care for patients
 7. Administrative requirements of completing data collection forms
 8. Interference with the usual patient–physician relationship
 9. Perceived conflicts between care offered patients in usual treatment versus that required by the protocol
10. Insurance issues that prevent or make it difficult for some groups of patients (e.g., those in a health maintenance organization) to enter certain hospitals and receive insurance coverage[a]
11. Level of financial reimbursement may seem inadequate
12. Overall value of the trial (e.g., additional information may have been obtained since the trial started, preference for one treatment)

A physician may experience a change in his or her:
 1. Personal life (e.g., new children, marriage, divorce)
 2. Commitments to other clinical trials
 3. Commitments to other activities or projects as a result of promotion, new responsibilities, or new interests
 4. Plans for vacation or upcoming sabbatical

Reprinted from Spilker (1991) with permission.
[a] Some insurance-related issues are discussed by Wood (1989).

gators, but be careful that their enthusiasm does not lead to enrollment of ineligible patients.

Overwork and Stress Do Not Allow Adequate Time for Recruitment

Overwork and stress on the part of the investigator and/or the person responsible for recruitment may result from trial-related activities, or from other activities. In either case a formula must be found to spend more time on patient enrollment. If the overwork is related to the trial, then shifting more efforts to recruitment should result in more positive entry rates.

If financial resources are available then help with recruitment may be sought by hiring medical contractor organizations or other groups to assist in recruiting activities. Without such resources, brainstorming sessions often are held to determine the group's optimal approach to improve recruitment.

Patients are Refusing to Sign the Informed Consent Form

Prepare a short guide for use by all staff who discuss the trial with patients, and request that the guidelines be followed, particularly when obtaining informed consent from patients. This guide should review:

1. The tone of voice and demeanor to use.
2. The pace to use in presenting information, and when to ask patients if they will sign the informed consent. Do not rush patients or their families.
3. When during the clinic visit to discuss issues. Consider when the patient will be alert and willing to discuss the trial.

TABLE 8.5. *Important principles for optimizing the chances of patients giving informed consent*

1. Do not rush patients at this time
2. Delegate this responsibility if you do not have the time, style, or patience
3. Provide privacy
4. Attempt to make it a positive experience
5. Give patients enough background about the trial and about the informed consent process before they read the consent form
6. Offer to provide patients with results of their own tests
7. Describe how the data obtained may assist the patient's physicians in planning for their health care
8. Offer to provide patients with published and unpublished material about their disease
9. Use large print informed consent forms for patients with visual problems

4. Who should be present during the discussion. Some patients desire that a relative or friend be present during discussions. Remember that privacy is important to many patients.

5. Who should present the information to the patient. Only specific personnel should be delegated by the investigator with responsibility for informing patients about the trial and obtaining the informed consent.

6. How to make the process of entering the trial as positive an experience as possible for the patient.

7. How much background information about the clinical trial is appropriate to present.

8. Whether other patient information sheets are available that discuss the trial and how or when to use them.

9. How long patients have to respond to the invitation to enroll.

10. How patients can obtain additional information about the trial or any implications about their participation.

Table 8.5 lists a few additional principles.

Brainstorming sessions could be held to identify additional information that could be provided to patients to help them decide whether or not to enroll in a trial. For example, Gelber and Goldhirsch (1988) state that a clinical trial could be considered as *the treatment of choice* for many types and stages of cancer.

A Sufficient Number of Patients Cannot Be Found to Screen, but Those Who Are Found Generally Enter the Trial

The answer to this problem is to increase the number of sources used to find patients. This may mean that new types of sources should be found or that a greater number of the same sources should be used. It may be uncertain initially which recruitment method(s) will prove most productive at each type of source used. Nonetheless, a plan can be developed that considers available resources and includes as many sources (see Chapter 3) and methods (see Chapter 4) as possible, within the economic and other constraints of the trial.

A few of the many methods available to increase awareness of the trial are to prepare and distribute:

1. Rolodex cards with the trial's name and contact telephone(s).
2. Post-it notes (i.e., pads of self-stick papers) with the essential message printed on each sheet.

3. Calendars printed on one sheet of heavy stock paper in attractive colors and laminated. The name of the trial and the inclusion criteria should be printed below the calendar, along with appropriate telephone number(s).
4. Sheets of heavy stock paper listing only the inclusion criteria and how to refer patients.
5. Small pads of paper with the trial information printed on each sheet.
6. Christmas holiday cards for potential referring physicians.

Too Few Patients Are Being Referred to the Trial

Monetary rewards are generally frowned upon to stimulate referrals (see Chapter 5). Standards can be established that a certain amount of money will be given for each patient referred who meets the entry criteria, whether or not the patient is willing to participate in the trial. Careful use of awards of textbooks or basic medical equipment is a more appropriate incentive that is both academically acceptable and well-liked by house staff. The books can be (1) placed in a general resident's office, (2) donated to a library, (3) placed in the on-call room, or (4) given directly to the person who made the referral. Each gift book should be inscribed with the name of the clinical trial from which it is received. Public presentation of each gift is a useful way to maximize the positive publicity for the trial as well as to recognize the people who made referrals.

Providing gifts and awards must not appear to create a conflict with the rule that perquisites must not be provided for any medical center staff person performing his or her regular job, or to affect the medical care provided to any patient.

Improving Patient Education to Enhance Recruitment Yield

Although some investigators have privately speculated that more informed patients are less likely to enroll in clinical trials, a few unpublished studies quoted by Llewellyn-Thomas et al. (1991) found the opposite to be true. Each investigator should carefully consider whether to provide special education and extra information before implementing it because of the potential that may exist for decreasing enrollment. Nonetheless, this highly ethical approach should be utilized as widely as practicable. Table 8.6 mentions some activities to improve relationships with patients.

TABLE 8.6. *Activities to improve relationships with patients*

1. Discuss the purpose of the trial
2. Discuss implications of the trial for patients
3. Discuss what goals the patient expects to achieve from enrolling
4. Send a note of appreciation to patients after their enrollment
5. Send a note of appreciation to patients at the end of their participation in the trial
6. Send a letter to patients' referring physicians at the start and end of the trial and inform patients that this was done

MODIFYING THE RECRUITMENT STRATEGIES DOES NOT ALWAYS WORK

Even successful diagnosis of the problem of poor patient recruitment and an appropriate prescription for the cure may be insufficient to solve the problem if the prescription cannot be fulfilled. If part of the prescription involves adding additional hospital sites, a sufficient number of hospitals of suitable quality must be available to add to the trial. Furthermore, there must be sufficient funds to pay for any proposals that require additional resources. Finally, a sufficient number of patients should be known to be available to enroll when inclusion criteria are relaxed. A long exercise that serves to relax criteria but does not improve results would be fruitless.

Various investigators and staff participating in a trial may have different concepts about which methods to implement; a consensus must be reached. This could be accomplished in a brief discussion or may involve many lengthy conferences. Long meetings may be necessary because (1) a variety of different approaches may be considered, (2) statisticians or others believe that changes to the inclusion criteria or other parts of the protocol may affect the integrity of the trial, (3) statisticians or others may not be willing to accept newly created (i.e., lowered) goals for patient recruitment, (4) clinicians may believe that proposed changes may (or will) lead to the enrollment of a significantly different patient population and would pose problems when data from the original and subsequent groups are combined, (5) the resources to implement the proposed changes may not be available or may represent a major cost to the sponsor or investigator, or (6) the likelihood of success of each of the proposed methods is uncertain and may not be agreed upon.

There is no question that all of these potential objections can be satisfactorily addressed, but this may require substantial time and effort by the group involved.

ENHANCING RECRUITMENT IN MULTICENTER TRIALS: GENERAL APPROACHES

When enrollment rates in large multicenter trials fall short of interim goals, planning committees face the question of whether to (1) increase the number of sites, (2) expand existing sites, (3) modify existing sites by changing staff, (4) extend the recruitment period, or (5) follow another course. Some of these choices depend on the sponsor's willingness to fund continuation or expansion of the trial. Many of the strategies to consider are listed in Table 8.7. Information on all aspects of the problems and pros and cons of each solution must be considered.

A specific reason (e.g., reimbursement of surgical fees) may be identified as the primary reason for recruitment problems. In such cases almost all the attention of the staff that is devoted to recruitment will focus on methods to address that issue (Jonas, 1986). However, the staff in most trials that have recruitment problems usually must deal with a variety of issues.

Add New Sites

When an additional trial site is invited to join a multicenter trial after its initiation, the invitee may feel this confers second-class status. In some cases, the new group

TABLE 8.7. *Strategies to consider when recruitment rates are lower than desired*

A. Site or staff related
  1. Add new trial sites
  2. Add more investigators or coinvestigators at existing sites
  3. Replace marginal or poor sites with better sites
  4. Hire a research coordinator at all sites
  5. Hire a recruitment coordinator at one or more sites or at a coordination center
  6. Threaten to terminate participation of a site
  7. Discuss the support for the trial with administrative staff
  8. Simplify the process by which patients are referred to the trial
  9. Hire a local (or national) public relations company to assist in recruitment
  10. Send a questionnaire to all investigators to learn their views
  11. Initiate a newsletter with information on the trial, recruitment tips and experiences, positive data
  12. Start a screening and enrollment log to monitor recruitment at each center
  13. Hire a behavioral scientist to advise on recruitment approaches
  14. Provide more frequent feedback to investigators and referring physicians about recruitment progress
  15. Provide feedback about status of patients to their referring physician
  16. Provide funds to a hospital for supporting meetings, dinners, or texts to be allocated at the hospital's (or investigator's) discretion
  17. Devote more time to recruitment and give it a higher priority in terms of efforts
  18. Ask the investigator's staff to review hospital admissions or clinic appointments to seek potential patients
  19. Increase financial incentives for the investigator
  20. Increase scientific/professional incentives for the investigator

B. Protocol or trial related
  1. Increase the duration of recruitment by a fixed length of time or leave it open
  2. Increase trial budget for specific recruiting activities
  3. Modify the inclusion criteria (e.g., age range)
  4. Use new sources and/or methods to recruit patients[a]
  5. Modify the trial's design (e.g., a parallel trial takes half the time of a cross-over trial)
  6. Modify the trial's requirements (e.g., concomitant medicines, number of failed treatments, number of clinic visits scheduled, eliminate some or all disagreeable tests)
  7. Modify the administration and management (e.g., lessen waiting time, provide escort service to one's car, give patients more feedback)
  8. Recalculate sample size needed based on an interim analysis
  9. Simplify the paperwork in quantity and complexity
  10. Add a continuation protocol so that patients may continue to receive a medicine if they have demonstrated clinical improvement in the trial
  11. Determine which techniques are working best at sites with high recruitment rates and utilize those techniques at sites with lower recruitment rates
  12. Have a major well-respected expert come to a site with low enrollment and encourage physicians to refer or enter patients into the clinical trial
  13. Combine approaches (e.g., have a newspaper article appear the day prior to a television appearance)
  14. Rescreen patients who had temporary reasons for exclusion
  15. Send reminders about the trial to referring physicians

C. Patient related
  1. Determine what factors are motivating patients to enter or not enter the clinical trial and attempt to address their needs (e.g., use a questionnaire)
  2. Talk to patients and provide printed information at the appropriate level of education
  3. Educate patients about the clinical trial before asking for their informed consent
  4. Show patients videotapes about the trial and their participation
  5. Provide a tour of the clinic for prospective patients and spend time answering questions
  6. Improve financial incentives for patients to enroll by reimbursing various costs (e.g., for meals, transportation, baby-sitting)
  7. Ensure that patients are informed about all of the important trial factors (e.g., they may receive treatments not otherwise available)

[a] See Chapters 3 and 4 on sources and methods of recruitment.

had been approached earlier but was unable to join the trial because of other commitments. Nevertheless, the new investigator must bring his or her research team into an ongoing trial without the luxury of the planning period and group conference that is usually held prior to startup of the trial. A full complement of staff, possibly including a recruitment coordinator and other support staff, must be readily available. Staff at the new site are often trained by the coordinating or primary center in a special session because they missed the initial multicenter group startup conference. Having gained the opportunity to meet staff from other sites and to hear about approaches used by other teams, the new group has the advantage of learning what has worked and what has not worked at other sites to this point. The new group can start in the trial with knowledge that should save them time in recruiting patients. A disadvantage of adding a new site is the inevitable time lag from the point at which the need for an extra site is recognized to the time when patient enrollment begins. It is not worthwhile to formally initiate a trial and enroll patients until all staff are trained and familiar with the trial.

Expand Existing Sites

An alternative to adding new sites is the expansion of existing sites to screen more patients from the same or a wider catchment area. The designation of a recruitment coordinator, if one did not exist, could result in redirection of efforts toward finding eligible patients. Expansion of the site may include not only initiating new techniques for patient recruitment but also spreading the trial's reach into distant communities and work sites. Problems may ensue if the clinical trial site where clinic visits must be held is distant from the area of patient recruitment, particularly if public transportation is poor. It is possible that immediate and nearby communities have already been depleted of readily available patients. Expanded screening may not yield reasonable numbers of potential trial candidates despite large screening efforts. Approaching distant communities may require establishment of a satellite trial site staffed by either part-time personnel from the central site or by a separate staff fully trained in the trial's procedures. Either approach usually presents a burden on the investigators because physicians generally are based at the central site and must travel to the satellite offices/clinics to see patients. As a result, expanding the trial to a satellite in a distant area may not be cost-effective. Selection of an alternate site in a new city may be more worthwhile.

Modify Existing Sites

Two types of staff changes at an existing site may dramatically alter screening and enrollment. One is a change in investigator and the other is a change in the trial or recruitment coordinator.

If the principal investigator steps down or leaves a site a new principal investigator is usually selected. The new investigator should be enthusiastic and a good manager of the research team. Different investigators are likely to have new contacts among his or her colleagues and new ideas about how to enhance recruitment. Having agreed to assume the role of principal investigator, he or she usually desires to succeed in this role. In addition, there is often a competitive urge to exceed prior screening and accrual rates. Whether or not any enthusiasm or competitiveness exists, the selection of a new investigator presents an excellent opportunity for him or her to reenter the community with a series of lectures to colleagues and to community groups to refocus attention on the trial and enhance recruitment. If the replacement investigator considers this role as an "assigned duty" and enters the program with little enthusiasm, site recruiting activity might slow significantly. This effect might be overcome if the trial coordinator maintains his or her pace based on independent enthusiasm to meet goals. This scenario is not uncommon if the trial is well underway and staff responsibilities are organized.

Trial coordinators often change during the course of a clinical trial. No matter what the screening and accrual rates had been with the previous coordinator, and no matter what rationale explained those rates in terms of size of the community, support from medical center staff, experience of the coordinator in recruiting, or personality of the coordinator, it is common for a new coordinator to initiate a surge in screening and enrollment. This may be attributed to the renewed vigor and eagerness to use methods that had not been as fruitful for previous staff or that had not been utilized for various reasons. Occasionally, this change does not result in renewed vigor, particularly if the new person is not inspired to take on the trial as his or her own responsibility but relies on the system developed by previous staff. In addition, there is always a period of unproductive time when the new coordinator is being trained. The site investigator and coordinating center must monitor the progress of a new coordinator until they are convinced about the quality and consistency of the new coordinator's performance. If the individual is inappropriate for the role, then he or she can be moved into another position.

Extend the Recruitment Period

A frequently employed method to allow a trial to reach its recruitment goal is an extension of the recruitment period (Fig. 8.7). Collins et al. (1984) list ten VA multicenter trials that suffered from insufficient patient enrollment during the original time period allocated for recruitment. Seven of the trials were extended for 6 to 18 months to randomize an adequate number of patients to complete the trial (Table 8.8). Pocock (1978) reported that a survey of oncology trials showed that slow patient accrual was a major problem. Extension of the recruitment period often is feasible

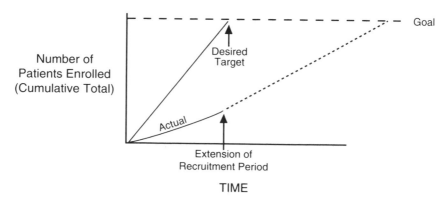

FIG. 8.7. Illustrating how extending the duration of patient recruitment achieves the total goal. The period of extension begins at the arrow.

TABLE 8.8. *Adjustments made for intake problems in selected VA trials*

Clinical trial	Adjustment
Antabuse	Early termination
Aphasia I	18-month extension
Aphasia II	12-month extension
Chronic brain	Early termination
Dental	6-month extension
Epilepsy	12-month extension[a]
Nursing home	18-month extension
Ulcer	Early termination
Ward milieu	12-month extension

Reprinted from Collins et al. (1984) with permission.
[a] Required because the sample size required was underestimated.

if extra funds are available for the additional time required (see Chapter 6 on Economics). However, this method is unsuitable for trials where maintaining the timetable to completion is of paramount importance. This is frequently the case in industry sponsored clinical trials.

Track Recruitment Activities Conducted through the Media

Advertisements in newspapers and magazines, and those on radio or television should be monitored to ensure that they were printed or presented correctly. The results of all advertisements in terms of patient contacts and the yield from each type of advertisement used should be evaluated. Analyses of size, frequency, duration, and content of advertisements may be made to improve their effectiveness.

Monitoring stories printed or aired as a result of press releases or other publicity may be important, but is more difficult and expensive than monitoring paid advertisements. If recruitment is progressing at an acceptable rate it is less important to monitor unpaid stories, and to obtain relatively complete feedback about a major trial.

In large national or multinational clinical trials, however, or in certain smaller ones, it may be important to obtain information on how often and in what ways news coverage mentions the ongoing trial as well as the geographical locations where it is or is not mentioned. While the trial organizers may collect some information to address this question their efforts are likely to be extremely limited if the trial is a large one and covers a wide geographical area.

The most desirable approach to this issue is to hire a professional service that can perform these activities comprehensively. These services are called "clipping services" and exist throughout the world. One major service in North America (Burrelle's, Livingston, NJ) covers 10,944 newspapers, 6,303 magazines, 450 television stations in 175 cities, and 57 radio stations in 25 cities, plus all major news services. They can provide a wide variety of services beyond merely clipping newspaper articles. For example, they monitor and provide typed transcripts of radio programs or video snippets of television programs where the clinical trial was mentioned (Fig. 8.8). The two major issues for the organizers of a clinical trial are to document a need for this type of service and second to determine if the fees for these services

BURRELLE'S

75 EAST NORTHFIELD AVENUE / LIVINGSTON / NEW JERSEY 07039
(201) 992-6600 / (212) 227-5570 / (800) 631-1160

RADIO
CLIPS

DATE   December 22, 1988   ACCOUNT NUMBER 56/767 G
TIME   3:05-4:00 PM
STATION KTRH 740 AM
LOCATION Houston
PROGRAM News

Tom Bacon reporting:

Houston's Baylor College of Medicine is testing a drug researchers say can slow the spread of chicken pox and make that disease less severe. Study co-director Dr. Leonard Goldberg says the college needs some child volunteers to take the oral drug *acyclovir*.

Dr. Leonard Goldberg: Now, we're looking for one hundred children. And we're going to be treating them within twenty-four hours of the first outbreak of the chicken pox. Seventy-five percent of the children will get the active medications, and twenty-five percent of the children that we enter into the study will get a placebo.

Bacon: In adults, this medication prevents further lesions and causes a quicker recovery. To volunteer children for this study, parents should call Baylor at 794-2508 or 798-2099. A nurse will come to your home to administer the drug.

FIG. 8.8. Transcript of a radio interview with a recruitment message. Reprinted with permission.

can be afforded. This type of service may appear expensive for a clinical trial budget, but if the information can help refine and direct a trial's recruitment strategy, it could be a cost-effective way of enhancing recruitment.

Improve the Attitudes of Staff Physicians, Patients, or Referring Physicians

When the problem is a lack of commitment to the clinical trial by staff physicians, the following approaches may be employed.

Involve the staff in the organization or management of the trial. For example, they could be asked to serve on a committee, or to act as coauthors of a manuscript. Site visits by the trial chairman or other experts may be made to review and (to the degree possible) laud the participation of the local group. This can sometimes be accomplished through public presentations (e.g., lectures to the medical and lay community). These presentations also inform potential referral sources about the existence and importance of the clinical trial.
Provide compensation to the staff for participating.
Provide other incentives to staff physicians.
Discuss resolutions among the staff (Figs. 8.9 and 8.10).

When a lack of interest is evident in the patients approached for screening, the following may be tried.

NEW YEAR'S RESOLUTIONS
PRINCIPAL INVESTIGATOR
CS#264

1. RESOLVED, IN 1989 I WILL SEARCH <u>ACTIVELY</u> FOR NEW PATIENTS INSTEAD OF WAITING FOR REFERRALS.

2. RESOLVED, I WILL SEEK OUT RESIDENTS <u>REGULARLY</u> TO REMIND THEM OF OUR SEARCH FOR PATIENTS AND THE BOOK AWARD AVAILABLE FOR ELIGIBLE REFERRALS.

3. RESOLVED, IN JANUARY I WILL <u>COMPLETE</u> <u>ALL</u> <u>LEFTOVER</u> FORMS TO START THE YEAR WITH A CLEAN DESK.

4. RESOLVED, STARING THIS WEEK I WILL <u>SCHEDULE</u> AN EXTRA HOUR WEEKLY TO SPEND WITH MY STUDY ASSISTANT TO REVIEW ISSUES AND PROGRESS.

5. RESOLVED, STARING IMMEDIATELY I WILL <u>FINISH</u> FOLLOWUP FORMS BEFORE LEAVING CLINIC AND PRE ENTRY FORMS BEFORE THE ONE WEEK VISIT.

6. RESOLVED, I RECOGNIZE THAT I AM <u>ACCOUNTABLE</u> FOR EVERY FACET OF CS#264 AT MY HOSPITAL, INCLUDING THE ACCURACY AND TIMELINESS OF DATA SUBMITTED BY MY STUDY ASSISTANT.

FIG. 8.9. New Year's resolutions for principal investigators in VA Cooperative Study #264.

Restate the purpose of the trial to define specific benefits for patients.

Clarify the importance of the trial for the advancement of science.

Laud the spirit of volunteerism using public relations releases in the media and in flyers distributed to prospective screenees.

Involve patients and their families in the trial through distribution of newsletters or progress reports about the trial. These can be shown to prospective screenees as an inducement to enroll. Other inducements are listed in Table 8.9.

If a lack of interest is shown by referring physicians or others,

Define the advantages of the therapies offered.

Clarify the special benefits their patients will receive.

Reassure referring physicians that they will not lose their patients; describe the procedures used to return patients after the trial is completed for each patient. Offer to provide progress reports.

NEW YEAR'S RESOLUTIONS
STUDY ASSISTANTS
CS#264

1. RESOLVED, IN 1989 I WILL SEARCH <u>ACTIVELY</u> FOR NEW PATIENTS INSTEAD OF WAITING FOR THEM TO FALL INTO MY LAP.

2. RESOLVED, IN JANUARY I WILL <u>COMPLETE</u> <u>ALL</u> <u>LEFTOVER</u> FORMS AND EDITS TO START THE YEAR WITH A CLEAN DESK.

3. RESOLVED, I WILL SPEND AT LEAST ONE HOUR A DAY WORKING QUIETLY IN MY OFFICE TO <u>KEEP</u> <u>UP</u> WITH FORMS AND EDITS.

4. RESOLVED, STARTING THIS WEEK, I WILL <u>FINISH</u> FOLLOWUP FORMS 8-15 THE DAY AFTER CLINIC AND MAIL THEM THE NEXT DAY.

5. RESOLVED, I WILL MAKE SPECIAL ARRANGEMENTS FOR <u>ADEQUATE</u> <u>TIME</u> TO ADMINISTER THE DRUG TOXICITY BATTERY AS SCHEDULED.

6. RESOLVED, I WILL ARRANGE TO ADMINISTER INITIAL, BASELINE DRUG TOXICITY BATTERY TESTING <u>PRE ENTRY</u> UNLESS THE PATIENT IS SEDATED OR POST ICTAL.

7. RESOLVED, I WILL FINISH ALL CS#264 TASKS <u>BEFORE</u> UNDERTAKING OTHER DUTIES.

8. RESOLVED, I REALIZE THAT I AM <u>RESPONSIBLE</u> FOR THE ACCURACY AND TIMELINESS OF DATA SUBMITTED FROM MY HOSPITAL.

FIG. 8.10. New Year's resolutions for study assistants in VA Cooperative Study #264.

TABLE 8.9. *Special inducements that may help enrollment among special groups*[a]

1. Free Papanicolaou tests
2. Transportation allowance
3. Food allowance
4. Baby-sitting service or allowance
5. Recruitment limited to warm seasons
6. Free cholesterol tests
7. Tests conducted at the patient's home
8. A staff member who provides social contact and accompanies the patient to clinic

[a] Including elderly, minority, those in poverty, or those living in the inner city. Not all of these could be considered in every country or jurisdiction (e.g., baby-sitting services or allowance might not be approved by some Ethics Committees/IRBs).

Use of Investigator Meetings to Enhance Recruitment

Regular meetings of all investigators and participating staff can be used to emphasize recruitment issues as well as other topics pertinent to the conduct of the trial. Single-site trials have the advantage of being able to conduct meetings frequently whereas site investigators in multicenter trials usually meet only once a year or less often because of the prohibitive travel costs. "The effect of annual investigator meetings on patient recruitment speaks to the importance of such meetings. They provided the opportunity for investigators to share experiences and suggest solutions for problems. In addition, a sense of camaraderie and dedication to the study was fostered" (The Brain Resuscitation Clinical Trial II Study Group, 1991). The cited group reported a distinct effect of investigators' meetings on patient recruitment as shown in Fig. 8.11. The anticipation of the meeting as well as the reinforcement of the importance of recruitment appeared to affect recruitment rates over the 3 years of the trial. Rates increased almost 40% after each meeting.

Use of Newsletters to Enhance Recruitment

Newsletters that describe the progress of the clinical trial to all participating staff often focus on recruitment problems and successes. Ideas for new or alternative sources and methods for patient recruitment can be described in detail. Dissemination of ideas in a newsletter is a convenient system for informing all participants, particularly in multicenter trials where the sites meet infrequently. Many trials use newsletters to list recent recruitment numbers or rates for each site, highlighting the leaders, and sometimes describing any special methods that have been highly successful. Possible contents of a clinical trial newsletter are listed in Table 8.11.

Assess Site-Specific Problems in a Site Visit

When one or several sites in a multicenter trial are far below the mean screening, enrollment, or completer rates observed at other sites, the trial organizers often step

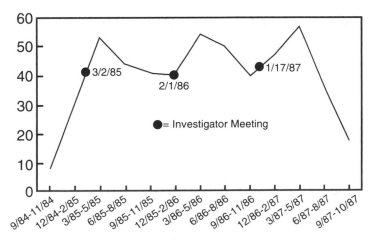

FIG. 8.11. An example of the positive effect that investigators' meetings may have on patient recruitment rates. Reprinted from the Brain Resuscitation Clinical Trial II Study Group (1991) with permission.

TABLE 8.10. *Issues to consider when evaluating whether to extend the period of recruitment*

1. *Length of time needed*
Extrapolate the current rate of recruitment to determine the length of time required to reach the target goal if the rate is maintained.

2. *Amount of money required*
Calculate the funds required and compare with available resources. What is the likelihood that any shortfall can be made up.

3. *Decision-making group*
The determination may be made by the investigator, a group of investigators, a sponsor (if any), an independent policy board, or another group.

4. *Statistical data*
Power calculations should be done for each of the major outcome variables using the reduced sample size if the trial were not extended. Trends in treatment differences that may have differed from pretrial expectations may or may not be considered. Estimates of variability based on actual data should be used.

in to assess local issues and problems. As described in Chapter 9 on goals and quotas, such a review often is mandated by established guidelines, newly devised quotas, or at the request of a data monitoring committee. Assessment should begin with (1) consideration of investigator and staff training and experience with the protocol, (2) evaluation of the catchment areas as a population base, (3) review of the sources, and (4) review of the methods used at the site. The next step is for an extended site visit during which an experienced recruitment coordinator (either from the coordinating center or from another site) works with the local staff for several days. The purpose of the site visit is to observe the typical daily schedule including (1) where, how often, and what techniques are used for screening; (2) type of follow-up of potential patients identified during initial screening; (3) how much information is gathered for recording in the screening log; and (4) how much time is spent on all aspects of screening. The recruitment coordinator can explore utilization of alternative sources for screening. For example, if local screening is performed only at

TABLE 8.11. *Contents of a clinical trial newsletter designed to stimulate staff and boost recruitment*[a]

1. Study update as a total number of sites and patients
2. Specific numbers of patients enrolled over the previous three (or other) months at each site
3. Cumulative total number of patients enrolled at each site
4. Any amendments to the protocol
5. Recruitment tips and new methods
6. Recruitment aids that may be ordered and whether Ethics Committee/IRB approval is required
7. Upcoming meetings
8. Presentations about the trial by investigators
9. Comments about problems or issues relating to the trial that monitors have observed
10. Tips on measuring values, using equipment, sending samples to a central laboratory
11. Graph of recruitment totals versus projected goals
12. Highlight a group or "Site-of-the-Quarter" and describe reason(s)
13. Highlight an individual or "Staff-Person-of-the-Quarter" and reason(s)
14. Names and telephone numbers of specific monitors and/or recruitment coordinator(s)
15. Best recruitment story of the quarter
16. Note any milestones in recruitment achieved (e.g., 100th patient enrolled, halfway point of the trial, all sites have reached a goal)

[a] This newsletter should provide positive feedback on the trial and should be written in a positive tone.

hospital clinics, the staff can be asked to try a demonstration of screening at the emergency room or on the wards during the site visit. The concept of the visit is to stress new approaches.

Next, the site visitor should observe the procedure used to explain the trial to a patient and family, and how the informed consent process is performed. No amount of reports or telephone calls can substitute for direct observation, which often reveals special problems that could have contributed to the slow enrollment at that site. Approaches by investigators and trial coordinators vary from being too high pressure to too low key, from expressing a sense of importance or urgency about enrollment to conveying a feeling of triviality or lack of motivation. Review the number of refusers listed in the screening logs for clues to this problem. Interviews with a few refusers, if acceptable, could be highly informative.

The number of drop-outs, particularly if they occur early in the patients' participation in the trial, is a clue to problems related to follow-up and completion. The site visitor should attend clinic to observe (1) how patients are scheduled, (2) how long they have to wait, (3) whether the tests (e.g., blood samples, vital signs) are performed together with the physician's examination or in separate locations, (4) how long the entire visit takes, and (5) the ambience of the clinic and the style of caring for patients exhibited by the investigator and all trial staff.

In addition to observing the patient-oriented activities, the site visitor should assess how much time is spent on administrative details. In particular, (1) Is the screening log maintained in detail? (2) Is there a plan for follow-up of initial contacts and how is it organized? (3) What activities take precedence during busy periods? Is screening stopped or is it considered a high priority? Numerous other administrative aspects of recruitment are observed during a site visit.

All of these aspects of day-to-day activity can be compared to the strategies and activities performed at other sites. The goal of the special site visit is to help the local staff discover new avenues for sources and develop new methods for recruitment of patients while streamlining their overall operations to allow more time to screen and enroll patients. Special site visits by a recruitment coordinator are a cost-effective means to enhance patient recruitment.

CHOOSING A METHOD TO ENHANCE RECRUITMENT

Selection of one of the methods described, or one or more other methods to enhance recruitment in a large multicenter clinical trial, often depends on available resources and timetable. No rule of thumb can be proposed to try one specific method before another because each clinical trial is unique. However, the decision can be based on some of the following observations.

1. Extension of the recruitment period is sometimes expensive (e.g., adding the cost of maintaining the entire clinical trial for extra months or years), although it is technically the easiest method to implement. The entire recruitment plan is extended at all sites for the desired number of months so the whole clinical trial "team" continues to work toward the recruitment goal. Criteria to use in evaluating whether to extend the recruitment period are listed in Table 8.10.

2. The next easiest method to implement is generally to change the staff at lagging sites. The peer pressure of seeing their low screening and enrollment rates frequently leads to staff resignations. Investigators who do not want to invest more time in the

recruitment process might be willing to add a coinvestigator, or transfer the leadership role to another physician in the group. Attrition, resignation, and transfers all bring in fresh staff at no extra cost and with a simple transition within the site.

3. The next easiest method to implement is expansion of a busy site. The addition of staff or facilities can be accomplished without adding to overall costs if the resources required are taken away from a slower site and transferred to the busy site.

4. Site replacement is often a tedious procedure because of the time required to document poor performance at a slow site using a quota system and a probation period. Thereafter, a new site must be selected and staff must be hired and trained before screening and enrollment begin. A further time lag occurs before the new site achieves the desired pace of activity. Addition of an extra site is faster (and more costly), but also incurs a time lag during selection, training, and startup before enrollments meet expectations. Anticipating the need for this step can greatly simplify its execution because potential sites can be evaluated and trained before their inclusion in the trial is confirmed.

Long-term multicenter clinical trials usually try to replace, add, or expand sites during the early years. Staff turnover is inevitable during long trials. In addition, it takes a while for the trial managers to realize that all the other recruitment methods will not increase the rate of enrollment. Merely modifying inclusion criteria is no guarantee that recruitment will be enhanced (Table 8.3).

RECRUITMENT ISSUES WHEN TOO MANY PATIENTS DESIRE TO ENROLL IN A CLINICAL TRIAL

A major recruitment effort that is "too successful" may overwhelm the system and result in too many patients arriving at a center for screening. This may often be controlled by scheduling appointments appropriately. But, if patients are asked to wait too long before their appointment occurs, or to wait too long in a waiting room, they may lose interest in the trial. In most cases, this is not a problem since patients who are not admitted to a trial continue with their usual forms of medical care. However, an excess number of available patients can be a major problem for a clinical trial when the patients actually demand entry into the trial. This has occurred in some clinical trials conducted with AIDS patients.

Major causes of this problem could be excess publicity about the trial; availability of a new, life-saving treatment; or availability of free care for otherwise expensive treatment that many patients want. Another cause could be a successful recruitment strategy that interests too many patients in enrolling in the trial. It is important to anticipate this issue whenever possible and to take steps to prevent its occurrence, or at least to minimize its implications. Nonetheless, there will be clinical trials where the problem occurs unexpectedly or occurs despite efforts to minimize it.

Several approaches to addressing this problem are straightforward and should be considered.

1. Increase the number of patients in the clinical trial. This makes sense particularly when the magnitude of the clinical effect resulting from treatment is uncertain and unknown and may be less than expected. There are practical limits as well as statistical considerations about how much this can be done. Precise details should be worked out with statisticians. Ensure that the difference between statistical significance and clinical significance is established in advance of the trial. This will prevent small treatment differences that are found to be statistically significant from being interpreted as clinically significant.

2. Limit Appointments. If the patient supply is expected to remain high, then the number of patients entering the trial every day (week or month) may be budgeted. If, however, the patient supply is only temporarily high (e.g., many students applying for entry in a trial are expected to return home from school) then an attempt should be made to increase or adjust the resources to handle the temporarily increased patient load.

3. Open more clinical trial sites. Although administratively more complex than the preceding items, this plan provides broad access to patients if new sites are in different locations.

4. First-come-first-served. This may be a fair way to solve the problem of screening order with large groups of patients. However, it is not an equitable method to use if patients entered the screening queue in an unfair order.

5. Lottery. A lottery could be used to choose patients for screening. This approach could create numerous problems, however, and would need careful review before being implemented.

6. Initiate new clinical trials expeditiously. If the investigator(s) were planning to initiate additional clinical trials, then one or more of these could possibly be expedited at the sites of greatest patient availability. New trials could be initiated either simultaneously or sequentially with the original trial.

7. Revise the protocol. The original protocol may include patients with mild, moderate, and severe symptoms. A rewritten protocol could limit participation to only those patients with a narrower spectrum of symptoms. A variation of this approach would be to divide the trial into two separate trials. For example, one trial could include patients with mild or moderate symptoms and the other could include patients with severe symptoms. Many other factors could be used as a basis to either restrict patient eligibility or to divide a trial into two or more independent trials.

9

Goals and Quotas for Patient Recruitment

DEFINITIONS AND CONCEPTS

After calculating the sample size needed to fulfill the trial objectives, and after determining the amount of time available (or necessary) to complete the recruitment phase, investigators should develop specific interim recruitment goals. The overall *recruitment goal* for a trial is the total number of patients (or total for each specific group of patients) needed to achieve the calculated sample size within a specified time frame. An *enrollment quota* is a minimum number of patients who must be enrolled weekly, monthly, or quarterly at each site for the group to reach its overall recruitment goal. A maximum total number of patients who complete the trial at each site is also part of the enrollment quota. A *recruitment quota* is the number of patients who must be screened during each recruitment period at each site to yield a sufficient number of patient entries. The *recruitment period* is the number of weeks or months during which the status of recruitment is assessed at each site. It should be divided into segments that last up to one-third the duration of the trial. This allows feedback to sites about slow recruitment. The *completer quota* is the number of patients who must complete the trial at each site. This completer quota is particularly important when the protocol mandates replacement of patient drop-outs. Each site in the same multicenter trial may have a different enrollment quota, recruitment quota, and completer quota.

All of these quotas are important for both single-site and multiple-site trials of any size. The recruitment quota influences the desired *screening rate* for each site. This rate is based on sample size, time available, and capacity of the staff to screen and enroll patients as well as conduct the trial. Availability of resources also affects the rate at which patients may be screened. A major influence on the screening rate is the estimated attrition as patients are contacted and undergo primary screening and then secondary screening and finally go through the informed consent process. Whether the trial is small or large, performed at a single site by the originator or in multiple sites with many coinvestigators, the principal investigator and staff generally monitor recruitment rates throughout the course of the trial.

This chapter addresses uses of recruitment quotas in both the initial planning and conduct of single-site and multicenter trials.

CRITERIA USED TO ASSESS THE PROGRESS OF RECRUITMENT EFFORTS

1. The Number of Potential Patient Contacts Per Specified Time Period

This may consist entirely of patients who contact a clinic, patients who are contacted by the clinic, or a mixture of both. If the number of patient contacts to a clinic decreases, it may become necessary to adopt a more proactive approach to stimulate more contacts, or to substitute staff-initiated contacts. A cut-off value (e.g., ten contacts per week for 2 weeks) may be established at which the latter process is initiated.

2. The Number of Potential Patients Screened Per Specified Time Period

This criterion may be subdivided into two, or more, stages of screening. For example, the number of patients screened on the telephone (i.e., primary screening), the number screened by physical examination and history (i.e., secondary screening), and those who are asked to undergo a third stage of more sophisticated laboratory tests (e.g., CT scans).

3. The Number of Prospective Patients Invited to Join the Trial Per Specified Time Period

This criterion is important because a large difference between this number and the number of enrollees indicates that the informed consent process is eliminating many patients. If that is true, then the various components of the informed consent process should be examined to assess which are responsible for the problem.

4. The Number of Patients Who Enroll in the Trial Per Specified Time Period

The trend of these data often are as important as the actual numbers obtained. For example, if any of these numbers are less than the established goals or quotas, but a positive trend is observed, remedial action may not be necessary.

The Coronary Primary Prevention Trial published data on three of these four criteria for each center. Undoubtedly, the fourth criterion is the most important. If the number of patients enrolled in the trial is satisfactory, but the first three are low, then there is less urgency to examine each of the preceding steps to determine how the numbers and rates can be increased. Any single step where a large fall-off occurs should serve as a warning to focus attention on identifying whether a problem exists, and if so, on how to improve the problem. Williford et al. (1987) discussed the value of using a constant intake rate model of patients into clinical trials or simply interim recruitment goals. They rejected the Poisson constant intake rate model and proposed a model of interim goals based on a Bayesian (updating) model. Given that the Bayesian model reflects the results obtained in real trials, their model makes both clinical and practical sense.

PURPOSES AND TYPES OF QUOTAS

Purposes of Quotas

The degree to which investigators would like the results of a trial to be generalizable will affect the level of homogeneity in patient characteristics that they strive for. That level of homogeneity is dictated by the inclusion criteria specified in the protocol. This goal is primarily achieved by adjusting the inclusion criteria that are specified in the protocol. In larger single-site or multicenter trials, recruitment should usually be completed as soon as possible because the type of patient enrolled, their disease characteristics, and the treatment options available might change over the course of an overly lengthy recruitment period. This goal is primarily achieved by adjusting the inclusion criteria that are specified in the protocol.

Establishment of minimum rates of patient accession are therefore important, even for small clinical trials conducted by a single investigator. In multicenter trials with approximately six or more sites, one or more sites typically lag far behind the mean accession rate for the group. Quotas are not only useful to document these problems, but also provide a basis for the trial organizers to determine if and when a site should be closed or replaced. Croke (1979) reported that in the National Cooperative Gallstone Study the threat of closing a site if quotas were not met often had a dramatic effect on increasing that site's recruitment rates.

Minimum and Maximum Rates

The majority of clinical trials use at least informal quotas to establish minimum rates of patient screening and enrollment because under-recruitment is an extremely common and important problem. Sylvester et al. (1981) reported that a predetermined minimal number of patients should be entered at each institution participating in a multicenter trial because sites that entered few patients did not perform as at high a standard of quality. In special situations, a maximum rate of enrollment can be established; this can help prevent the problem of patients entering too rapidly to allow for adequate evaluation, or at a rate that strains staff resources. Burns et al. (1990) reported losing 200 potential enrollees who had called the site in response to a newspaper advertisement, because of the staff's inability to process the inquiries. Scheduling special pre-entry testing, arranging clinic space for follow-up visits, or asssuring the ability of trial staff to maintain the administrative work load are factors that must be considered in determining a maximum recruitment rate or maximum quota.

A separate issue is the establishment of a maximum number of patients who may be enrolled at a particular site in a multicenter trial. This number may be calculated simply by dividing the total sample size required by the number of sites. In many cases various factors (e.g., investigator enthusiasm, patient availability, previous enrollment history) changes this number for one or more sites. On occasion, a multicenter trial attempts to use maximum quotas to maintain a more even distribution of total patient enrollment across all sites and not allow any site to far exceed its overall total number. In most cases, it is acceptable to increase the maximum number of patients for one or more sites to account for under-recruitment at other sites, but this should be discussed with a statistician because a great imbalance may affect the ability to pool data (e.g., if unbalanced blocks are obtained at some sites, if patients recruited differ in important ways from those at other sites, if data obtained are quite different in terms of the amount of missing data). If randomization is balanced within sites, pooling of the data generally should not cause any problems.

Whether a maximum quota should be imposed depends on the design and size of a trial. For extremely large trials (e.g., over 1,000 patients), including major multicenter trials with over 5,000 patients, it makes little sense to impose an upper limit of patients at any site. For small trials, however, if one site totally dominates recruitment because an upper limit was not established, there could be major implications for the statistical validity of combining data and of reaching a valid clinical interpretation.

Types of Quotas

Screening Quotas

Screening quotas are more difficult to establish than enrollment quotas, particularly if novel protocols (i.e., those for which no prior experience exists) are used. Prior experience with similar inclusion criteria usually provides an estimate of the degree of difficulty (or simplicity) of finding patients to screen. In such cases, screening quotas can be readily established in advance. Both naive and experienced investigators often have great difficulty guessing how extensively they will have to comb the community to find patients to screen, particularly for rigorously defined patient populations (i.e., trials with strict inclusion criteria). In these situations, a pilot trial may be initiated that is either part, or independent, of the main trial. In either case the screening goals and/or recruitment methods can be redefined as experience with the recruitment campaign develops.

Enrollment and Completer Quotas

Quotas for patient enrollment and completion usually can be established easily simply by dividing the required sample size by the number of sites. It is common

TABLE 9.1. *Patient intake characteristics of nine Veterans Administration multihospital clinical trials*

Study	Number of hospitals	Initial patient enrollment target	Target rate of enrollment per hospital per month	Number of randomized patients	Final rate of enrollment per hospital per month	Lowest monthly site enrollment rate	Highest monthly site enrollment rate	Number months extended
Aphasia I	5	160	1.33	68	0.32	0.1	0.6	18
Ulcer	15	600	1.67	81	0.34	0.1	0.8	0—Terminated
Antabuse	6	216	3.00	82	0.35	0.4	1.0	27—Terminated
Chronic brain	10	600	4.29	89	0.64	0.1	1.4	0—Terminated
Sleep	3	113	1.26	102	0.87	—	—	10
Aphasia II	5	135	0.75	122	0.51	0.6	0.8	12
Diabetes	11	456	1.90	231	0.59	0.3	0.9	16
Nursing Home	8	1200	5.00	403	1.20	0.5	2.5	18
Epilepsy	10	480	1.21	569	1.19	0.3	1.8	12

Adapted from Williford et al. (1987) and from Collins et al. (1984) (lowest and highest monthly site enrollment rate columns) with permission.

TABLE 9.2. *Recruitment data for 13 studies funded by NHLBI*

| Study | Number of subjects recruited | | | Recruitment time | Person-years in planned recruitment period |
	Actual	Planned	Actual/planned	Actual/planned	Actual/planned
AMIS	4,524	4,250	1.06	1.00	0.83
BHAT	3,837	4,020	0.95	1.21	0.82
CAPS	502	500	1.00	1.08	0.82
CARDIA	5,182	5,100	1.02	1.00	0.86
CDP	8,345	8,380	1.00	1.22	0.55
CSSCD	3,241	3,220	1.01	1.13	1.16
HDFP	10,940	10,500	1.04	1.50	1.02
LRC	3,843	3,550	1.08	1.54	0.34
MILIS	985	1,200	0.82	2.71	0.35
MRFIT	12,866	12,000	1.07	1.13	0.81
POSCH	838	1,000	0.84	1.58	0.25
SHEP pilot	551	500	1.10	1.17	0.71
TIMI-I	316	340	0.93	0.96	0.98

From Probstfield et al. (1987) with permission.

practice, however, for sites with larger population bases or more extensive referral patterns to be assigned higher than average quotas, and vice versa for smaller sites. Additional resources (e.g., trial coordinator or assistant) can be provided to sites that exceed their recruitment goals, or these resources can be shifted from less productive sites. This system can be used to balance recruitment activities across all sites in a multicenter trial without overwhelming some of the smaller sites with unrealistic requirements. Two numbers for completed patients may be assigned to each site. The first is a quota that represents a *minimal number* and the second is a *maximum number* that is the largest number of patients that may be enrolled and complete the trial. Table 9.1 describes the recruitment characteristics of nine multicenter trials that fell behind the originally planned enrollment rates. The recruitment period was extended in seven trials by 10 to 27 months and six of these trials were completed. Three trials were terminated because of the apparent inability to reach the goal. Similar experiences for trials sponsored by the National Heart, Lung, and Blood Institute are listed in Table 9.2. Recruitment fell short of established goals in four of 13 trials, although the recruitment period was extended in ten of 13 trials to reach the goal.

Sequential trials represent a special case in patient recruitment because the total number of patients to be enrolled is unknown at the start of the trial and depends on the results obtained. Statistical textbooks describe the methods to determine when enrollment may be considered complete. Nonetheless, the principles of the methods to recruit patients and the use of screening, enrollment, and completer quotas is the same as for more traditional trials. These goals of specific rates of patients screened, enrolled, or completed per week, month, or 3 months are as helpful and important in these trials as in others. Only the total number of completed patients is unknown during most of the clinical trial.

USING QUOTAS

Use of Quotas to Measure Progress

Dividing the recruitment period into time periods of equal lengths with specific quotas for patient screening and enrollment in each provides a simple method to measure recruitment progress. Lower screening rates or smaller numbers of patients enrolled usually signal problems that should be investigated immediately. When quotas are consistently unmet, the ability to complete the trial may be jeopardized.

Quotas are an important method to determine the adequacy of screening and whether the trial as a whole, or an individual site, should proceed or be terminated. If a site is terminated, a determination must be made about follow-up of the already enrolled patients. Although a monitoring committee often makes these decisions in multicenter trials, single-site investigators must also assess the viability of their trial based on their ability to enter eligible patients. Each investigator recognizes that failure to meet minimum recruitment quotas month after month means that their trial will not be completed within what they originally defined as a reasonable time period. The waste of one or more investigator's time as well as other resources may be greatly increased when a trial is extended unrealistically in one or more centers in the vain hope of finding and enrolling a sufficient number of patients.

Relationships Among Types of Quotas

In most circumstances, screening large numbers of potential enrollees is the optimum method for finding and enrolling appropriate patients into a trial. If the typical enrollment rate for a specific trial is 10% of screenees, then at least ten times as many patients must be screened to fulfill enrollment quotas. If 5% of randomized patients drop out of their own volition and fail to complete the protocol, an extra 5% of patients may have to be enrolled (if stated in the protocol) to meet the completer quota. These obvious numerical relationships among types of quotas make it relatively straightforward and possible (1) to adjust and refine specific quotas at any point during the trial, (2) to compare recruitment results between different periods of the trial, and (3) to compare recruitment data with similar trials where recruitment data are known. Relationships among the types of quotas are illustrated in Fig. 9.1. This figure also presents a number of options to consider when a specific quota is not being achieved.

Predictions of Recruitment Rates

Trials usually begin with an estimate of the recruitment rate needed to reach the goal by a specific target date. Some trials continue to accrue patients without any time limit until their recruitment goal is fulfilled. The majority of trials specify an amount of time allocated for patient recruitment because of financial considerations and the necessity of establishing an overall or estimated budget for the trial (see Chapter 6, Economic Issues). Although the length of the recruitment period may be based on conjecture, optimum conditions in a pilot trial, or prior experience, there is no way to know with certainty how long it will take to recruit and enter the required number of patients.

Calculation of the availability of potential patients in the catchment area is a first step in estimating whether quotas can be met for many types of trials. Zifferblatt (1975) described a simple formula to calculate the net fraction of the total population in an area that would meet enrollment criteria for a trial. This number is that fraction of patients who meet age, sex, and physiological entry criteria, and who have no exclusionary characteristics, multiplied by the fraction of patients screened. An im-

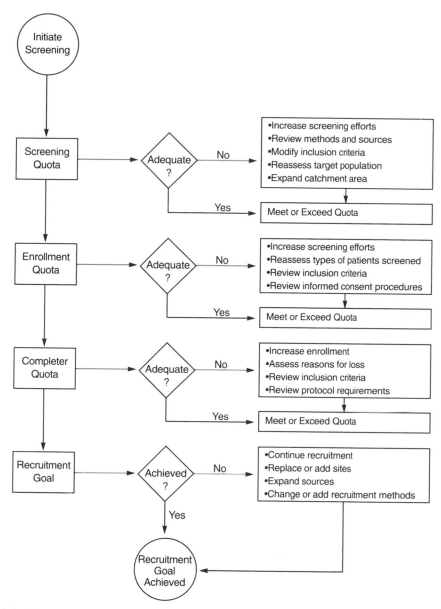

FIG. 9.1. Relationships among the several types of quotas. A number of options to consider are also shown if a quota is not being met.

portant caveat to the use of this formula is that the fraction of patients who pass the screening can be estimated only after experience is accrued with the particular inclusion criteria.

Moussa (1984) developed a computer program to predict the course of recruitment. Again, the accuracy of these projections is enhanced when the recruitment rate is established or readjusted in an ongoing trial. Among other considerations, Moussa described how to: (1) calculate the constant and nonconstant recruitment rates, (2) develop a monitoring plan for interim goals, (3) determine the likelihood of meeting the overall goal based on earlier recruitment rates, and (4) determine the length of an extension period needed to meet recruitment goals.

A periodic report of patient recruitment at different sites in a clinical trial may be shown graphically (Figs. 7.11 to 7.15) or in a table (Table 9.3).

Planning to Achieve Minimum Screening Quotas

The following are seven steps to be used in the planning process for establishing minimum screening quotas:

1. Review the experience of other investigations using similar protocols that recruited populations resembling the one you wish to use.
2. Estimate the number of patients screened in other trials to yield an adequate number of randomized and completing patients.
3. Compare the differences between the current protocol and others in terms of eligibility criteria, time constraints to completion, and incentives to patients, as well as changes in the local population.
4. Extrapolate how the differences between previous trials and the ongoing trial will affect recruitment for the current trial.
5. Select a system of screening based on achieving the expected yield (e.g., screen ten times as many patients as needed in order to yield one randomized patient), or based on expected activity at the site (e.g., expect to screen all patients seen at weekly clinics plus all ward patients daily, or use a combination of both systems).
6. Review the screening system(s) monthly or quarterly to assess its outcome and productivity. Use current data to develop the yield data for the ongoing trial. Plot changes in yield over time for lengthy trials and note the time points at which changes to the recruitment system were made.
7. Adjust the screening quota and systems used based on actual enrollment and the level of activity at the site.

Planning to Achieve Minimum Enrollment Quotas

Similar to the concepts described above for screening, three steps for establishing the enrollment quotas are listed.

1. Determine the amount of time available to perform the trial and the maximum

TABLE 9.3. *Sample layout for a periodic recruitment report*

Site number	Number of patients screened during previous period (e.g., month)	Number of patients enrolled during previous period (e.g., month)	Number of patients projected to be enrolled	Total number of patients projected for enrollment
1				
2				
3				
4				
5				
. . .				
n				

length of the recruitment phase. Calculate the number of patients who must be entered monthly or quarterly to reach the recruitment goal.

2. Consider the staff time (e.g., physicians, nurses, research assistants, secretaries), facilities (e.g., interview or examining rooms, office space and telephone, pharmacy space for investigational medicine), and other resources (e.g., printing and distribution of flyers or posters, cost of advertisements) needed to maintain the trial at a low or high pace. Is a specific person hired to work full-time on patient recruitment for this program? Is sufficient space allocated to this trial? Are adequate funds designated for supplies? If staff resources are underutilized when recruitment is low, can they be redeployed to other projects? If inadequate staff time spent on recruitment is a reason for low enrollment, can it be expanded? For example, part-time attention to recruitment can usually be expanded with additional time from the investigator, research assistants, clinic staff, and ancillary personnel (e.g., laboratory technicians, housestaff).

3. Determine if the minimum enrollment quota can be achieved with available resources of time, money, and facilities. Is the trial utilizing excessive resources relative to the number of patients screened, entered, and actively participating? Is the trial understaffed, underfunded, or given inadequate facilities to process the number of patients available? How much effort can the staff spend on difficult patients (e.g., those who are less cooperative, more tardy in completing tasks, do not maintain diaries, do not comply with the protocol, do not return for follow-up) and how many total patients can realistically be handled each month? Consideration of these questions helps ensure that minimum enrollment quotas are met for each recruitment period.

SCREENING LOGS

Records should be maintained that describe the characteristics of patients who are entered into the trial as well as those who are eliminated from further evaluation and the reason(s) for their elimination. These data provide important information not only for the ongoing trial but also for future trials run by the same group, and, if published, for other investigators as well. Screening logs provide the basis for assessing and evaluating progress toward the recruitment goal of the trial. This is achieved by tabulating the number and type of patients screened and randomized in the trial. For the screening log to be an effective tool, it is essential that trial staff record all patient screenings, even if an individual is obviously ineligible, and use a consistent method both inter- and intra-site. Whether 1% or 30% of patients screened meet the inclusion criteria and enter a trial, the details of those screened but not entered are an important part of the trial record. Charlson and Horwitz (1984) consider that trials should not be criticized for lack of generalizability because of the high ratio of patients not entered, as long as screening data document the differences between the groups. The purposes and uses of screening information are described below.

Purposes of Screening Logs

1. Screening data may be used to quantify the productivity of each site. This is done by counting the number of prospective participants evaluated and also the

number of patients enrolled during each recruitment period. Screening data readily show whether sites are screening enough patients to meet their quotas, and also illustrate if each site has an unusually high or low rejection rate.

2. Screening data may be used to define the types of patients who are initially contacted and reviewed, and whether they do or do not meet all of the inclusion criteria. Contacts may be patient or site initiated, or both approaches may be used.

3. Screening data may be used to document the overall population assessed and can allow comparisons to be made between those patients enrolled and those who did not enter the trial.

4. Screening data allow an assessment to be made of the potential to extrapolate trial results. This evaluation is based on a comparison of major characteristics of the population enrolled versus those of the general population screened (see Chapter 12, Extrapolation of Results).

5. Identifying every potential trial candidate allows tabulation of the number of patients in the catchment area who have the type of disease being evaluated. These data may help provide the denominator for epidemiological studies.

6. Screening data can be used to determine the prevalence of various problems that result in ineligiblity for the trial.

7. The number of patients screened is a direct measure of the efficiency of a specific recruitment method to interest patients in the trial. This assumes that all patients screened during a specific period were recruited using a single method. Different methods could be compared over time. For example, the amount of screening activity after implementation of a new technique (e.g., letters to local physicians) can be used to evaluate the value of that effort.

8. The amount of staff activity devoted to recruitment, and the productivity of that staff may be measured indirectly using screening records. However, the size of the local population base is a major determinant of the possible quantity of screening and must be considered if different sites are compared.

9. One of the primary uses of screening logs *during* a trial is as a source to search for clues as to why patients are being rejected from the trial. If an excessive number of patients are discontinued for the same reason and enrollment is low, then consideration should be given to whether the inclusion criteria or some other factor should be modified. The log that lists the reasons why patients refuse to sign the informed consent may demonstrate various requirements in the protocol that patients find onerous and which possibly could be modified. For example, the problem could be that there are too many clinic visits scheduled, too many tests scheduled at each clinic visit, no chance for patients to receive the new medicine after the trial if it is found to be active, or too great a chance for patients to receive placebo.

10. After a trial is completed, screening logs are used to compare medical characteristics of various patient groups to assess the extrapolatability of data obtained to other groups.

Information to Include in a Screening Log

Screening logs usually are organized as questionnaires. They should include a variety of questions that are pertinent to defining the patient population (e.g., demographic information, presumed diagnosis, reasons why the individual is excluded from further evaluation or continues toward enrollment). Examples of screening logs are shown in Figs. 9.1 to 9.4 and in a reference by Swinehart (1991). The basic types of information that should be collected in a screening log include the following:

1. An accession number is assigned to every person who is considered a potential trial candidate, even if disqualifying factors are obvious. The series of patient numbers used for this process is generally different than the patient numbers used for randomized patients. To prevent confusion, the screening code numbers could use a prefix letter or number (e.g., S001 or 9001 would be assigned to the first patient screened and 001 for the first patient enrolled). Accession numbers should be assigned in chronological order.

2. The date of screening should be listed. Changing patterns or trends in the population's medical characteristics can be identified more easily if this is done.

3. The person's name or other personal identification number (e.g., social security number, hospital unit number) is listed so that no individual is screened more than once. Although the full name and social security number are preferable, privacy regulations sometimes prohibit their use. Initials and date of birth are an alternative, albeit less effective, method of patient identification.

4. The demographic characteristics including date of birth (rather than age), sex, race, level of education, level of employment, and employment status, are recorded to describe the population being screened. Not all of these items are usually known at the time of initial screening, or are even available for the clinical trial staff.

Protocol Number _____ Title _____

_____

Month: _____ 19 _____

Date In Month	Number of Patients Contacted re: Clinical Trial	Number of Patients Contacted But Not Screened	Number of Patients Screened
1	2	1	1
2	3	0	3
3	0	—	—
4	4	4	0
5	2	1	1
6	1	0	1
7	6	3	3
8	2	1	1
•••	•••	•••	•••
31	7	7	0
TOTAL =	N	X	Y

FIG. 9.2. Sample logsheet of potential patients contacted about a clinical trial. Reproduced from Spilker (1991) with permission.

Protocol Number ______________ Title ______________________________ Month & Year ______________

Date In Month	Number of Patients Screened	Number of Patients Disqualified at Screen	Reasons for Disqualification of Patients at Screen[a]												
			1	2	3	4	5	6	7	8	9	10	11	12	Other:
1	2	1			✓										
2	4	0													
3	4	4					✓			✓		✓			✓ Pain resolved spontaneously ✓ Primarily due to anxiety
4	2	1													
5	0	0													
6	3	3					✓✓				✓				
7	6	1			✓										
8	1	0													
•	•	•													
•	•	•													
•	•	•													
31	11	7			✓		✓				✓		✓	✓	✓✓ Pain in wrong location
TOTAL =	Y	Z	A	B	C	D	E	F	G	H	I	J	K	L	M

[a] 1 = Patients age or weight outside of inclusion criteria
2 = Previous medical history unacceptable
3 = Alcohol or drug abuse
4 = Recent surgery
5 = Insufficient severity of symptom
6 = Insufficient duration of symptom
7 = Presence of concomitant medicine
8 = Previous participation in clinical trial
9 = Medicine allergies
10 to 12 = Other defined reasons

FIG. 9.3. Sample logsheet of potential patients disqualified during the screening process. Reproduced from Spilker (1991) with permission.

5. The disease characteristics pertinent to the inclusion criteria including current and prior medical diagnoses, current medicines (including doses), date of onset of pertinent diagnosis, date of onset of present episode, and type and duration of treatment(s). These data provide information about the medical status of the screening pool. All major inclusion criteria described in the protocol should be listed on the screening log as a definition of the eligibility of enrollees. There are some exceptions to this rule, e.g., a screening log for a telephone screen of only the most major inclusion criteria, listing of only identifiers and reasons for exclusion on the screening log, and using data collection forms to check off the inclusion criteria.

6. Prognostic characteristics of the disease are critical to ascertain. These would include identification of all risk factors, aspects of the past history of treatment that influence response to new treatment, and characteristics of the disease that influence patient outcome. The same exceptions and caveats exist as for point number five.

7. Reasons for rejecting each patient (e.g., inappropriate diagnosis, inappropriate current medication or other therapy, too long or too brief a duration of the illness, too mild or too severe symptoms) provide information that is helpful in understanding the ability to extrapolate data.

8. The referral source or method of recruitment that reached the patient may be listed to provide information about the effectiveness of each recruitment method (e.g., media, poster, individual letter). Obtaining details on which specific letter, advertisement, or poster location usually can help in designing which recruitment methods should be emphasized.

How to Develop a Screening Log for a Specific Trial

Deciding what to include in a screening log will depend on the complexity of the disease itself, the size of the trial, the importance of the trial, and the protocol used. The amount of information to be collected should be determined after considering the eight categories described above. Apart from basic demographic data and patient identifiers (e.g., patient code), it is most important to collect prognostic characteristics and the reason(s) why patients are excluded at each stage of recruitment. Computer screens may be designed to enter these data, or paper forms may be used. A single separate log should be created for each major step of recruitment, rather than attempting to collect all data on a single form. For example, the reasons for patient exclusion relating to informed consent are collected separately from reasons why some patients fail to pass specific inclusion criteria. It is possible to combine data and summarize the number and percent of patients who did not pass each step of the recruitment process. This subject is discussed further in Chapter 11.

When to List a Patient in the Screening Log

Direct contacts to patients (e.g., with letters) may be used to specify that all patients contacted are given accession numbers at the time of the mailing. Alternatively, only patients who respond or complete a preliminary screen may be given accession numbers. This may occur at the time of the telephone or mail response. Another approach is to give accession numbers only to those patients who attend the screening visit at the clinic (at the time of the screening visit).

For *indirect* contacts with patients (e.g., advertising), it is possible to list all patients who respond to the advertisement and to give them accession numbers (at the time of the telephone, mail, or personal response). Alternatively, only patients who complete the primary screening phase may be given an accession number. This occurs after the telephone, mail, or personal response to the advertisement is reviewed. Finally, only patients who pass the primary screen and attend the secondary screening visit at the clinic may be given accession numbers (i.e., at the time of the clinic visit).

Use of Screening Logs to Assess Recruitment Efficiency

Screening logs can be used to demonstrate apparent enhanced or diminished site and staff efficiency, particularly in multicenter trials. If screening logs are maintained assiduously so that every patient approached who is walking down the hospital's corridor is listed, the site and recruitment coordinator will appear to be active. However, this large amount of apparent activity can be deceptive, depending on whether the actual enrollment rate and number is low or high. Conversely, if screening logs are not completed for many patients who are casually reviewed and rejected, but the number of entries at that site is average, the site will appear to have a deceptively high ratio of entries.

The real effectiveness of recruitment, however, must be judged by the number of patients enrolled and not by the number of patients screened or by the apparent yield. The major purpose of a screening log is as a tool to aid in enrollment. Thus, it is important to prevent the use of the log from interfering with the recruitment effort. Nonetheless, the other purposes of the log (e.g., to aid in extrapolatability of results) must not be ignored if a decision to discontinue use of the log is considered.

Scrutiny of screening logs by the coordinating center and conversations with the recruitment coordinator and other staff about their system for recording screening data may reveal practices that are rather unusual or inconsistent with the national standard. For example, some sites may ignore selected questions on the screening log because the answers are not readily available without a careful chart review or patient interview (e.g., marital status, or age of onset of the disease). Lapses in recording data on screening logs can be detected by finding gaps in entries. In single-site trials, inconsistencies in the style of collecting information either between staff (e.g., different styles to determine patients' current functional level, or different level of searching for a list of medicines previously used for the disease) or because of cyclical pressures, can cause the same artifacts as described for multicenter trials.

The number of patient contacts in various screening logs can provide misleading information. Staff may casually review patients and not record them on a screening log because of their obvious ineligibility. Further, the same single-line entry in a patient log is usually given to an individual rejected from the trial after an extensive and expensive evaluation as is given to someone whose rejection is based on a 2-minute review of a medical chart. Patients who are fully eligible for the trial and reach the point of invitation to participate but decline to enter at the point of informed consent are listed as refusers because they are a separate group. Another issue is that unusually high refusal rates require an investigation to determine whether the trial is being presented to patients in an appropriate manner by staff, or whether other factors are causing a negative reaction in potential candidates (e.g., trial site location, clinic hours).

ASSESSING PATIENT "YIELD" AT EACH SITE

The relationship between screening and enrollment is usually similar at different sites in a multicenter trial so that an average yield of enrollees to screenees can be calculated. This yield could be expressed as one patient randomized in the trial for every so many (e.g., ten) patients who undergo the primary screen (1:10). Some sites will probably have a higher (e.g., 1:5) or lower (e.g., 1:20) yield. Some sites may exceed the number of patients required to be screened during each period but fail to meet enrollment quotas, or vice versa. Because screening is usually required to enroll patients, low screening rates are acceptable if adequate numbers of patients are enrolled and randomized to treatment. However, this pattern would suggest a rich pool that might yield even higher enrollment rates if patients were screened more effectively. This pattern could also indicate complacency at the site about screening because staff understand that they can readily meet monthly recruitment goals.

Sites that screen many patients but find few appropriate trial candidates to enroll might need to examine their approach to patients and seek the reason(s) for their problems. If this problem occurs at most or all sites it could indicate problems with protocol requirements or inappropriately restrictive inclusion criteria.

ESTABLISHING A FAIR QUOTA SYSTEM

Steps to Avoid Lasagna's Law

Avoiding the trend described by Lasagna's Law (actual enrollment is approximately 10% of that anticipated) should be a major goal of all clinical investigators. To achieve this goal requires knowledge of the pitfalls to avoid plus knowledge of the factors to consider in achieving successful recruitment.

1. Assess whether the inclusion criteria expected to exclude most patients may be relaxed.
2. Assess whether the staff have sufficient time, equipment, facilities, and interest in screening the number of patients required to yield the necessary number of enrollees.
3. Assess how much effort the staff can spend on difficult patients (e.g., those who are less cooperative, are tardy to complete tasks, do not maintain diaries, do not comply with the protocol, do not return for follow-up) and how many total patients can realistically be handled each month.
4. Assess the motivation of patients to enter and to complete the clinical trial.
5. Assess the number of staff available to conduct the trial and those required to process the requisite number of patients.
6. Do the investigators have experience recruiting the types of patients to be entered in the clinical trial? If so, how much experience do they have?
7. Can the investigators document their capability to enroll the required number of patients?
8. Conduct reviews of charts prior to making a commitment to including a specific investigator. Use the inclusion criteria to evaluate the number of patients who meet all of them and then discuss them with the investigator to evaluate the number who are likely to pass all screens and would enroll. While this may be

done for patients in the investigator's practice for chronically ill patients, if the trial studies acute disease or emergency cases, it will not be possible. In that case, review all patients seen over the last 3 to 6 months to determine the number who would have been eligible. In some countries only the investigator or his or her staff may review actual patient medical records and patient names must be held confidential through use of initials or a code.

The Value of Experience

Extensive experience in recruitment does not necessarily mean that the same investigators conducting the same type of clinical trial a few years later will have the same experiences. Many factors may differ, some obvious and others more subtly. For example, replicating a protocol to evaluate epilepsy medications in sequential VA Cooperative Studies, Mattson et al. (1985 and 1992) had to screen more than twice as many patients to randomize one-third fewer participants compared with their own earlier trial. In another example, the initial marketing of cimetidine drastically reduced the number of patients being referred to ulcer surgery trials (Collins, 1980). Far fewer patients were interested or willing to join a surgical trial when an alternative medical treatment was available. A similar situation occurred with the testing of other medicines for ulcers. Now that most ulcer patients are well treated with medicines, it is extremely difficult to conduct that type of trial today, either for surgical treatment or to evaluate a new medicine.

Quotas should not be taken from one trial and used in similar trials for many reasons. There are also reasons why quotas should be changed during the course of a clinical trial.

1. More patients may have moved into or outside of the catchment area. The demographic distribution of patients with a specific disease may change markedly within a short time period in any catchment area.
2. Investigators and staff may have changed positions; referring physicians may no longer be seeing patients suitable for referral, or their attitudes about referral may have changed.
3. New medicines or other treatments may be available and patients may therefore be less interested in the treatment options offered in the proposed trial, as in the above example of ulcer medication.
4. By chance, more patients attending a clinic or referred to it may have mild or severe disease symptoms. For example, more public attention may have led many patients to receive an earlier diagnosis and treatment than in the past. As a result, fewer patients with severe problems can be found.
5. A similar trial may be underway in the same community. This trial could be led by the same, or other, investigators. It will undoubtedly draw patients from the same pool of eligible patients, and make quotas unattainable that would have been reasonable a short time before.
6. The protocol may be slightly different from that used in the prior trial or in a pilot trial.

Developing a Quota System in Single-Site Trials

Trials performed at one site range from unfunded projects undertaken by a solitary investigator to large trials carried out by a consortium of investigators and research staff supported by major grants or contracts. The ability to monitor recruitment goals is facilitated with a quota system no matter how small the trial. Some of the major considerations for the investigator are:

1. Consider what can be done if the quota is not met once, occasionally, or regularly. Is it feasible or necessary to alter any aspect of the recruitment process or the protocol? Can resources used for recruitment be increased? Can the time period for recruitment be extended? Can additional recruitment methods be implemented?

2. Determine at what point the investigator should determine whether the trial is still viable. For example, establish a time at which to evaluate whether the trial should be continued or be terminated. This could be a fixed time (e.g., one year after the first patient is recruited) or at a fixed percent completion (e.g., when 40% of patients are enrolled).

3. Could the resources allocated for this trial be redistributed to another clinical research activity rather than maintaining a weak recruitment program for a trial that probably will not fulfill its recruitment goal? Discontinuing a nonviable trial early allows alternative plans to be implemented by the sponsor or the consortium of investigators (e.g., initiation of a different trial, refining the clinical methodology in a new pilot trial).

The use of quota systems may create problems. Table 9.4 gives examples of various types of problems, their results, interpretation, and possible outcomes. For example, the second example indicates that although the number of patients screened is below expectations, adequate numbers of patients are enrolling and completing the trial. No real problem exists because the screening quota is higher than necessary.

Developing a Quota System in Multicenter Trials

Multicenter trials are amenable to use of screening, enrollment, and completer quotas because of their central organization and monitoring procedures. The major steps to develop a quota system are as follows:

1. Establish the timetable to use for a specific number of monthly or quarterly quotas. For example, trial sites could be asked to screen a minimum of 20 patients monthly and to enroll a minimum of 3 patients monthly for the duration of the recruitment period. Each site could be contacted prior to an annual review and asked to complete a specific number of patients within the next 3-month period to meet their recruitment goal for the year.

2. Define exactly what will happen to a site if their quota is not met for one or two recruitment periods. Explain whether the site will be put on probation with a more exacting screening or enrollment quota, or whether it will be summarily closed down a certain number of months after the target date. It is far better to determine and communicate all of the consequences prior to the trial's initiation and ensure that all investigators understand this issue.

3. Consider what will happen to patients who are already participating in a long-term trial if their site is closed down. Will enough staff be retained to continue long-term follow-up? Will only recruitment be stopped at that site but follow-up activities continue, or will there be a total closure of the site? Will patients be transferred to an alternate site? If so, where will it be located? Can long-term patients be followed by mail and telephone contacts from a remote site? When

TABLE 9.4. *Types of problems in meeting quotas*

Type of quota					
Number screened	Number enrolled	Number of completers[b]	Issue or problem	Possible reasons	Possible outcome
+	+	+	No problem	Large or rich population base Special recruitment methods	Successful recruitment
−	+	+	No problem	Screen quota too high or irrelevant	Lower screening quota
+	−	+	No problem	Enrollment quota too high Special retention techniques	Lower enrollment quota
−	−	+	No problem	Screen and enrollment quotas too high	Lower quotas
+	+	−	High loss rate during trial	Protocol too arduous	Must replace losses Need tighter inclusion criteria to reject patients unable to complete trial
−	+	−	High loss rate	Enrollees unable to finish protocol	Must replace losses Review informed consent procedures Change methods of screening Close site
+	−	−	Low enrollment rate	Screening ineligible population	Review informed consent procedures Close site
−	−	−	Non-performing site	Insufficient local population Inadequate recruitment plans Staff inefficient or unenthusiastic	Have an emergency meeting to discuss options Place on probation Close site

[a] Adequate number of patients completing the trial to reach overall trial goal.
+, conducted successfully; −, not conducted successfully.

256

will patients be told that their site is being closed and that their participation in the trial is being discontinued? Even if all safety data are usable, what efficacy data from that site will be considered usable in the trial's analyses?

4. Firmly maintain the probation and termination procedures for investigators who do not meet recruitment quotas. Establishing and defining a quota system requires that the trial organizers consider all of the above issues in advance of the trial's initiation and develop an equitable and reasonable quota system. The plan should be reasonable and agreed to by all investigators. At that point it should be implemented and proceed without backsliding despite various internal or external pressures. Closure of a site unfortunately affects the salaries of trial staff more frequently than those of the investigators. Nonetheless, few sponsors can afford to support a trial site that is not contributing adequately to the overall recruitment plan.

Establishing a Probation System

An interim step in a quota system is to place sites on probation if they do not meet quotas. The length of time of unacceptable recruitment that places a site on probation must vary depending on the total period of recruitment, urgency of completing it on time, and duration of the trial. If recruitment is divided into periods, then failing to achieve quotas for two consecutive periods is one measure that could place a site on probation. Probation gives the site an extra period to address local problems and to increase recruitment. This tactic is most successful when the trial managers think that the principal investigator or staff are not sufficiently motivated or are not giving sufficient attention to recruitment. Many trial sites show a miraculous turnaround after the attention of investigators and staff is refocused and pressure is applied through placing them on probation (or merely indicating that this will occur). For example, increased enrollments may occur prior to or shortly after (1) a meeting of investigators, (2) a quota is imposed, (3) probation is decreed, or (4) a site visit is scheduled. Investigators or staff who work on multiple trials simultaneously are most likely to be influenced by this approach.

The probation system (or its threatened imposition) might need to be maintained to sustain the pace of enrollment in a trial. However, if a site has a continuous record of low enrollment, further delays allowed by a probation period may not be productive. If enrollment has fluctuated widely and appears to be correlated with staff efforts, the patient population probably is available for screening and enrollment. In this case, probation might provide the necessary stimulus for some sites to maintain higher rates of recruitment. However, a site should not be allowed to remain on probation indefinitely. It might be decided, for example, that if a site is on probation for 6 continuous months or a total of 10 months, it will be closed. Criteria for a site to be removed from probation must be clearly stated (e.g., one or two adequate recruitment periods).

Implementing a Quota System During an Ongoing Trial

A quota system should be designed during the clinical trial planning process and included as part of the protocol. Nonetheless, a quota system can be added to an ongoing trial. Implementation of a quota system while a trial is in progress generally will be perceived as a punitive measure occurring in response to a problem. Such a focus on slow sites exposes them to peer pressure and heightens concern for their viability. The protocol must specify whether a site that has entered twice its quota in one recruitment period must enter its quota in the next period to avoid probation, or whether a carryover system (i.e., future credit for past enrollment) will be used. A carryover system is recommended because if there is no carryover system, then even sites with high rates of accrual will feel concern over their ability to retain the necessary recruitment rates. Quota plans that are implemented as a crisis management technique are extremely delicate matters that should be undertaken with the understanding that some sites will probably fail and have to be closed, and that the morale of others *could* be negatively impacted. A carryover system will help assure active sites that they do not have to stockpile patients for subsequent recruitment periods.

Trial organizers, investigators, and staff should be convinced (insofar as possible) not to perceive quotas as punitive measures. Instead, quotas should be viewed as an effective method to improve recruitment after standard recruitment methods have proven inadequate or failed. The two most important principles in implementing a quota system are that (1) quotas are designed to aid the clinical trial by stimulating patient recruitment, and (2) quotas should not damage the trial (e.g., destroy staff morale, remove sites that are recruiting the maximum number of patients in their catchment area). Public exposure and peer pressure are the major factors that force investigators to bring forth an influx of patients after a quota is imposed during an ongoing clinical trial. Such stories are plentiful among experienced clinical trial managers, although few are published to provide comfort to others facing the same dilemma.

Suggestions for implementing a quota system during an ongoing multicenter trial include:

1. Calculate the total number of patients still needed from all sites to meet the screening, enrollment, and completer goals in the remaining weeks, months, or years of the trial.

2. Plan what type of quota system to implement. Decide whether to ask high accessioning sites to continue to recruit at their previous above-average rate, thereby allowing for a smaller quota to be implemented at currently slow sites, or whether to establish a uniform quota for all sites. This latter approach is not generally recommended because the sites will have already shown differences in recruitment, and the trial organizers should take advantage of these differences. If the slow sites enroll at least a reasonable number of patients, there are no critical statistical problems with an unbalanced quota system.

3. Assess whether a site has low screening or enrollment rates because of a small population base that will never provide an average or adequate number of eligible patients. If so, consult with statisticians and other experts to decide whether maintaining the site with lower expectations is wiser than closing or replacing it.

4. Identify the slow-accessioning sites that are likely to fail to meet their quotas. Usually, a few sites in a large group will lag far behind the mean and others will far exceed the mean. Slow sites may be made aware of their "poor" performance through newsletters and periodic reports, as well as anxious telephone calls from the coordinating center and trial chairman.

5. One or more people should be appointed to counsel slow sites about a variety

Protocol Number _____

Title: _____

Week	Dates	Number of Patients Screened	Number of Patients Passing Screen	Number of Patients Enrolled In Trial	Reasons for Nonenrollment by Successfully Screened Patients					
					No Interest	Insufficient Inducements	Informed Consent Not Signed	Inadequate Time	Lives Too Far	Other (List)
1	Jan 14-20	17	12	10			1	1	1	
2	Jan 21-27	24	20	14	1	2	2			
3	Jan 28-Feb 3	14	14	13		1				
4										
5										
6										
7										

FIG. 9.4. Sample logsheet of potential patients entered in a clinical trial. Reproduced from Spilker (1991) with permission.

of methods that may be used to enhance screening and recruitment in general (see Chapter 8) and to inform them of some important issues that may be pertinent to their locale. Try to resolve any special problems that exist in the trial before implementing a quota system. Examples of such problems include a temporary lack of an overall recruitment coordinator, inadequate telephone lines that temporarily hinder recruitment, and other problems discussed throughout this volume. It behooves the trial organizers to work with slow sites before considering probation or termination. Sites should have a chance to work out their specific local problems and to establish a workable system to screen and enroll patients.

6. Decide what action will be taken when a site fails to meet a quota and how long to wait before taking action. Because the trial is ongoing, the records of *actual* screening and enrollment rates can be used to estimate whether to act in 1 or 2 months or to wait for 6 or more months. Choices of actions range from merely chiding the slow site, to putting a site on probation, to direct closure of a site. Quotas should not be used merely to apply pressure and to harass the staff. Those techniques soon lose any degree of effectiveness they might initially have.

Announcement of a Quota System During a Clinical Trial

The proposal to announce a final quota that must be met or face closure of the site, and the issue of probation should be discussed with principal investigators before the general announcement is made. Be sure that trial staff are fully aware of the ramifications of using a quota system because they may be personally affected by staff cutbacks or site closure. Staff should be made aware if their prior or current recruitment strategies are not working. They need to consider all methods to enhance recruitment (see Chapter 8), including strategies previously used without success (for reasons now known), or strategies that they have never tried.

Explain that the new quota system and patient log data will help identify reasons why recruitment remains slow. A "last chance" quota plan can be used to demonstrate to all sites and to a monitoring board (if one is present) that the slow sites cannot perform at the necessary level of recruitment and can be closed without damaging the program.

Simultaneous with the announcement of the quota plan to all participants, trial managers should be prepared to comfort staff at sites that are not clearly in danger, but whose staff might worry excessively. The quota system should be handled with great care to avoid alarming staff into resigning prematurely from the trial. It should rather heighten their sensitivity to the the need for expanded recruitment plans. Average and superior recruiting sites will have been watching slower sites and wondering how their suboptimal performance affects the trial as a whole. Anxiety generated at sites put on probation lead some staff to look for more secure jobs elsewhere. This action would be most damaging to fragile sites on probation that have a good team in place but need to improve their pace of recruitment.

DRAWBACKS TO THE ESTABLISHMENT OF QUOTAS

Some investigators of high recruiting sites become complacent and divert their attention to other clinical projects, feeling comfortable with their initial recruitment rate. Such complacency is difficult to discourage. In ongoing trials, a new quota system is designed to spark these groups to renew their enthusiasm for the trial and to maintain a good enrollment rate. Nevertheless, sites that are not leaders in recruitment often begin to feel comfortable if they slip for a few months because they are ahead of the cumulative average. This attitude is potentially damaging to a trial because these sites may have lost patients that they could easily have handled. Sites with erratic enrollment should feel pressured knowing that slipping for more than a month or two might put them in the dangerous position of being put on probation for having missed their quota.

Undoubtedly, the imposition of a quota system during an ongoing clinical trial is more problematic than a quota established during the planning of the trial. The issues include problems of implementation as well as psychological impact on all staff. It is difficult to avoid the appearance (intentional or unintentional) of targeting one or several slow sites that could cause embarrassment, anxiety, frustration, or anger when initiating a system in the middle of a trial. If the decision to use a quota system is made prior to starting a trial, investigators and staff can more readily accept the democratic aspects of the rules, even if strict, because most sites expect to perform well and not to be penalized by a quota system.

ACCOLADES FOR HIGH RECRUITMENT

Sites that exceed their recruitment goals deserve a reward. Most commonly, a listing in a newsletter or being at the top of the table listing recruitment rates is all they receive. Such good work on behalf of the trial should sometimes be rewarded in other ways. Compliments for all those involved should be expressly written in trial reports sent to all investigators as well as in individual letters from the trial chairperson to all responsible trial staff. If resources are pulled away from slow sites, funds could be reallocated to hire additional staff at busy sites as an alternative to opening a replacement site. Investment in high capacity sites often is worthwhile because of the large amount of time it takes to fund and staff a new site. Initiating a new site also requires staff training and time to work through initial problems. In contrast, an ongoing busy site may be expanded relatively rapidly with the hiring and training of one or more staff who will learn quickly from coworkers who are already skilled in the process.

One traditional reward for the principal investigator of the busiest site is to be asked to write the final manuscript or to be placed high on the list of coauthors. If the list of coauthors of a manuscript is not alphabetical, it is commonly assumed that the sequence is determined by the number of patients entered. Compliments for the staff could include inviting them to help train new staff from other sites or to make training visits to teach their techniques to other sites.

10

Specific Patient Populations, Diseases, and Issues

A variety of special situations occur in the development of recruitment plans for individual trials. Many of these topics are addressed in this chapter under eight broad headings. Numerous patient populations that require special recruitment approaches are listed in Table 10.1.

RECRUITMENT IN VARIOUS THERAPEUTIC AREAS AND DISEASES

The original intent of the authors was to prepare a detailed chapter focusing on special recruitment issues appropriate for particular therapeutic areas and specific diseases. *After carefully evaluating the published literature and discussing this issue with numerous clinical investigators, we are convinced that with few exceptions, the appropriate recruitment techniques to use and strategies to develop are specific to the nature and requirements of a particular clinical trial rather than to a specific disease or therapeutic area.*

The perspective of the investigator who specializes in oncology, cardiology, or another area may initially be that recruitment techniques must be different for each therapeutic area. However, the principles and golden rules of patient recruitment

TABLE 10.1. *Selected patient populations that require recruitment approaches*

Population	General approach
Illiterate	Offer to read informed consent and any other material "if they would like some help"
Visually impaired	Print all brochures and informed consents in large size print
Demented	Discuss enrollment with guardian or appropriate person
Non-native speaking people	Identify languages most likely to require translators
Debilitated	Offer physical assistance (e.g., transportation)
Very sick	Offer to go to their home (if possible) to collect data
Terminally ill	Discuss the trial with family as well

are common to virtually all trials (e.g., loose inclusion criteria facilitate patient enrollment, and restrictive inclusion criteria make enrollment more difficult). The various sources of patients and various methods can be used by all types of trials. Therefore, this chapter addresses general issues that are pertinent to most clinical trials because we do not consider that recruitment techniques and strategies are specific to a disease or therapeutic area. For example, if a trial of an antidepressant is conducted with inpatients, the recruiting principles would differ from those used if outpatients are enrolled. If a trial is conducted in the frail elderly, the recruiting principles would differ from those used if young adults are sought. This same concept may be replicated for many other factors: a small trial versus a large one, single site versus many sites, a relatively safe medicine versus a toxic medicine, a difficult trial for patients to complete versus a relatively easy trial for patients to complete, a 50% chance of receiving placebo versus no chance, stringent inclusion criteria versus broad inclusion criteria. This list could go on and on, but it makes the point that the factors influencing patient recruitment do not depend on the nature of the specific disease, but on the details of the specific clinical trial that make it more difficult or easier to enroll patients. A number of generalizations about recruitment in 23 different therapeutic areas are presented by Swinehart (1991).

Surgical Trials

A surgical trial's recruitment experiences are described by Buchwald et al. (1987), and a valuable literature summary with an annotated bibliography of recruitment experiences in all types of clinical trials is presented by Hunninghake et al. (1987).

Is Cancer a Special Therapeutic Field for Patient Recruitment?

In reading the literature on patient recruitment it is easy to convince oneself that cancer represents a unique therapeutic area. After all, there are many clinical protocols available and several authors have documented the low rate of patient recruitment in cancer trials (Wittes and Friedman, 1988). This therapeutic area *is* somewhat unique in that there are a relatively large number of established trials into which oncologists in private practice as well as those in academic centers are encouraged to enter patients. Methods used by the NCI to stimulate patient recruitment are reviewed by Wittes and Friedman (1988). Other approaches are presented by McCusker et al. (1982). The American Medical Association Council on Scientific Affairs (1991) recently reviewed several reports in this area and described recruitment rates ranging from 1% to 3% of the available patient population in trials for cancers of the breast, colon, and rectum, and adjuvant treatment. Although various concerns by patients led to their refusing to enter a trial, the major factor in several evaluations was found to center on the physician. Several of the reasons that physicians are reluctant to enroll patients, or to suggest enrolling patients, are presented in Chapter 2. The American Medical Association Council on Scientific Affairs (1991) commented that "the interesting part about these attitudinal studies is that they involved established physician investigators. Across studies, there was a recurring theme that the obligation of caring for an individual patient at a point in time supercedes the societal need to evaluate therapies that might be used more widely for future patient populations."

An alternative perspective on oncology trials is possible when considering patient recruitment into academic versus industry sponsored trials. Most reports of oncology trials are based on extremely large trials sponsored by the National Cancer Institute (NCI) and enlist both community and academic physicians to refer and enroll patients. Pharmaceutical company sponsored oncology trials usually are much smaller in size and all investigators are individually recruited to join the trial. Industry sponsored trials do not have the same problems enrolling patients, which suggests that the real issue lies in the nature of the clinical trial (e.g., size, sponsor) and not in the therapeutic area studied.

RECRUITING YOUNG AND OLD PATIENTS

Recruiting Pediatric Patients

Approaches to children are not particularly different from others as far as principles of recruitment are concerned. The special keys to successful recruitment of children are:

1. Pay particular attention to details of the recruitment strategy that may be necessary to modify for use with children (i.e., use common sense in dealing with children).
2. Include staff who are experienced in working with children. If children are members of a minority group, it is desirable to have staff of the same ethnic or racial group.
3. Allocate sufficient time to spend with each child and parent (or guardian) during recruitment and during the trial.
4. Avoid demands that could be viewed as excessive or bothersome. This means having as simple a trial design and requirements as practical to address the objective.
5. Be aware of children's short attention span when talking or explaining information (i.e., keep it brief).
6. Carefully train children in trial procedures prior to enrollment to ensure that they are willing and capable of participating.
7. The same physician should see each child at each screening visit (as well as during the trial) and an alternative physician should be available if the relationship is not positive.
8. Question the children and parents in a nonthreatening manner about their con-

cerns or problems. Have a private comfortable room available for these discussions.

9. Reinforce the importance of the concept of the trial and maintaining the protocol with the parents and the child.
10. Have appropriate toys and games available and a suitable play environment for the children's use while waiting, and for siblings while the children are being examined or tested.

Two articles that discuss recruitment issues in children are by Gómez-Marín et al., 1991, and by Collet et al., 1991.

Recruiting Elderly Patients

Age per se does not create special recruitment problems. The same principles apply for the elderly as for younger adults. The steps to follow are listed in Table 10.2. However, many factors are more commonly found to occur in older patients (e.g., social isolation, poor diet, poor hygiene, debilitation) and many of these have significant implications for recruitment. In addition, Kirkpatrick (1991) reported that the elderly respond better than younger adults to altruism as a motivator and less to money.

Considerations for recruiting elderly patients include:

1. Involve the patient's own physician if one is present; his or her endorsement of the clinical trial is often essential to obtain the patient's enrollment. Many elderly patients have developed a long-term relationship with a physician and have become dependent on this person's advice in medical matters.
2. Family members or friends should be involved in the patient's recruitment and participation if the family members or friends play an active role in the patient's life. One of these people may have power of attorney.
3. Social isolation is commonly found in elderly patients and must be considered. For example, social interaction among patients and between patients and staff may be a strong motivation for some elderly patients to enroll.
4. Arranging for transportation to and from the clinical trial site is often essential to encourage an elderly patient to enroll. Other areas of possible inconvenience should be considered and efforts made to minimize their impact on the patient.
5. The fewest number of clinic visits necessary to achieve the trial's objectives should be scheduled for patients. Each visit should be as brief as possible.
6. In a trial that lasts for more than a few weeks, periodic assessments of patients'

TABLE 10.2. *Steps in recruiting elderly patients*

1. Obtain permission from the primary physician to approach the patient and indicate that endorsement to the patient; for example: "Your doctor suggested that I talk with you about this program." "Your doctor thinks that you would benefit from participation in this program."
2. Assess in advance and during the conversation whether the patient is able to understand the protocol and provide informed consent
3. Answer all of patient's questions, and offer to explain the trial to the family as well
4. Explain the logistics of the protocol with special emphasis on accommodations for transportation and the type of tests to be performed
5. Allow adequate time for the decision to be made voluntarily, even if this means waiting for a relative to visit and assist the patient to reach a decision

emotional status should be made. Their views about the trial should be discussed. Attention to these personal aspects may help prevent patients from dropping out, which in turn creates the need for more recruitment.

7. If elderly patients are being recruited through any of the institutions listed in Table 10.3 or other organizations, reimburse that group for all reasonable costs, including protection for malpractice and liability.

Elderly patients are more likely than younger patients to enter a trial that offers direct medical benefit (Lipsitz et al., 1987). Morgan et al. (1974) reported that many nursing home patients were reluctant to enroll in a clinical trial of a hypnotic medicine because of (1) fear related to changing their currently used and effective regimen, (2) fear related to the newness of the medicine, and (3) annoyance at the likelihood of being asked questions on a daily basis. Nonetheless, the authors found that a more aggressive approach describing the trial to potential patients in another nursing home yielded better recruitment results. However, Zimmer et al. (1985) noted that geriatric patients need extra time to decide whether to participate in a trial; placing pressure on the elderly for a rapid response about enrolling led to a higher likelihood of refusal.

A more assertive approach to recruitment was also found to yield higher recruitment rates by Leader and Neuwirth (1978). This study had several methodological flaws (e.g., one approach was used prior to the other rather than simultaneously, and the authors tailored their approach to senior citizen clubs). It is unknown whether the same results would have been obtained had one or both social clubs been divided into two groups and each assertive approach used with a different group within the same broad population. It would also be possible to design a trial where a second type of assertive approach is used on all elderly who refused the trial after the first type of approach.

Conducting a trial in a nursing home presents additional problems. Lipsitz et al. (1987) suggested that preferential treatment of nursing home patients who participate in a clinical trial can cause jealousy or resentment in some nonparticipants. These authors recommended avoiding the use of material reward to participants because even the extra attention provided by the trial represents a special feature for elderly participants.

TABLE 10.3. *Selected sources for recruitment of elderly patients[a]*

1. Nursing homes[b]
2. Retirement centers
3. Adult day-care centers
4. "Meals on Wheels" and other food programs (e.g., government food distribution)
5. Geriatric clinics
6. Patient support groups
7. Religious organizations and churches
8. Pharmacies
9. Health fairs
10. Civic organizations
11. Social clubs for the elderly
12. Local cable television community bulletin boards
13. Newspapers or magazines directed to the elderly
14. Associations of the elderly (e.g., American Association of Retired Persons)

[a] Investigators should contact the medical or executive directors of such organizations/institutions and seek assistance in recruiting activities. Additional sources and details are given by Petrovitch et al. (1991).
[b] See Annas and Glantz, 1986; Yu et al., 1990.

General references to recruitment issues for elderly patients are by Vestal (1985) and Smith et al. (1985), and attitudes of the elderly about clinical research were reviewed by Kaye et al. (1990).

RECRUITING DIFFERENT RACES INTO CLINICAL TRIALS

The general sources, methods, and strategies of recruitment do not differ for one race or another, providing that a suitable patient population pool is available. Nonetheless, different social classes, religions, or cultures within a race may have different beliefs that influence recruitment. Most clinical trials do not attempt to set quotas for different races, nor use any methods to ensure the presence or absence of different races. Trials in hypertension are an important exception and have sometimes been designed for one race or to compare responses between races.

Svensson (1989) examined the representation of American blacks in clinical trials of new medicines. He did this by evaluating information in the methodology section of studies published in *Clinical Pharmacology and Therapeutics* during 1984 through 1986. Of 50 trials that met his predetermined criteria for inclusion in his study, only ten included data on the races of enrollees. This finding is particularly noteworthy because of the high proportion of pharmacokinetic trials published in that journal and the importance in these trials of specifying all demographic data and many other details (e.g., diet) of enrollees. Moreover, members of the American Society for Clinical Pharmacology and Therapeutics, a group that should be particularly attuned to methodological issues are subscribers to that journal. Svensson (1989) was able to obtain (through correspondence) full racial data for an additional 25 trials, or 35 of the 50 trials. He noted under-representation of American blacks in the trials compared to their proportion in the cities in which the trial was conducted and of the entire country and discusses possible reasons for his observation.

To recruit patients of specific race(s) investigators must devise a strategy to be initiated at the outset of a trial. Efforts required may or may not be substantial, but a periodic review of the numbers screened and enrolled versus goals for each race should serve to trigger concern if appropriate numbers are not being achieved. Specific sources or even methods should be identified (e.g., advertising in specific newspapers, speaking to specific organizations, seeking referrals in specific hospitals) that would increase enrollment of specific racial or ethnic groups. Tielsch et al.(1991) discuss recruitment methods where obtaining racial balance was a critical factor in the trial.

One issue is whether new medicines should be evaluated in all major racial groups to ensure that any unusual or unexpected responses are observed prior to marketing. While several pros and cons can be presented on this point, this book is limited to recruitment issues. If a racial quota is imposed or if a racial balance of some type is desired, then recruitment strategies must be adjusted to ensure this is done. One of the most important components should be to include at least one member of each race on the investigator's staff. If this is not feasible because of the expense, then help of a part-time worker, or even a volunteer may be enlisted. This person should ideally be from the same social and economic level of the targeted group so that he or she understands the culture and beliefs of the screened population, or at least is attuned to these issues.

Some men with strong ethnic or racial upbringing are particularly concerned about their virility and are more hesitant to enter and remain in clinical trials (Cramer et al., 1988). Dealing with this issue is made more difficult if the patient is not comfortable with the trial staff (e.g., a black male patient recruited by a young, white nurse, or an Hispanic patient recruited by a physician who does not speak Spanish).

RECRUITING INPATIENTS VERSUS OUTPATIENTS

Inpatients

There are two types of inpatient trials. In the first, patients are recruited and enrolled as outpatients and then enter a hospital for some or all of the trial. In the other type, patients already in a hospital are recruited to participate in a clinical trial. These patients may have just entered the hospital or have been in the hospital for a few days or longer. Investigators conducting a clinical trial in which current inpatients are recruited must be sure to consult with each patient's primary care physician before discussing the trial with patients or attempting to enroll them. The purpose and scope of the clinical trial should be explained to the physician so that he or she can participate in the decision of whether the trial is appropriate for the patient at this time.

Recruitment occurs in some trials at a time when the patient is severely ill. At such times, the need for a rapid decision on enrollment places pressure on the patient, who in turn usually relies on the advice of his or her physician. Recruitment becomes an ethical issue in these instances because of the special trust the patient and family has placed in the treating physician.

In many trials, the inclusion criteria preclude entering patients who are ill enough to be hospitalized, making inpatient recruitment inappropriate. Koenig et al. (1989) discuss this issue in terms of the type of inclusion criteria that commonly require current good health aside from the specific disease of interest. In addition, many inpatients are too ill to allow for possible randomization to a placebo (Rowlands, 1987). Trials in which an active control (e.g., comparing two potentially effective medicines) is used would be acceptable for this population.

Volunteer Inpatients

Some inpatient trials admit patients to evaluate special procedures or tests. Patients and normal volunteers who have a stable or unstable medical condition usually are screened prior to the hospitalization. Recruitment for this type of trial often has a low yield with people who work or have responsibilities that would interfere with their being hospitalized.

Special incentives might be offered to volunteers to enhance recruitment. The following might be adequate compensation to a patient for the intrusiveness and bother of an inpatient protocol.

1. *Compensation for time.* This compensation might be in lieu of lost pay from time away from work and could involve hiring of a caretaker for a family during the hospitalization.
2. *Medical evaluations.* Various tests and evaluations can be provided during hos-

pitalization as part of the protocol that are of interest to patients, particularly if there is no charge.

3. *Evaluation of the disease.* This is usually conducted as part of the protocol.

Healthy volunteers are often concerned about indemnification in case of injury during their participation in a clinical trial (Macrae et al., 1989). Information on this subject should be given to these volunteers and to patients.

Recruiting Patients with Organ Dysfunction

Patients with organ dysfunction (e.g., end-stage renal disease) often are easy to find but not necessarily easy to recruit into clinical trials. Such patients usually are managed by a select group of specialists so that identification is usually limited to specific physicians. These patients often are extremely cautious about taking an investigational medicine without a strong endorsement from their primary physician. Some patients have concerns that participation in a clinical trial could interfere with their ability to receive an organ transplant when a suitable donor is identified. On the other hand, these patients are particularly tied to their physician with an emotional bond that enhances the likelihood of their recruitment into a trial if encouraged by that physician.

Recruiting Patients Versus Symptomatic Volunteers

A distinction has been made in recent years, particularly in psychiatric and psychological research, between true patients and symptomatic volunteers (see Fig. 1.2). *Symptomatic volunteers* are people from the general population who respond to advertisements or publicity about clinical trials. *True patients* are those people with medical problems that are already involved in a relationship with the health care system. Questions have been raised regarding (1) whether clinically significant differences exist between these two groups, and (2) whether data obtained in one group are extrapolatable to the other group. Both groups usually are included in the single term *patient*; this distinction is rarely used except for clinical trials.

Clinically important differences do not exist between these groups in most disease areas. Symptomatic volunteers with rare diseases generally are not sought through advertisements and publicity, but usually are found as patients through specialized clinics and medical specialists. True patients with common diseases are usually found in adequate numbers in the medical practice(s) of the investigators. Screening tests, medical history, and an overall evaluation can usually assess whether the patients and symptomatic volunteers are similar.

A comparison of true patients versus symptomatic volunteers in bulimia nervosa research (Mitchell et al., 1988) found that 40 patients who presented for treatment were similar to a group of 40 symptomatic volunteers recruited through newspaper advertisements. The authors of the study examined pertinent aspects of medical histories and found few differences between the groups. They are conservative in their interpretation of the results, which are strongly supportive of the generally held view that relevant differences between patients and symptomatic volunteers are uncommon in clinical trials.

Covi et al. (1979) found so few depressed patients for a clinical trial that they initiated advertising to seek symptomatic volunteers. They noted that recruitment should include a system to refer volunteers who are ineligible for a trial to receive appropriate medical care. Clinical trials of antidepressants usually can be conducted in hospitalized patients or outpatients. The choice of patients is sometimes based on the perceived ability of staff to recruit patients, particularly if outpatients have to enter a hospital to conduct the trial.

Although advertisements can detail some or all inclusion criteria for a clinical trial, Shtasel et al. (1991) chose to use a simple, one-sentence newspaper advertisement to recruit normal control subjects for a brain function trial: "Healthy people ages 18–45 are needed at the Hospital of the University of Pennsylvania for paid research." They evaluated 1,670 callers using a structured screening performed by trained interviewers. This process excluded 252 people with a psychiatric diagnosis and 303 people with medical or neurological disorders. An additional 76 volunteers were found to have a psychiatric disorder during secondary screening interviews. This report underscores the need for careful delineation of the characteristics of a control group. The issue of how the advertising was carried out is discussed in Chapter 4.

RECRUITING PATIENTS WITH SYMPTOMATIC VERSUS ASYMPTOMATIC DISORDERS

Symptomatic Disorders

Patients who have an established diagnosis are often well aware of their treatment options and have undertaken therapy suggested by their physician. Adverse reactions to therapy often are superimposed or interact with disease symptoms, creating a situation where the origins or causes of some symptoms are unclear. Some patients discontinue treatment, preferring to endure continuous or cyclical symptoms rather than take chronic medication, particularly if adverse effects are as problematic, or more so, than the symptoms. Other patients search for complete control of their disorder and request alternative medication when they experience adverse events or poor disease control. Various types of patients with symptomatic disorders may be identified in the records of their long-term care provider. Appeals to recruit such volunteers or patients are simplified in that the individuals reading an advertisement or hearing about a trial are able to identify themselves immediately as potential candidates for the program. The direct appeal to these patients is usually an efficient recruitment technique that is likely to bring a high yield of accrual. However, a burdensome protocol can defeat the advantage of having a readily identifiable population. Quick et al. (1989) screened 1,388 glaucoma patients and found only 15 patients willing to participate in a trial requiring three day-long testing sessions in addition to other visits.

Asymptomatic Disorders

Finding patients who have not yet been diagnosed with the disease of interest is problematic in that such individuals do not recognize themselves as potential participants. Various mass screening techniques are one means of locating such patients (Table 10.4). These screening methods require:

TABLE 10.4. *Approaches to screening for selected asymptomatic disorders*

Disorder	Technique	Population sought
Lung cancer	Chest x-ray	Smokers
Breast cancer	Mammogram	Women aged 40–60
Colon cancer	Fecal blood test	Adults aged 40–70
Hypertension	Blood pressure test	Adults possibly of specific races (e.g., blacks)
Hyperlipidemia	Cholesterol blood test	Adults and children
Glaucoma	Intraocular pressure	All adults

1. Education that encourages the targeted population to come forward for testing. However, these people will volunteer if they believe that they are susceptible to the disorder.
2. The desire, on the part of some individuals, to be tested to assure themselves that they are not afflicted.

When the small number of patients with positive tests are identified, subsequent recruitment steps must provide the patient and his or her family physician with a full understanding of both the medical disorder and the treatment option provided within the framework of the research program.

Problems in Recruiting Asymptomatic Patients

Some patients who have heard the appeal and offer of free testing respond by visiting their own physician for the test, thereby eluding the screening network. Many asymptomatic patients identified as positive by screening tests prefer to have their treatment with a private physician rather than participate in a clinical trial (Baines, 1984). Similar problems are seen in trials of preventive measures. Weintraub et al. (1980) list a variety of reasons why families declined to enroll their children in fluoride treatment trials.

RECRUITING PATIENTS WITH NEW VERSUS ESTABLISHED DIAGNOSES

New Diagnosis

After diagnosis of a disease, patients often undergo a period of adjustment in which they slowly come to accept (or not) the diagnosis. Some patients choose to deny that they have a specific disease, prefer to ignore their signs and symptoms, and refuse treatment. If recruited into a clinical trial at too early a point in this acceptance phase, such patients tend to refuse entry or to drop out after enrolling. They may feel that they have been pulled into the treatment program without their full understanding of the consequences involved. Screening must proceed carefully with such patients because they (and, often, their families) are not yet adjusted to accepting the diagnosis. Such patients often feel that they have become a "guinea pig." As an example, Jack et al. (1990) described the refusal of women diagnosed with breast cancer to enroll in a breast conservation trial. The recruitment of patients into a clinical trial during the throes of a personal dilemma is usually inappropriate; furthermore, it is relatively less productive if other more suitable patients are available.

During the acute emotional period of learning that they have a new disease and hearing the physician's recommendation for treatment, many patients initially agree to do whatever the physician suggests, whether it is a standard or experimental treatment. On reflection and consultation with family and friends, some people change their minds, preferring to alter their lifestyle instead of accepting standard therapy, or accepting standard therapy instead of enrolling in a clinical trial. For example, some patients deny that they have epilepsy and think that if they obtain adequate sleep, avoid drinking excessive amounts of alcohol, or significantly reduce their stress, no more seizures will occur. This conclusion is often reinforced by the episodic nature of seizure disorders. Similarly, hypertensive patients may promise to diet and avoid salt in their food rather than take medication. Even patients with life-threatening disorders such as cancer often deny the existence of their disease or continuously postpone their treatment. Breast cancer patients fearing disfigurement sometimes postpone or decline a mastectomy and diabetic patients sometimes refuse limb amputation. Paskett et al. (1990) report that more than 40% of the women informed about abnormalities seen on Papanicolaou smears do not return for proper evaluation. This observation was made in a group of mainly indigent women who came to a gynecology clinic for a cervical cancer screening program but did not respond to multiple contacts for follow-up care.

Some patients who have felt intermittent chest pain on exercise understand that they may have angina, although it has never been diagnosed. Similarly, some who have experienced abdominal distress rightfully believe that they have ulcers. Women with undiagnosed stress incontinence were recruited into a trial by advertisements that listed the signs and symptoms of the disorder (Burns et al., 1990). These symptomatic volunteers had been embarrassed by their incontinence but did not realize that it is often a treatable medical condition. Whether or not they participated in the trial, the screening process enabled them to understand their problem and to seek appropriate treatment. On the other hand, many patients who have had intermittent chest pain, gastric pain, or incontinence do *not* have angina, ulcers, or treatable stress incontinence.

Acute Disorders

Clinical trials of emergency medical problems (e.g., acute infections, stroke, trauma surgery) present special recruitment problems because the investigator must wait for specific types of patients. Clinical trials that require such patients often screen for patient eligibility in the emergency room, or even in the ambulance during transport to a hospital. Assessment of eligibility must be made "immediately," often with very little information. Assistance in screening is provided by emergency medical technicians, triage nurses, as well as emergency physicians. Once a patient has been treated with medication, he or she becomes ineligible for some trials. LaRue et al. (1988) were able to recruit only one patient over two years for an acute stroke trial because of the strict entry criteria. The ability to (1) rapidly screen and determine eligibility of patients, (2) notify the clinical trial staff about the patient, and (3) then recruit the patient as rapidly as possible are essential ingredients for such trials. The ability to obtain informed consent in these urgent circumstances is discussed in various textbooks on ethics.

Established Diagnosis

Chronic Disorders

Patients whose diseases are well controlled and who are comfortable with an established treatment may see no reason to change their therapy. To recruit these patients into a clinical trial one must educate them about the potential benefits of the experimental treatment. Some patients whose disease has not been controlled despite treatment with a variety of medicines might consider themselves "sensitive" or "nonresponders" to any investigational medicine. These patients need special attention and education during the recruitment process. They need information about the adverse effects anticipated from the experimental therapy as well as the potential advantages (e.g., greater efficacy). Barofsky and Sugarbaker (1979) described the difficulty of recruiting sarcoma patients into a clinical trial because of the expected severity of treatment options. The patients reported that they anticipated a diminished quality of life if they enrolled.

Patients whose diseases are poorly controlled with existing therapies often eagerly await the development of experimental treatments and usually accept them readily, no matter what risks are described. Such patients perceive the opportunity for a thorough evaluation of their disease by the expert investigator as a major benefit. Other advantages may include evaluations using more modern technologies and expensive new tests.

Secondary Prevention

Unlike patients whose chronic disease symptoms provide repeated reminders (e.g., arthritis pain), patients who have recovered from a myocardial infarction or stroke are usually treated for prevention of a recurrence. Recruitment into a prevention trial is often more difficult than for a therapeutic trial where symptoms are treated. An education program often is necessary for patients entering prevention trials. This education should include information on medical controversies about whether or not to use prophylactic treatment. Patients' perceptions of risk, and their psychological accommodation to their prior recovery, are factors to consider when screening individual patients for prophylactic trials.

Disorders That Already Are Adequately Treated

Recruitment of patients for evaluation of a new antiulcer medicine was not a problem for sponsors in the mid-1970s, but by the late 1980s finding enough patients to study became a major issue. Most patients with ulcers are currently well-maintained on regimens using one of several available medicines. Thus, ulcer patients usually have little motivation or need to enter a clinical trial to evaluate a new therapy today that does not offer hope of a significant advantage. Physicians also have little motivation to refer such patients for a clinical trial of yet another H-2 antihistamine. The same situation has occurred in several other therapeutic areas as well. It is clearly a positive event for society when a medicine introduced on the market adequately treats most patients with a particular disease. Nonetheless, sponsors often attempt to find populations of patients or methods of recruitment that address this issue. Some of the approaches are to eschew tertiary care centers and to approach primary practitioners, to approach health maintenance organizations, and to conduct clinical trials in other countries where patients are inadequately treated, or are treated with other types of medicines or therapies.

RECRUITING PATIENTS WITH COMMON VERSUS RARE DISEASES

Common Diseases

Clinical trials involving common medical problems, such as hypertension or hyperlipidemia, usually use restrictive inclusion criteria. Thus, although the patient population eligible for screening is enormous, relatively few patients may actually meet the restrictive entry criteria and agree to enroll. Descriptions of stringent entry criteria in advertisements or in written comments to potential referring physicians are usually brief, decreasing the likelihood for obtaining appropriate referrals. In some cases, it is possible to make a partial determination of eligibility (e.g., elevated blood pressure during the initial screening visit) when the results of the test are immediate. On the other hand, tests for elevated cholesterol require a laboratory analysis, professional review of the report, and notification of the patient or referring physician, followed by subsequent invitation to participate in the trial. Plans may be made to refer ineligible patients to other physicians for follow-up of a medical problem previously unknown to the patient. Patients who attend a screening visit can become an important source of referrals by asking them to search their network of family and friends for other potential screening candidates.

Rare Diseases

Recruiting patients with uncommon medical disorders may require virtually unrestricted or minimally restrictive inclusion criteria. Once they are identified, a large percentage of screenees will be eligible for the trial. In some cases, the diagnosis made during the referral visit or during the initial screening visit may be difficult to make with certainty. For example, the cancer cell type or stage of a disease often is not defined at the time of the screening evaluation. With rare diseases, it is important to deal mainly with medical specialists who are best able to diagnose and treat the disease to be studied. Registries of lay and professional societies may have information about potential enrollees that can be provided, as long as patient privacy is assured.

RECRUITMENT DEPENDENT ON THE PHASE OF A NEW MEDICINE'S DEVELOPMENT

The type of patient or volunteer recruited into clinical trials for a new medicine generally differs from one development phase to another (i.e., Phase I versus Phase IV). Nonetheless, the important recruitment issues relate to the other factors discussed in this book and not to the phase per se. The nature of the protocol, which in turn is often dependent on the phase of development, is the major factor that influences sources and methods to consider in creating a recruitment strategy.

How is Recruitment Affected by the Phase of a Clinical Trial?

In Phase I trials, the type of volunteer to be recruited should be discussed in advance of recruiting efforts. The best place(s) to find the volunteers should be discussed in advance. Advertising for volunteers is often necessary (see Chapter 4, Methods).

In Phase II trials it is necessary to determine characteristics of disease to focus on for recruitment strategy. It may not be relevant to build the strategy around the (1) type of disease, (2) severity of disease, or (3) prognostic criteria (e.g., risk factors). This choice may lead toward a specific strategy. For example, if enrolling patients with mild disease is the key, turn to private practice physicians. If enrolling patients with severe disease is key, turn to tertiary care centers.

In Phase III trials it is necessary to determine where the best sources are to meet the enrollment goals in terms of rates. Assess how inclusion criteria affect the recruitment. In Phase IV trials, if few patients are receiving the medicine, then efforts may be best directed toward boosting use of the medicine before a trial is undertaken to follow a large cohort.

Follow-up Trials

Follow-up trials present a very different problem in recruiting patients in that a specific cohort that participated in a previous program is now invited to participate in the follow-up evaluation. The Natural History Study of Congenital Heart Defects (O'Fallon et al., 1987) is an example of a trial in which follow-up was attempted for 2,408 patients who had been evaluated between 1958 and 1973 for congenital heart defects during childhood. The first activity was to determine the current address of all individuals who participated in the earlier trial. Before contacting a patient, the most recent physician was informed of the study and asked to assist in recruiting the patient. Thereafter, a mail program was set in motion for contacting the patients. Mailed packages included a reminder of earlier participation in the pediatric study, a questionnaire on current health, a medical records release form, and a card requesting or refusing more information or participation. Most importantly, a stamped, addressed return envelope was included with the package to enhance the return rate of information. Thereafter, follow-up mail and telephone contacts were utilized.

11

Publishing Data on the Recruitment Process

REASONS TO PUBLISH DATA ON PATIENT RECRUITMENT IN A CLINICAL TRIAL PUBLICATION

Inclusion of patient recruitment data in the publication of clinical trial results or in another report of the trial is an essential aspect of the reporting of clinical trials. Depending on the type, amount, and quality of the recruitment data published, the reader learns:

1. The number of patients screened and enrolled.
2. Whether original recruitment goals and quotas were met or whether changes had to be made to the protocol or trial before it could be completed.
3. The number of patients who reached each of the stages of the recruitment process and whether the funnel effect (see Chapter 1 for definition and discussion) was marked or mild.
4. Characteristics of patients in groups 1,2, and 3 above, including basic demographic and prognostic criteria. Other types of clinical characteristics may be included in the presentation.
5. The comparison of patient characteristics of those entered in the trial with those who were not. Comparisons with patients in the reader's medical practice, or with all patients with the disease being tested, enables the reader to make a judgment about the extrapolatability of the data obtained in the clinical trial.
6. The identity of problems that occurred during the recruitment process that should be avoided, or cannot be avoided but should be considered during the planning process.

7. The identity of sources and methods that were and were not useful in recruiting patients.
8. The costs required to enroll each patient and which methods were most cost effective.
9. The nature of the recruiting strategy used and whether it was successful.

Finally, readers planning or contemplating a similar trial will be able to judge on what aspects of recruitment to focus on and how.

THREE LEVELS FOR REPORTING RECRUITMENT DATA

Three levels of reporting of recruitment data are found in the medical literature. These levels are defined below on the basis of the quantity of recruitment data presented, as well as the type of data.

Level One: Superficial Details

Reporting the number of patients entered in the clinical trial is usually presented as a percent of those screened who were entered in the trial (e.g., 650 patients were screened for the trial and 125 were enrolled) (Table 11.1). In some cases the sources of patients and methods of recruitment are not fully described or may not even be mentioned. Also, the reasons for patient exclusion (e.g., ineligible, refused) frequently are not given.

Level Two: Funnel Effect and Description

Reporting the number of patients who were or were not entered in a clinical trial may be done using a flow diagram, table, or text that itemizes several categories of patients at various stages of the recruitment process. Additional categories of patient numbers that arise during the trial's conduct may be presented in the same or other

TABLE 11.1. *Number of patients screened, excluded, and randomized by medical center in VA Cooperative Study #75*

VA medical center	Number screened	Number excluded	Number and (%) randomized
1	148	104	44 (29.7)
2	246	219	27 (11.0)
3	369	317	52 (14.1)
4	529	480	49 (9.3)
5	263	192	71 (27.0)
6	282	219	63 (22.3)
7	304	259	45 (14.8)
8	236	186	50 (21.2)
9	107	96	11 (10.3)
10	4	0	4 (100.0)
11	82	72	10 (12.2)
12	85	78	7 (8.2)
13	32	28	4 (12.5)
Total	2687	2250	437 (16.3)

Reprinted from Martin et al. (1984) with permission.

TABLE 11.2. *Categories of patients that may be described in the recruitment section of a publication[a]*

1. Patients potentially available for entry into a clinical trial (i.e., the total pool of patients in a given area)
2. Patients available for initial verbal screening (e.g., many patients are unavailable for a variety of reasons)
3. Patients preliminarily excluded because of failure to meet basic inclusion criteria
4. Patients available for initial interview and screening tests
5. Patients available for interview and informed consent discussion (e.g., some patients are not suitable because of language problems, personality traits unsuited to a clinical trial, physical impairments, mental impairments, severe allergies)
6. Patients who pass screening tests who are offered informed consent
7. Patients verbally consenting to enter the clinical trial
8. Patients signing informed consent statements
9. Patients who enter the active baseline period of a clinical trial
10. Patients who receive treatment in a clinical trial

Reprinted from Spilker (1991) with permission.
[a] Entry into a clinical trial may be defined as the time of signing the informed consent statement (point 8), entry into an active baseline (point 9), or as the moment when treatment is initiated (point 10). Each of these may be appropriate in different clinical trials. In this book, the first definition is used.

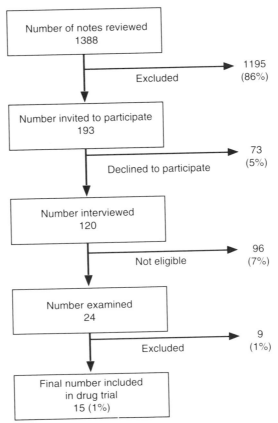

FIG. 11.1. Summary of the number of patients recruited and excluded during the recruitment process. Reprinted from Quick et al. (1989) with permission.

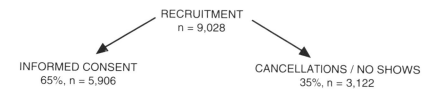

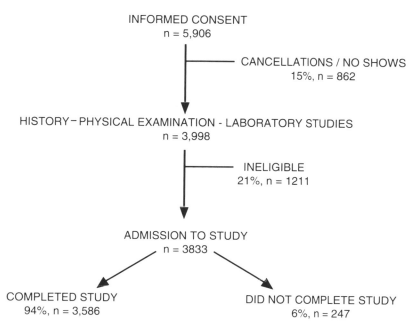

FIG. 11.2. Disposition of patients from recruitment through trial completion. Reprinted from DeVries et al. (1989) with permission.

formats to show patient dropouts and discontinuers (Table 11.2 and Figs. 11.1.to 11.6). Additional numerical data or information in the text should describe the characteristics of the population screened and the nature of the screening process. Level two data usually illustrate the funnel effect (see Chapter 1). Figures 11.7 and 11.8 show the funnel effect for both screening and postscreening visits before enrollment. Figure 11.9 illustrates more graphical presentation of the funnel effect. Other examples may be found in Prout (1981), Tielsch et al. (1991), Gomez-Marin et al. (1991), CASS Principal Investigators and Their Associates (1983), and Buchwald et al. (1987).

Level Three: Detailed Discussion or Presentation of Recruitment Data

Reporting the number of patients who were or were not entered in the clinical trial with detailed reasons and descriptions for some or all of the steps described in level two is defined as level three. Tables 11.3 to 11.9 show examples of level three publications. Extensive descriptions of recruitment experiences, methods used, or

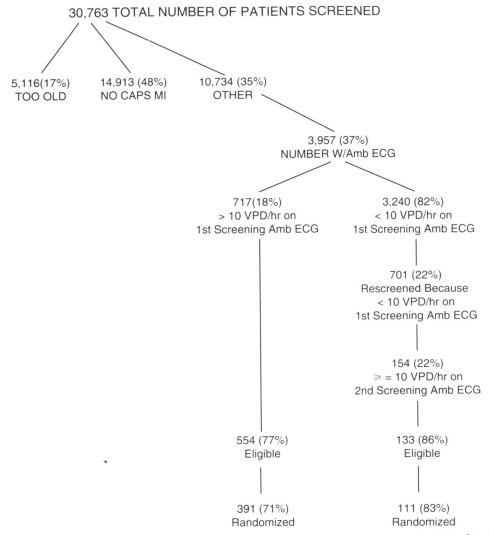

FIG. 11.3. Screening patients for enrollment in the Cardiac Arrhythmia Pilot Study (CAPS). ECG, electrocardiogram; MI, myocardial infarction; VPD, ventricular premature depolarizations. Reprinted from CAPS Investigators (1988) with permission.

other recruiting topics are the most common examples of level three data presented in the literature.

RECRUITMENT DATA THAT SHOULD BE REPORTED IN A CLINICAL TRIAL PUBLICATION

The amount of information described in level one is inadequate on its own for any full publication about a clinical trial. Although this amount of data is all that is commonly found in many clinical publications, it is an unacceptable practice in the 1990s. Journal editors should ensure that more information is presented. Researchers should assure that if not published with the results, the full information is published

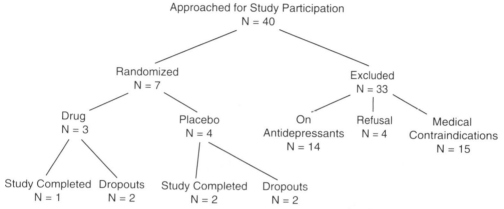

Medical and Neurological Service Admissions over 10 Months
N = 964

Eligible Patients after Exclusions
N= 773

Patients with Complete Evaluations
N = 680

Patients Scoring above Cutoff on the GDS
N = 81

Patients Evaluated by Psychiatrist
N = 79

Major Depression
N = 41

Approached for Study Participation
N = 40

Randomized
N = 7

Excluded
N = 33

Drug
N = 3

Placebo
N = 4

On
Antidepressants
N = 14

Refusal
N = 4

Medical
Contraindications
N = 15

Study Completed
N = 1

Dropouts
N = 2

Study Completed
N = 2

Dropouts
N = 2

FIG. 11.4. Patient flow diagram. GDS, Geriatric Depression Scale; AD, antidepressant. Reprinted from Koenig et al. (1989) with permission.

TABLE 11.3. *Illustration of the funnel effect in a postoperative pain trial evaluating a new medication[a]*

8,027	Inpatients potentially available for the clinical trial
−3,103	Patients unavailable during hours scheduled for 4,924 interviews (e.g., late admissions, referral to specialty clinic)
−4,254[b]	Preliminary exclusions
670	Available for interview
−21	Patients not screened for various reasons
649	Patients screened and reviewed in detail prior to interview
−258[b]	Rejected prior to interview
391	Patients interviewed
−53[b]	Rejected after interview
338	Patients asked for consent to enter trial
−92[b,c]	Patients not consenting
246[c]	Patients consenting to participate in the trial
−146[b,d]	Patients not medicated
100[d]	Patients given medication

[a] Table created from data in a paper by Calimlim and Weintraub (1981). Reprinted with permission. Table 11.3 to 11.9 are based on a trial originally published by Calimlim et al. (1977).

[b] Reasons (i.e., level three) are listed in Tables 10.3 to 10.10.

[c] These two groups were compared for age, sex, social class, and anticipated pain severity after surgery. Only age differed significantly. (Nonconsentees were older with a mean age of 41 versus 35 in the consentees.)

[d] These two groups were compared (data were only available on 134 of nonmedicated patients). Age and social class did not differ but more females were in the nonmedicated group ($p = 0.01$). The anticipated pain severity after surgery was greater in the medicated group than in the nonmedicated group ($p = 0.02$).

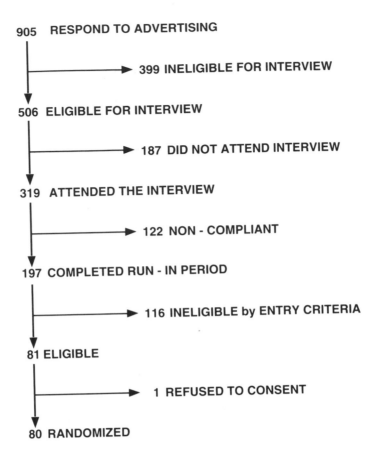

905 RESPOND TO ADVERTISING

→ 399 INELIGIBLE FOR INTERVIEW

506 ELIGIBLE FOR INTERVIEW

→ 187 DID NOT ATTEND INTERVIEW

319 ATTENDED THE INTERVIEW

→ 122 NON - COMPLIANT

197 COMPLETED RUN - IN PERIOD

→ 116 INELIGIBLE by ENTRY CRITERIA

81 ELIGIBLE

→ 1 REFUSED TO CONSENT

80 RANDOMIZED

REQUIRED SAMPLE SIZE 128

FIG. 11.5. The Concerned Smoker Study: Flow through the steps in the recruitment pathway. Reprinted from Arnold et al. (1989) with permission.

TABLE 11.4. *Reasons for preliminary exclusions*

Below 21 or above 65 years	1921	45%
Insufficient postoperative pain	1155	27%
Excluded surgical procedures	718	17%
No physician consent	337	8%
Short-term admissions	123	3%
Total	4254	100%

Reprinted from Calimlim and Weintraub (1981) with permission.

TABLE 11.5. *Patients available for interview*

Total number	670	
Patients not screened	21	
Patients screened	649	
	670	
Patients interviewed	391	60%
Patients rejected before interview	258	40%
Total	649	

Reprinted from Calimlim and Weintraub (1981) with permission.

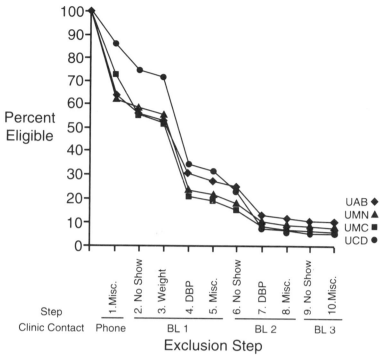

FIG. 11.6. Percent remaining eligible after completion of each exclusion step by clinic. Reprinted from Borhani et al. (1989) with permission.

elsewhere. *Controlled Clinical Trials* has published more information on recruitment than any other journal.

The data described in level two are considered both appropriate and necessary for full publications of clinical trials. This represents the standard that should be used in all journals.

The level of detail described in level three is rarely presented in the literature. The examples shown in Tables 11.3 to 11.9 were presented in a paper dealing with recruitment issues and were not part of a publication on results of a clinical trial.

TABLE 11.6. *Reasons for rejection prior to interview*

Multiple medical problems	82	31%
Overweight or underweight	60	23%
Sensitivity to study medication	28	11%
Emotional overlay	20	8%
Chronic analgesic intake	17	7%
Active peptic ulcer disease	16	6%
Psychiatric history or illness	10	4%
Language problems	8	3%
Multiple allergies	6	2%
Physical impairment (deaf, blind)	4	2%
Refused surgery	4	2%
Mental retardation	3	1%
Total	258	100%

Reprinted from Calimlim and Weintraub (1981) with permission.

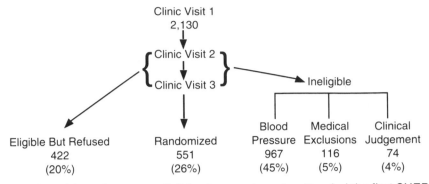

FIG. 11.7. Disposition of persons eligible at screening who attended the first SHEP clinic visit, with reasons for ineligibility and proportion who refused participation. The "Clinical Judgement" exclusion was made in cases where the physician believed the individual was not likely to be a reliable participant. Usually, this related to suspected alcoholism. Reprinted from Vogt et al. (1986) with permission.

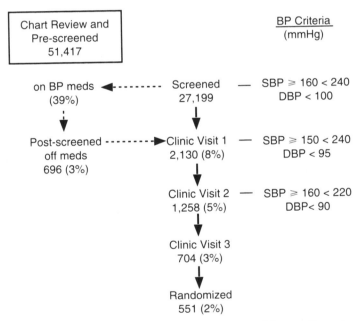

FIG. 11.8. Number of persons seen at each level of the SHEP recruitment process. "Pre-screened" refers to individuals on whom blood pressure information was obtained prior to screening through routine blood pressure checks, medical records, etc. Persons likely to be eligible from such information were selectively invited to screening. "Post-screened" refers to those persons who discontinued antihypertensive medicines after screening in order to determine if they were eligible for the SHEP. BP, blood pressure; SBP, systolic blood pressure; DBP, diastolic blood pressure. Reprinted from Vogt et al. (1986) with permission.

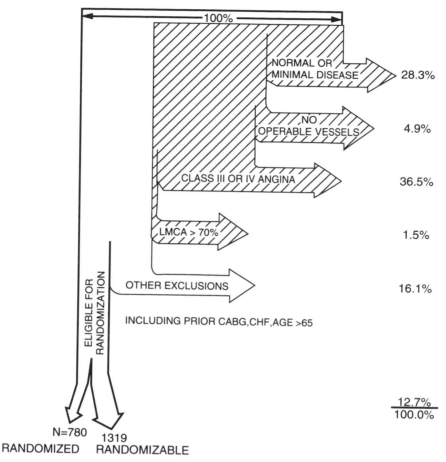

Fig. 11.9. Allocation of patients in CASS registry at randomizing sites. Reasons for exclusion of patients from the study. Width is proportional to the number of patients in each category. LMCA, left main coronary artery; CABG, coronary artery bypass graft; CHF, congestive heart failure. Reprinted from CASS Principal Investigators and Their Associates (1983) with permission.

TABLE 11.7. *Patients interviewed*

Number of patients interviewed	391	
Number interviewed but rejected	53	
Reasons for rejection		
Multiple allergies	14	
Medical problems	13	
Very apprehensive	13	
Overweight	7	
No relief from trial medicine	3	
Language problem	3	
Patients asked for consent	338	
Patients consenting	246	73%
Patients not consenting	92	27%
Total	338	100%

Reprinted from Calimlim and Weintraub (1981) with permission.

TABLE 11.8. *Reasons for not consenting*

Prefers intramuscular injection	65	71%
Cannot decide	10	11%
Trial medicines not effective in past	9	10%
Family refuses	5	5%
No reason	3	3%
Total	92	100%

Reprinted from Calimlim and Weintraub (1981) with permission.

TABLE 11.9. *Reasons for nonmedication*

Consenting patient		
Not medicated	146	
Data not available	−12	
Total	134	
Insufficient pain when oral medication allowed	47	35%
Oral medication not permitted and the patient is then discharged on day 1	35	26%
Oral medication not permitted on days 0, 1, 2, 3	29	22%
Patient dropped from trial by request of patient or surgeon	10	7%
Medical complications occurred after surgery	9	7%
Surgery canceled	4	3%
Total	134	100%

Reprinted from Calimlim and Weintraub (1981) with permission.

TABLE 11.10. *Patients who entered or refused entry into one of ten clinical trials as a percentage of those screened in selected DVA studies*

Clinical trial name	Percentage of patients who entered	Percentage of patients who refused entry
Antabuse	19.2	29.0
Aphasia I	6.3	1.1
Aphasia II	6.3	2.0
Chronic brain	28.6	20.3
Dental	69.7	21.5
Diabetes	41.0	7.6
Epilepsy	13.6	3.8
Nursing home	20.9	26.1
Ulcer	32.0	6.7
Ward milieu	32.6	9.6

Reprinted from Collins et al. (1984) with permission.

TABLE 11.11. *Screening checklist data summary for potential participation in DVA lithium treatment in alcohol dependence study–Hines VA Medical Center*

Number of admissions	97	100%
Number ineligible	38	39.2%
Number eligible	59	60.8%
Reasons not eligible		
Demographic	22	22.7%
Not alcoholic	3	3.1%
Psychiatric	15	15.5%
Medical conditions	11	11.3%
Other	15	15.5%
Refused	16	16.5%

Reprinted from Collins et al. (1984) with permission.

TABLE 11.12. *Adjustments made for intake problems in selected VA trials*

Clinical trial	Adjustments
Antabuse	Early termination
Aphasia I	18-month extension
Aphasia II	12-month extension
Chronic brain	Early termination
Dental	6-month extension
Diabetes	16-month extension
Epilepsy	12-month extension[a]
Nursing home	18-month extension
Ulcer	Early termination
Ward milieu	12-month extension

Reprinted from Collins et al. (1984) with permission.
[a] Required because the sample size required was underestimated.

In fact, the same authors published a separate article on the clinical data obtained (Calimlim et al., 1977). The paper by Calimlim and Weintraub (1981) is the most detailed description of the funnel effect found in the medical literature. A full publication of clinical trial data should include the amount of detail listed in Table 11.2. This could be presented as either a figure, table, or even as a statement in the text. The specific, more detailed information shown in Tables 11.3 to 11.9 should be collected on patient logs for analysis (if necessary) during clinical trials, but is not necessary to publish in most instances.

Other examples of level three publications are by Lee and Breaux (1983), Koenig et al. (1989), and Detrc et al. (1977). Recruitment issues in multiple trials that were published by Collins et al. (1984) are shown in Tables 11.10 to 11.13. Level three reporting of recruitment data is given in Tables 11.14 to 11.20.

Generally, the amount and type of data that should be reported in a clinical publication fit level two. The publication of a clinical trial should state in the text, tables, or figures, the following information:

1. The overall recruitment plan or strategy.
2. The original recruitment goal per site and the total goal for all sites combined in terms of number of patients and time period allotted to recruitment.
3. The sources of patients used and the methods used to recruit patients.

TABLE 11.13. *Drop-out rates in selected VA trials*

Clinical trial	Percentage of drop-outs
Antabuse	42.7
Aphasia I	50.0
Aphasia II	22.4
Chronic brain	21.3
Dental	39.0
Diabetes	1.3
Epilepsy	36.3
Nursing home	10.6
Ulcer	10.3
Ward milieu	50.7

Reprinted from Collins et al. (1984) with permission.

TABLE 11.14. *Reasons for exclusion of patients from VA Cooperative Study #75*

Exclusion reason	Exclusion n	Reason (%)	Percent range[a] for VAMCs
1. Patient has advanced disease: bedridden, poor general condition, expected survival less than 2 months	715	(24.0)	17.0–43.3
2. Other conditions related to patient's cancer: multiple malignancy, histologic type not properly identified, etc.	412	(13.8)	8.1–33.4
3. Patient unable to follow instructions to keep appointments	412	(13.8)	8.2–20.5
4. Patient on other protocol[b]	350	(11.7)	3.1–14.9
5. Physician prefers another (nonprotocol) treatment for patient	284	(9.5)	4.4–20.2
6. Patient with prior or current bleeding	256	(8.6)	5.1–13.6
7. Patient prefers another treatment or no treatment	228	(7.7)	3.3–12.4
8. Patient has other serious medical condition, not related to malignancy[c]	208	(7.0)	3.0–8.3
9. Patient is moving or feels he cannot make regular appointments	73	(2.5)	0.5–6.4
10. Patient already on warfarin	43	(1.4)	0.3–3.0
Totals	2981	(100.0)	

Reprinted from Martin et al. (1984) with permission.
[a] Low and high percent of times reason was selected across all medical centers.
[b] National protocols (56%), local protocols (42%), unspecified (2%).
[c] The medical problems included cardiovascular disease, liver disease, pancreatic dysfunction, thrombocytopenia, and prolonged prothrombin time.

4. Recruitment results obtained (e.g., Figs. 7.10, 7.11, 7.13, 7.14) and how they compared to the goals.
5. Measures taken to modify recruitment strategy, sources, or methods during the trial.
6. A statement of whether the data for patients recruited after modifications to the protocol (e.g., inclusion criteria) or strategy (e.g., three new methods were used, including television advertising) were made (e.g., efficacy, demographic, prognostic factors) and analyzed separately and compared to the original group. If this step was done before the data were pooled, what was the result?
7. Other noteworthy events related to patient recruitment that occurred during the course of the trial, and the implications of these for the trial's data, and the interpretation and extrapolation of those data.

The Practice of Excluding Some Recruited and Entered Patients from Data Analyses and Publication

There are well known biases that arise when patients who do not meet certain entry criteria are excluded from the data analyses. While this practice often makes the analyses easier to conduct and interpret, it takes them further from reality. This practice is particularly unacceptable if the criteria used to exclude patients are not identified in the protocol prior to initiating the trial.

Even if it is determined, prior to conducting the trial, that certain patients should be excluded from one or more efficacy analyses, the publication should fully describe all patients recruited. This principle was substantiated by the Toronto Leukemia

TABLE 11.15. *Sample size determination made during the planning phase of VA Cooperative Study #75*

Disease: Tumor category	Average number of patients expected to be screened/site/yr. A	Distribution of patients within each stratum (%) B	Number of patients to be randomized C	Average number of patients expected to be randomized/site/yr. D = A×B×C	Patient entry needed/yr. E	Number of sites required F = [E/D] + 1
Lung						
Non-small cell	69					
Limited		16.0	70.0	7.73	24.24	4
Disseminated		38.1	70.0	18.35	23.76	2
Post "curative" resection/radiation		27.7	70.0	13.38	41.28	4
Small cell[a]	15	18.2	70.0	8.79	23.76	3
Colorectal[a]						
Disseminated		16.0	87.0	2.09	30.36	15
Resected		71.1	87.0	9.28	79.20	9
Prostate, disseminated[b]	28	38.0	73.0	7.77	49.32	7
Head and neck[b]	21	50.0	70.0	7.35	36.72	5

[a] Reprinted from Martin et al. (1984) with permission. References in footnotes refer to original publication.

[b] One hundred percent of the patients were not accounted for in each of the disease categories—for the colorectal category, histologic confirmation of disseminated disease was not available in 12.7% of the patients randomized in the study report in reference 3. Only 38% of the patients reported with prostate cancer reported in reference 7 had documented disseminated disease and only 50% of the patients reported in reference 6 with epidermoid tumors in the head and neck had evidence of progressive disease.

TABLE 11.16. *Number of patients actually accrued to CSP #75 versus expected accrual*

Disease: Tumor category	Number of actual center months of accrual	Screened patient distribution within disease type expected[a]/actual (%)		Number of patients randomized expected[b]/actual		Actual (%)	Number of patients required for entire study
	A	B	C	D	E	F = (E/C) × 100	G
Lung	377	2168	1659 (100)				
Non-small cell							
Limited		347	415 (25.0)	243	64	(15.4)	73
Disseminated		826	932 (56.2)	577	133	(14.3)	71
Post "curative"		600	122 (7.4)	421	44	(36.1)	124
Resection/Radiation							
Small cell		395	190 (11.4)	276	50	(26.3)	71
Colorectal	363	396	431 (100)				
Disseminated		73	336 (78.0)	64	68	(20.2)	91
Postresection		323	95 (22.0)	281	13	(13.7)	238
Prostate, disseminated	288	255	268 (—c)	186	24	(9.0)	148
Head and neck	306	268	329 (—d)	188	41	(12.5)	110
Total		3087	2687	2236	437		926

Reprinted from Martin et al. (1984) with permission.

a Expected number of patients screened = [(Col. A, Table 11.15)/12] × (Col. B, Table 11.15) × (Col. C, Table 11.16).

b Expected number of patients randomized = (Col. B, Table 11.16) × (Col. C, Table 11.15).

c All prostate cancer patients were not screened. Thus, the percentage with disseminated disease was not determinable.

d All head and neck cancer patients were not screened. Thus the percentage with recurrent disease was not determinable.

TABLE 11.17. *Sources of patients used in the Coronary Prevention Trial phase 3 recruitment*

Hire recruitment coordinator
Identify potential sources
  Industry
  Health fairs
  Athletic events
  Shopping centers
Screen entire town
Send mass mailings
Write feature articles
Contact local organizations
  Blood bank
  Heart association
  Other trials

Reprinted from Prout (1981) with permission.

TABLE 11.18. *Patient recruitment trial of acute myocardial infarction*

Percent of the total population	Protocol category	Percent of the previous category
100	Patient admitted	100
65	Suspect acute myocardial infarction	65
52	Age eligible	80
19	Clinical myocardial infarction	35
17	Alive five days	90
13	"Study" acute myocardial infarction	75
5	Exclusion criteria	40
4	Physician consent	85
3	Patient consent obtained and patient randomized	75

Reprinted from Prout (1981) with permission.

TABLE 11.19. *Recruitment model near, average, and far areas*

	Near	Average	Far
Population	2,376,000	4,301,000	10,526,000
Population in cooperating hospital area	1,758,000	2,881,000	6,421,000
Names	1,260	1,710	3,230
Logged in	133	158	245
Screening/baseline	87	103	160
Randomization	12	12	12

Reprinted from Buchwald et al. (1987) with permission.

TABLE 11.20. *Distribution of reasons given by children for nonparticipation in cardiovascular examination by race, sex, and age group, Bogalusa, Louisiana, 1978–1979*

Race, sex, and age group (years)	Nonparticipants (no.)	Child refused (%)	Child afraid (%)	Parent refused (%)	Medical problem (%)	Absent or away (%)	Too many times (%)	Lost form (%)	Other[a] (%)
Whites									
Boys									
5–9	57	19.3	8.8	21.1	24.6	3.5	0.0	7.0	15.8
10–14	78	26.9	20.5	20.5	7.7	5.1	3.8	1.3	14.1
15–17	157	38.2	10.8	4.5	2.5	11.5	4.5	9.6	18.5
Girls									
5–9	51	17.6	23.5	21.6	21.6	2.0	2.0	0.0	11.8
10–14	116	28.4	23.3	19.0	7.8	1.7	0.0	0.9	19.0
15–17	155	39.4	16.1	5.8	9.0	5.8	0.0	3.9	20.0
Blacks									
Boys									
5–9	11	9.1	9.1	18.2	18.2	0.0	0.0	9.1	36.4
10–14	21	19.0	9.5	14.3	19.0	4.8	0.0	4.8	28.6
15–17	46	26.1	2.2	6.5	4.3	15.2	2.2	19.6	23.9
Girls									
5–9	10	0.0	40.0	20.0	0.0	0.0	10.0	10.0	20.0
10–14	8	0.0	12.5	50.0	0.0	0.0	0.0	25.0	12.5
15–17	51	35.3	9.8	3.9	7.8	7.8	2.0	13.7	19.6

Reprinted from Croft et al. (1984) with permission.

[a] Reasons included too busy, did not want to miss school, bad experiences, transportation problems, felt threatened, advised against program, did not understand program, and unknown.

Study Group (1986) when they found that the complete remission rate ranged from 44% to 85% depending on the specific exclusion applied. These investigators concluded that both the interpretation and extrapolation of data require presentation of data on all patients, even those not given chemotherapy or those who received aborted courses of treatment because of infectious complications leading to death.

ADDITIONAL APPROACHES TO PRESENTING RECRUITMENT DATA IN A PUBLICATION OR REPORT

When percents rather than numbers are used to describe the proportion of screened patients who enroll in a clinical trial, it is important that the specific items referred to are clear. This clarity can best be achieved by including a description of the specific categories referred to in the text as well as in footnotes to tables. This practice is particularly essential when percents are used in two or more different ways in the same table or figure—a rather common occurrence in the recruitment literature.

A few additional ways of presenting data are listed. Several of the figures and tables shown throughout this book illustrate novel approaches for presenting results of recruitment.

1. List the number of patients at each stage of the recruitment process and alongside each list the most common (or all) reasons why drop-outs occurred. Show the number (and percent) affected by each reason.
2. Table of costs in money and staff time to enroll a patient using different methods.

3. Table or graph of goals or quotas for each center and how well each performed. Overall data or data for each recruitment period could be shown.
4. Graph of time versus cumulative number or percent of patients enrolled, indicating important changes as arrows under the abscissa (e.g., point at which inclusion criteria were modified, time when an investigators' meeting was held).
5. For rare diseases the percent of all patients with the disease, either in the catchment area or in the entire country, could be indicated.
6. In epidemiological studies, it is useful to present the percent of the entire population sought or present in the catchment area.
7. In addition to illustrations about the funnel effect that start at the number of patients contacted or screened, it is sometimes useful to know what percent of the total population these people represent.

While most journals rarely allow authors to publish extensive details about recruitment experiences and results in an outcome paper, this type of information should be considered for inclusion in ancillary papers that focus on patient recruitment or clinical application of the findings.

A Caution

Some authors report and publish interim trial results in "clinical alerts," consensus conferences, meta-analyses, or other formats. Chlebowski et al. (1989) describe how this type of summary outside traditional "peer-reviewed" procedures may lead to changes in a protocol design and may also influence patient recruitment. Premature disclosure of any clinical trial results may markedly affect recruitment in either a positive or negative manner.

PART III

Consequences and Summary
of Recruitment Issues

MUENCH'S LAWS

Law 1. No Full-Scale Study Confirms the Lead Provided by a Pilot Study.

Anyone who has ever set out to confirm such leads will recognize the universal applicability of Law 1.

Corollary 1.1 (Due to R. Werdin, DVM) When working toward the solution of a problem, it always helps if you know the answer.

Corollary 1.2 (Due to R. Werdin, DVM) Provided, of course, that you know there is a problem.

Corollary 1.3 Anytime that things appear to be going well, you have overlooked something.

Corollary 1.4 Studies can be called pilot studies and so avoid criticism for poor design.

Corollary 1.5 Pilot studies are a waste of time, money, and effort.

Law 2. Results Can Always Be Improved by Omitting Controls.

The Second Law is the most fruitful law.

Corollary 2.1 Placebos are a hindrance in research.

Corollary 2.2 Randomization is a useless procedure.

Corollary 2.3 Statistics is the curse of medical research, since it takes the interpretation of results away from "personal impression" and thus makes interpretation of studies infinitely more difficult.

Corollary 2.4 The amount of monkeying with the data is inversely proportional to the quality of the data.

Corollary 2.5 The data are never as the investigator says they are.

Corollary 2.6 The more and more closely you look at the data, the bigger trouble you are in.

Corollary 2.7 People who insist on controls, randomization, or masked [blinded] evaluation are nitpickers and should be ignored.

Law 3. In Order to Be Realistic, the Number of Cases Promised in any Clinical Study Must Be Divided by a Factor of at Least Ten.

The Third Law produces several interesting corollaries.

Corollary 3.1 (Due to JR Assenzo, PhD) The length of time estimated as necessary to complete a study must be multiplied by a factor of at least ten.

Corollary 3.2 The sum of money estimated as necessary to complete a study must be multiplied by a factor of at least ten (without inflation).

Corollary 3.3 (Due to J Berkson, MD, DSc) But *never* collect more than ten times the amount of data you are going to use.

Corollary 3.4 (Due to LE Hollister, MD) The difficulty in dealing with the data from any study is expressed by the function, $D = a + bt^{10}$, where D is the difficulty, a and b are constants each greater than 1, and t is the time interval since gathering the data.

Corollary 3.5 The difficulties arising from the administrative aspects of research are at least ten times the magnitude of the scientific ones.

—Bearman et al. (1974)

12

Extrapolation of Clinical Trial Results

Its Dependence on Recruitment

TYPES OF CLINICAL EXTRAPOLATIONS

Dimensions Used for Extrapolating Results

Extrapolation of clinical trial results is the process of extending the conclusion from one (1) group of patients, (2) disease, (3) set of conditions, or (4) other aspects of a trial to a new set of circumstances or conditions. The degree of extrapolation is the same as the generalizability of the results (i.e., the predictive value). Extrapolations may be made by the person who has planned and conducted the trial, the person who has analyzed and interpreted the results, or by anyone who has read a published article about the trial. The latter person is at a disadvantage because he or she does not have immediate access to all of the data or details of the clinical trial that might be necessary to extrapolate the results to a new situation. Results can be extrapolated to (1) different patients, (2) other investigators or physicians, (3) other medical practice settings, (4) other periods of time, and (5) other levels of biological organization (e.g., physiological, cellular, molecular levels). Each of these dimensions and the entire topic of extrapolating data from clinical trials are discussed in Chapter 90 of *Guide to Clinical Trials* (Spilker, 1991). This chapter reviews extrapolation issues related to recruitment.

Primary, Secondary, and Tertiary Extrapolations of Clinical Results

The types of extrapolations discussed in this section (i.e., primary, secondary, and tertiary extrapolations) focus on patients, their disease, and the disease's characteristics. This classification ignores three of the other dimensions mentioned above (physician, medical practice setting, and time period). This is believed acceptable because in many cases those other dimensions are either constant or are not believed to markedly affect particular cases where the results are extrapolated. This classification is not meant to replace the one based on the five dimensions, but supplements it when one is extrapolating the data from one group of patients to another. Figure 12.1 illustrates the three types of patient extrapolations.

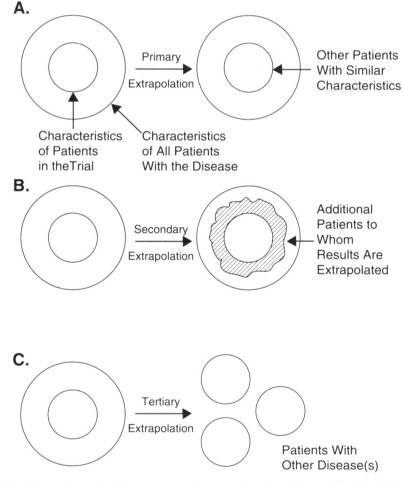

FIG. 12.1. Illustration of primary, secondary, and tertiary types of patient data extrapolations. The circles are representative schematics of the range of demographic and prognostic characteristics. The inner circles in panel A could both be larger or smaller, as long as they were the same size. In panel B the same point could be made, and the stippled area would generally be larger when their inner circle is larger. In panel C the number, type, and size of the circles on the right would depend on the specific case (see text for specific examples). There is no significance to the smaller size of the circles on the right in panel C, and they represent different circles (i.e., diseases) than those on the left in panel C.

Primary Extrapolations. Extrapolations of clinical results to patients not enrolled in the trial but who have similar disease characteristics as defined by trial eligibility criteria.

Secondary Extrapolations. Extrapolations of clinical results to patients with the same disease, including those with different disease characteristics.

Tertiary Extrapolations. Extrapolations of clinical data to patients with other diseases.

Some of the types of tertiary extrapolations are discussed below.

Types and Examples of Tertiary Extrapolations

Type 1. Tertiary Extrapolation: For Beneficial Effects

Assume that patients with arthritis respond to an anti-inflammatory medicine. The results are then extrapolated to patients with other rheumatological diseases and to patients with nonrheumatological diseases that have an inflammatory component (e.g., asthma).

Type 2. Tertiary Extrapolation: For Adverse Reactions

Assume that patients with a given disease take a medicine and develop an adverse reaction. The presence of that adverse reaction is then extrapolated for consideration as a beneficial effect in other diseases or conditions.

Example 1. Female patients with hypertension develop excessive unwanted hair growth. The medicine then is tested in men with baldness.

Example 2. Patients with hayfever take histamine antagonists and become sedated. The medicine is then studied as a sleep promoting agent.

RELATIONSHIP BETWEEN RECRUITMENT AND EXTRAPOLATION

The types of patients to whom clinical trial results may be extrapolated depends primarily on the type of patients entered in the clinical trial and also on the nature of their disease. Recruiting patients into a clinical trial who meet the inclusion criteria enables the results to be extrapolated to similar patients (i.e., primary extrapolation), and possibly to others with the same disease (i.e., secondary extrapolation). Extrapolating data to patients with other diseases or conditions is more problematic.

Extrapolation of data may be considered either narrowly or broadly when determining the types of patients to recruit. For example, if one desires to extrapolate the data from a clinical trial narrowly to a specific subtype of patients with explicit risk factors and characteristics (e.g., renal failure), then that is the sole type of patient that should be recruited and enrolled. The opposite is also true (i.e., to extrapolate broadly the data from a trial it is best to have a heterogeneous patient population). In that type of trial it is more reasonable to extrapolate the results to most, if not all, patients with a disease.

This suggests that the type of patients one should recruit depends on the type(s) of extrapolations one wishes to make. This is generally true, although there are exceptions, such as for a Phase I pharmacokinetic trial. In that type of clinical trial, a narrow range of patients is studied but the results of absorption, metabolism, and elimination are usually extrapolated broadly. If the appropriate group and numbers of patients are unavailable for a trial, then serious consideration must be given to either changing the clinical trial's objective, canceling the trial, or finding a solution to the recruitment problem. A less restrictive objective, such as a larger minimum detectable difference or larger Type I error rate, could allow a smaller sample size to be required and thus enable the trial to be conducted. This situation is sometimes faced when marked problems in recruiting patients are encountered. Even when a smaller sample size is used and the trial conducted, something is usually forfeited (i.e., a larger Type I error rate is accepted) and the modified design is less rigorous than the original one. Sufficient funds to open new sites or advertise widely could represent a solution to recruitment limitations.

Broad eligibility criteria are encouraged by Yusuf et al. (1990). Yusuf et al. state that not only is a heterogeneous population unlikely to reduce treatment effects, but it also is not worthwhile to characterize patients precisely with precise baseline variables. Recruitment of sufficient numbers of patients to balance the groups is more important in reducing random error. "The wider the types of patients enrolled, the greater the applicability of the trial and the greater its impact on public health." This concept is an important one for most large trials but does not apply to many smaller ones.

Influence of Yield on Extrapolation

The "yield" (i.e., number of enrolled patients divided by the number screened or contacted and multiplied by 100) is rarely included among the information published at the conclusion of a trial. This is probably because editorial space restrictions and other factors (see Chapter 11, Publishing). The lack of information on recruitment in published reports contributes to the uncontrolled, and often imprudent, extrapolation of results. A small yield is not a problem *per se*; but a small yield is more likely to mean that the enrolled population is nonrepresentative of either the total group of patients screened or the hypothetical population to which one might extrapolate results. If the small yield can be shown to be representative of the patients screened (by using patient screening log information), then the small yield is not a particular problem, just a lot more work for the trial staff than a large yield. The Study of Left Ventricular Disorders (SOLVD) trial is a good example of a trial where a small yield was no impediment to extrapolating results, because they not only had a log of screened patients, but they also recorded some laboratory data on nonenrolled patients.

The most widely believed generalization about yield is that the lower the percent yield, the more questionable is the practice of extrapolating results obtained. Even a primary extrapolation of results to patients with apparently similar disease characteristics is sometimes questioned if the yield is low, because it is quite possible that the patients enrolled differ from the group to whom results are primarily extrapolated in one or more important factors. To demonstrate that this is either true or false, one may compare the demographic and prognostic characteristics of patients who met the inclusion criteria but did not enter the trial. This is best done by using the screening log, indicating the importance of collecting appropriate data in the log, particularly on prognostic characteristics.

Comparison of Randomized and Nonrandomized Patients Who Met Randomization Criteria

To evaluate whether a trial's results may be extrapolated to other patients with similar inclusion criteria it is desirable to compare the clinical outcomes of patients who were randomized with those who declined participation in the same trial. This was done in the Coronary Artery Surgery Study (CASS Principal Investigators and Their Associates, 1984). A 5-year follow-up was conducted on 780 patients who entered the trial and 1,315 patients at the same sites who met randomization criteria but declined to join the trial. The clinical outcomes were similar in each group both for the overall results and for all subgroups examined. This excellent study is a rare example of this type of comparison in the clinical literature. The trial authors caution against the temptation to combine results of these two groups to provide a larger data base.

ROLE OF SCREENING LOGS IN THE EXTRAPOLATION OF RESULTS

To determine whether data may be extrapolated to patients with other disease characteristics (i.e., a secondary extrapolation), one could search the screening logs for data of patients who did not meet inclusion criteria. The disease characteristics, including prognostic criteria, of that group could be compared with those patients who were enrolled. Statistically and clinically important differences would also be sought, apart from that reason(s) that excluded the patient from the trial. Since the intervention was not tested in these patients, there is a certain leap of faith in guessing how they would have responded. Still, the type of patients to whom the results may be extrapolated may be described better. These considerations must be made prior to the trial, when steps can be taken to ensure the appropriate design and use of screening forms at all trial sites.

If a screening log has been maintained, it should document the characteristics of those patients who did not enroll. These data should be compared with the same data from those who enrolled. A comparison of important prognostic and demographic characteristics will indicate the degree of similarity between those patients who were enrolled and those who were not. Similarity of data between these groups does not necessarily mean that the trial results may be extrapolated with confidence to a larger population of patients. There may be various unmeasured parameters (e.g., psychological, social, behavioral) that could affect the extrapolatability of the results. However, if the two groups are similar in their clinical, demographic, and prognostic characteristics, there is greater probability that the data obtained from the group enrolled in the trial are not strictly limited and may be extrapolated to a matched population. Significant differences in important characteristics between enrollees and nonenrollees does not necessarily mean that the trial results cannot be extrapolated further. Each clinical trial must be reviewed individually before deciding how broadly the results may be extrapolated.

The minimal data to collect in a screening log on all patients contacted and screened that would enable the above analysis to be conducted are (1) basic demographic data, (2) known and/or potential prognostic characteristics, (3) pertinent past medical history, and (4) reasons(s) for nonenrollment. Of these, prognostic characteristics are most important and past medical history is generally least important. Examples of screening logs are shown in Figs. 9.2 and 9.3.

When only a small and nonrandomly selected percentage of suitable patients actually enroll in a clinical trial, it usually means that the responses in either treatment group may not be typical of most patients with the disease. This indicates that changes in the disease observed in the control group may not be used to study the natural history of the disease (Chalmers, 1982). As discussed above, a small yield is not necessarily a problem for extrapolation.

SAMPLE SIZE AND POWER

Major problems can be created when the total number of patients enrolled in a clinical trial is less than the projected sample size required to achieve an appropriate power to address the trial's objective(s). This issue was addressed by Charlson and Horwitz (1984), who presented a list of 41 multicenter clinical trials from the National Institutes of Health that had a projected sample size ranging between 250 and 200,000 patients. Of these 41 trials, only 14 achieved 100% (or more) of their sample size.

1. Narrow Inclusion Criteria Used in Protocol A

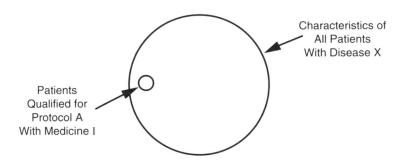

2. Broad Inclusion Criteria Used in Protocol B

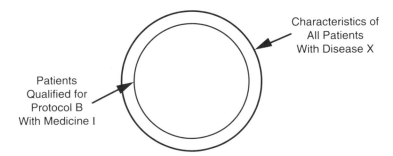

FIG. 12.2. The scope of patients in a trial depends on the protocol's inclusion criteria. In the top panel, narrow inclusion criteria in the protocol restrict enrollment to a highly limited group of patients. In the bottom panel, almost all patients with the disease would qualify for the trial. The upper panel is characteristic of many Phase I and II trials, and the lower panel is characteristic of many Phase III trials.

Another six trials achieved 90% to 99%. The authors discuss these and other data in some detail and document various failures of these large trials (e.g., to maintain screening logs). They raise the important question of whether the results from a trial may be extrapolated from those who entered the trial to those who have similar disease but were disqualified from entry or refused to enter the trial.

The total amount of data used to demonstrate efficacy of a new medicine should be from patients who have a wide range of clinical characteristics, including almost

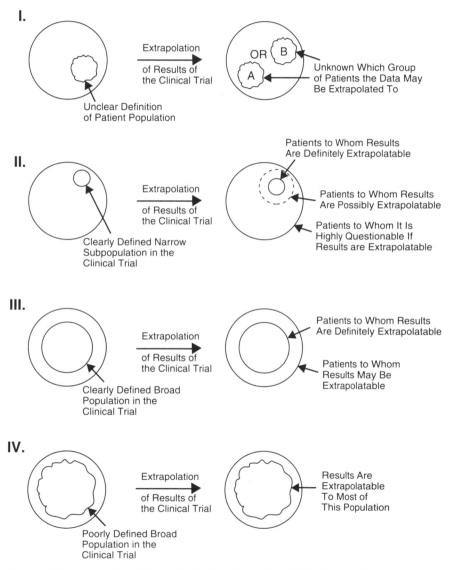

Medical Characteristics of the Total Patient Population With Disease X Are Included in the Outer Circle (i.e. outer circles of I to IV are the same).

FIG. 12.3. Schematic diagrams of various patterns of extrapolation. Medical characteristics of the total patient population with the disease are included within the outer circle. Thus, the outer circles of I to IV are the same.

all types and characteristics of patients with the particular disease being evaluated. Most Phase III clinical trials are designed to include a broad range of patients. If all Phase III trials only enroll a narrow patient subgroup, practicing physicians and regulators will be more skeptical of the results, which could lead to restrictions being placed on the medicine's labeling. These principles are illustrated diagramatically in Figs. 12.2 and 12.3.

Some clinical trials are specifically designed to enroll the highest-risk patients to maximize the probability of detecting treatment differences. This practice sacrifices extrapolatability of results. This is an "insider's" viewpoint and some clinicians outside the trial group may extrapolate the results "broadly." This was the rationale used for restricting some heart disease trials to males only, and has resulted in the recent effort to eliminate restrictions on enrollment of women in NIH-funded trials.

DO DIFFERENT RECRUITMENT SOURCES AND METHODS RECRUIT DIFFERENT TYPES OF PATIENTS?

The obvious answer to this question is "it depends." If recruiting methods change significantly during a clinical trial, then the investigator(s) should always compare data obtained with each group of patients prior to pooling the data. Demonstrating that demographics, prognostic characteristics, and patient responses are similar provides confidence that the two groups are sufficiently homogeneous so that their data may be pooled.

Royce and Arkowitz (1977) compared two groups of volunteers used in a study— classroom enrollees and subjects recruited by newspaper advertisements. They found no differences in the characteristics of the two groups. Their study involved social anxiety treatment research. They quote a study by Little, Curran, and Gilbert where the same two recruiting methods enrolled two patient groups with important differences in their characteristics. Thus, there is conflicting evidence about whether these two groups of volunteers recruited by different methods can be considered equal in terms of the data they provide.

Patients recruited via three quite different approaches (i.e., traditional, semitraditional, and nontraditional) for a depression trial were compared. Breckenridge et al. (1985) found no significant differences (by recruitment method) in the 112 patients for (1) duration of the depressive period, (2) precipitating stressful event, (3) perceived relation of stressful event to development of the depressive episode, (4) number of symptoms related to depression, (5) pretreatment and post-treatment scores on the Beck Depression Inventory, (6) ratings on a suicide question and pretreatment scores on the Hamilton Rating Scale for Depression, (7) expectancy of treatment outcome, (8) demographic details, (9) psychiatric history, and several other factors. This is clearly a demonstration that the two populations were close enough in their clinical characteristics to justify pooling their data.

Comparison of Solicited and Unsolicited Patients as the Basis of Extrapolating Results

Krupnick et al. (1986) evaluated 14 trials of psychotherapy and psychopharmacological treatments in solicited and unsolicited patients. Pretreatment variables were comparable in these trials, and Krupnick et al. (1986) reported that results from solicited volunteers can be extrapolated to other patients, at least in the diseases and types of trials studied. Whether these results can be extrapolated to other diseases is doubtful, without specific studies to provide additional evidence.

Duration of Recruitment

The validity of extrapolating data from a clinical trial to other patients becomes more questionable when the recruitment period is dragged out. One question is whether the population's characteristics have changed. It is necessary to ensure that patients recruited at the end of a trial are similar to those recruited early in the trial. It is also necessary to compare each patient groups' prognostic characteristics and demographics whenever major changes in recruitment are initiated (e.g., modification of inclusion criteria, use of additional recruitment methods that differ from the original methods). This comparison may be done on an ongoing basis for an open-label trial. Even for a double blind trial an ongoing comparison may be made. This is done by combining data from all patients enrolled via a single recruitment method and comparing them with data from patients recruited with other methods. This comparison may be made before or after a trial is completed for any trial design. The danger of waiting until the trial is completed before comparing prognostic characteristics of patients recruited with different methods is that any problem observed cannot be rectified.

EPIDEMIOLOGICAL USE OF SCREENING DATA

Collection of appropriate screening logs allows investigator(s) to formulate a demographic profile of their clinic population. If this population is large enough, investigators may be able to construct a profile of most patients with a specific disease or problem in that community. These profiles are valuable to a local investigator even when they are collected for a nationwide trial because they provide important comparisons between the local site and other areas.

Prognostic information collected from the screened population can be used to construct a general estimate of the type of patients with the disease and the severity, incidence, and prevalence of the disease in the catchment area. These logs provide valuable pilot data for future clinical trials of similar diseases in the same or other communities by establishing the types of patients with specific problems. Screening data also can be used for ancillary analyses or as the basis for a justification of need for other trials. The data may serve as a quasi-census of the medical status of those patients with a particular disorder in the community. These data may therefore have important uses in planning for current and future medical studies. Figure 12.4 illustrates a comparison of a large clinical trial (Systolic Hypertension in the Elderly Program, SHEP) and a community sample for cognitive impairment, depression, and activity limitation. This demonstrates the degree to which the SHEP population is representative of the community. It does not, on its own, indicate the degree to which results may be extrapolated, because it does not compare the characteristics of the two groups. It is quite possible that they differ in one or more important factors.

Wilhelmsen et al. (1976) compared participants and nonparticipants in a large cardiovascular trial in Goteborg, Sweden. They commented that "a fundamental prerequisite in all epidemiological work is that the selected sample really represents

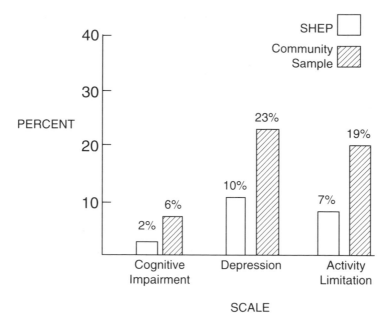

FIG. 12.4. Comparison of Systolic Hypertension in the Elderly Program (SHEP) participants and community sample with respect to the proportions having cognitive impairment, depression, or activity limitations according to behavioral assessment package used in the SHEP study. Reprinted from Vogt et al. (1986) with permission.

the population one wishes to characterize.'' They found that the total incidence of coronary heart disease was 1.6% in nonparticipants and 0.9% in participants. They mentioned that a trial for pulmonary tuberculosis in Denmark also demonstrated the same result. The authors quote some of their own work and that of others about social factors of nonparticipants. Nonparticipants were found to be more likely to be (1) unmarried, (2) divorced, (3) alcoholic, (4) on a low pension, and (5) have a negative attitude toward medical care. One of the consequences suggested by these results is that the magnitude of alcohol as a risk factor for disease and death in some (or many) epidemiological studies may be underestimated.

CAUTIONS ABOUT EXTRAPOLATING SUCCESSFUL RECRUITMENT METHODS FOR USE IN A NEW CLINICAL TRIAL

There is a tendency, among clinical trial investigators or planners, to read or hear about successful recruitment techniques used by other investigators and believe that those method(s) will work in one's own trial. This belief may be correct. Nonetheless, before adopting and incorporating their sources or methods into your trial it is essential to assess the likelihood of successfully extrapolating the recruitment approach to your trial. This can be done by asking the following questions about the published or completed trial and your planned one.

1. Is the disease being evaluated the same in the two trials? If it is not, caution needs to be used, though it is still possible that the recruitment method is extrapolatable.

2. Are the inclusion criteria for the patients being recruited comparable?
3. Are the social and economic levels of the patients comparable?
4. Are the degrees of physical and mental debility of the patients comparable?
5. Are there approximately the same total number of patients in the catchment area(s)? If there are fewer patients present in the area, are proportionally fewer required in the trial?
6. Are there any special features about the protocols, requirements that patients might object to more in the planned trial (e.g., lumbar punctures)?
7. Are there any special features about the setting, staff, or facilities of the clinical trial sites that patients might object to more in the planned trial (e.g., duration and frequency of follow-up)?
8. Are there any additional informed consent issues in the new trial?

If answers to all of these questions indicate that the new trial is comparable or more "patient-friendly" (i.e., less onerous for patients to participate in), and patients are as able to participate, then extrapolation of the methods should be acceptable. If the two trials differ in several major ways, then careful review and discussion are needed to assess whether extrapolation of methods is warranted. Of course, any method may be used, but an investigator normally wants to choose those with the greatest chance of success that are within his or her budget and resources. Consider calling or writing the investigators of the other trial to discuss their recruitment experiences. If all answers to the above questions suggest that the currently planned trial involves more difficulties, the method(s) used in the successful trial might still be the best ones to choose for the new trial. However, additional staff time, and possibly money, may be required to make those methods work successfully.

13

Golden Rules of Patient Recruitment

A broad overview of issues and standards of patient recruitment shows that numerous principles exist that can be applied to most clinical trials. Most of the principles have been stated in other chapters of this book and are summarized below in six major categories based on the chronological order of the steps involved in a clinical trial. This list is not meant to be complete and other principles could also be described as golden rules of patient recruitment.

PRIOR TO WRITING A CLINICAL TRIAL PROTOCOL

1. Assemble a group of individuals with different types of expertise to discuss recruitment issues.
2. Identify both the actual and potential pool(s) of patients (or volunteers) to be approached.
3. Identify the disease and nondisease characteristics of those patients likely to enroll in the clinical trial. This is often based on clinical experience of the investigators, and sponsors, if any.
4. Calculate and agree on the rate of patients to be recruited, being careful to caution strongly against overoptimism.
5. Create a clearly articulated and fully developed recruitment strategy. Be as realistic and conservative as possible in creating this plan.
6. Have the recruitment strategy critiqued by appropriate personnel (i.e., friends or colleagues who are knowledgeable about recruitment).
7. Identify additional methods that could be used if necessary. Even a method that works initially may not work later on, and vice versa.
8. Identify means of increasing efforts on each of the methods chosen to recruit patients and identify when those additional efforts would be implemented.

DURING THE WRITING OF A CLINICAL TRIAL PROTOCOL

1. Carefully evaluate how each aspect of the trial (e.g., number of clinic visits, duration of each visit, demands at each visit) is expected to affect patient recruitment.
2. Carefully evaluate how each inclusion criterion is expected to affect patient recruitment.
3. In all multicenter trials and in all sponsored trials, visit the potential investigators and assess insofar as possible (e.g., chart reviews, previous trials conducted) their ability to recruit a sufficient number of patients within a specified time period.
4. Ensure that people recruiting patients for double-blind trials will have no means of guessing which treatment will be assigned to any prospective enrollee (see Chalmers et al., 1983 for a discussion on this point).
5. Appoint a recruitment coordinator at each site. The investigator may assume the role or select a staff person who may or may not have other responsibilities for the trial.
6. Establish interim goals for the number of patient contacts, screens, and enrollees per week, month, or other time period.
7. Devise a contingency plan to enhance patient recruitment.

ASSESSING THE LIKELIHOOD OF RECRUITING AND ENROLLING A SUFFICIENT NUMBER OF APPROPRIATE PATIENTS

1. Check the medical records of potential patients to assess the number and percentage that meet all entry criteria.
2. If medical records are inappropriate to evaluate (e.g., for an acute treatment trial where patients do not yet have their problem such as acute backache) assess the number of patients with the condition of interest treated at the clinic(s) over the previous X number of months or years.
3. If a very large clinical trial is being considered or planned, conduct a formal pilot trial. Assess the value, success, and cost of each recruitment method used.
4. Determine which change(s) in the protocol's inclusion criteria would enable enrollment of the largest number of additional patients, with the least negative effect on achieving the trial's objective(s). Assess the possibility of making these changes.
5. Confirm the necessary agreement and support of all relevant institutions and professionals involved in the recruitment strategy.
6. Consider and make allowances for normally slow periods for recruitment (e.g., summer vacations, winter holidays).

DURING THE INITIATION OF A CLINICAL TRIAL

1. Obtain adequate personnel for answering telephones, scheduling clinic visits, and conducting each type of screen.
2. Train all personnel appropriately and evaluate their skills. Assure that aggressive approaches to patients are not used.
3. Conduct a cost-benefit analysis of each recruitment method considered and

choose the one(s) that are most desirable and most comfortable for the staff and institution to implement.

4. Develop guidelines, questionnaires, and forms for telephone interviews and screening examinations.
5. Develop a screening log to record the age, sex, race, and prognostic characteristics of all patients who are contacted, screened, and entered. Indicate the major (and all other) reasons why nonentered patients were not enrolled.
6. Contact health professionals or physicians who will provide patients or who operate facilities at which patients will be recruited. Provide feedback to these people throughout the trial.
7. Discuss important trials with the medical community in the catchment area before any large media recruitment is initiated. Seek agreement to the recruitment approach considered and also seek cooperation in obtaining referrals.
8. Plan for a slower initial recruitment period if potential problems are anticipated in the early phase of a trial. Work problems out of the referral system before it is widely used.
9. Take whatever steps are necessary to implement contingency plans that may have to be used at a later stage of the clinical trial (e.g., visit potential sources of patients and discuss recruitment issues with relevant personnel).

DURING THE CONDUCT OF A CLINICAL TRIAL

1. Maintain logs of all patients contacted, screened and enrolled in the clinical trial.
2. Track the recruitment of patients at each site in a multicenter trial on a frequent basis (e.g., weekly or monthly) and plot the number of patients enrolled versus the anticipated (expected) rate of enrollment. Provide the graphs or tables of actual versus projected recruitment to all sites. Provide positive feedback (e.g., awards to investigators meeting goals, "milestone" celebrations).
3. Monitor the trial's conduct to ensure that potential enrollees are not kept waiting for long periods and are treated with appropriate care and respect.
4. Investigators and their staff must spend sufficient time with all patients and their families to answer all questions and to explain the nature of the clinical trial. This explanation should use whatever educational level the family desires and is able to understand.
5. When the actual rate of patient enrollment is less than the expected rate by a predetermined amount for a predetermined length of time (e.g., below quota), investigate the causes of this issue.
6. If the number of enrollees does not achieve a minimum standard per week or month or other period, then take steps to evaluate the number of patient contacts and screens and also to modify the recruitment strategy as discussed in Chapter 8.
7. Investigate each recruitment issue thoroughly to develop a counterplan and to initiate a response.
8. When major problems in recruitment occur, call a meeting of all relevant personnel to address the problem.
9. In modifying the recruitment strategy, alter one method at a time if it is important to know which particular change has an effect on recruitment. Changing two or

more methods together will complicate the interpretation of which is responsible for any change observed.

10. Adjust (if necessary) the goals used as targets for patient recruitment.

AFTER A CLINICAL TRIAL IS COMPLETED

1. Prepare a funnel chart, table, or diagram to document recruitment data that will be included in a clinical trial report or in another publication.
2. Provide feedback to all sites and investigators about how well they recruited patients. Provide pointers to help them with future trials as well as cumulative graphs on their projected versus actual recruitment and graphs for the trial as a whole.
3. Publications of clinical trial results should describe recruitment data using level two (see text for discussion).

PATIENTS WHO MAY BE RECRUITED INTO CLINICAL TRIALS

1. No person should be approached for enrollment in a clinical trial as a volunteer or patient if there is a superior–subordinate relationship (c.g., teacher–student, supervisor–employee, advisor–graduate student).
2. Extreme caution should be used in deciding whether to approach people working in the facility where the research is to be conducted.
3. No person should be approached for enrollment if there are substantial doubts over the use of free will to sign an informed consent (i.e., prisoners, mentally retarded patients). Exceptions may be made by ethics committees under unusual circumstances.

The effectiveness of patient recruitment must be judged by the number of patients enrolled and not by the number of patients screened, or even by the apparent yield of the method(s) used. A high percentage yield may not enroll a sufficient number of patients within a reasonable period. Nonetheless, it is important not to push recruitment so much that inappropriate patients are enrolled or patients are inappropriately enrolled. These practices may raise ethical issues or the problem of the bad data collected being actually worse than having no data.

Appendix

COMMON RECRUITMENT PROBLEMS

This Appendix presents a number of common recruitment problems that arise in clinical trials as well as basic answers. These exercises on patient recruitment issues are intended to stimulate discussion by clinical trial planners and managers of either small or large trials. They are written for less experienced individuals who wish to read additional examples that present common recruitment problems. Various approaches to address recruitment problems are presented throughout this book. Therefore, only brief suggestions or approaches to each problem are outlined in this appendix.

Problem: I have very few resources to initiate and conduct a single site study. What type of recruiting strategy do I need to develop?

Answer: If you know that you have ready access (e.g., in your own practice) to all the patients you need, then you do not need any strategy. If you anticipate problems, then you certainly should evaluate how you will attract a sufficient number of patients of the right type at the right time. These are the three major elements of any strategy—a plan to enroll the right *number of patients*, the right *type of patients*, and at the right *time*. Refer to Chapter 7 on the steps to develop a recruiting strategy.

* * *

Problem: We weren't getting any referrals from our physician colleagues who we hoped would send us the patients we needed. When we called a few of these physicians they claimed that they either had forgotten or were unaware of the trial.

Answer: Periodic reminders that avoid harrassing prospective sources are a good method to keep the trial in their minds. Those who were unaware of the trial need to be properly informed. In addition, you could advertise in local medical journals, speak at medical meetings, post notices, and send letters to your contacts. However, avoid being too persistent with any one source.

* * *

Problem: We weren't getting any referrals from our physician colleagues who we hoped would send us the patients we needed to enroll in our trial. When we called several, they all gave feeble excuses. Clearly, they did not want to go to the trouble to refer their patients or they were concerned that the patients would be lost to their practice. What can we do?

Answer: If the physicians truly have no suitable patients then you should reexamine the premises on which you approached them. Also, consider switching to other sources. The easiest option may be to provide reassurances to the physicians about their concerns of potentially losing the patient and the associated financial benefits. Another approach is to visit different groups of physicians to encourage them to send patients. Show the physicians that you truly believe in the trial, by providing them with feedback on their patients. If the problem is the amount of work needed for physicians to refer patients, determine what you could do to decrease this aspect of the referral. Define exactly how the clinical trial staff will interface with referring physicians and their staff, particularly in terms of work load related to patient recruitment.

* * *

Problem: My practice has about 125 patients who appear to qualify for a trial, but none seem to want to enter. Why, and what can I do?

Answer: Have you asked them why they do not want to enter? Is there a general theme or do all the reasons seem to differ? Are there points in the protocol that are difficult for patients to accept? What would encourage your patients to want to enter? How are patients approached and by whom? Is the approach positive and upbeat? Are they given adequate information about advantages as well as other informed consent issues? If they say the protocol is too arduous or complex, can it be altered?

* * *

Problem: We've tried to find the reason for low patient enrollment in a multicenter trial but can't. What can we do?

Answer: Bring all the investigators together to share experiences and opinions. Find out what works at sites where enrollment is best. Ask the trial coordinators or recruitment coordinators what they think are the problems and possible solutions. Use open, roundtable discussions to identify the problem(s), and brainstorm for solutions.

* * *

Problem: I am running a trial both through my private office and through my clinic at the hospital. I am enrolling almost all the patients through the hospital, but no one from my practice seems to want to join, why?

Answer: Are the social and economic levels of the patients different? Is their disease severity different? Have you asked the patients why they do not want to join the trial? What about their incentives to join? Are you asking private patients to attend follow-up visits at the hospital (which might be less convenient than the private office)? Are you presenting the trial equally strongly at each site?

* * *

Problem: I'm organizing a multicenter trial to enroll 100 patients over one year. How many sites do I need to reach this target?

Answer: The number of patients enrolled per site depends on many factors. How many patients can each site comfortably enroll in the target period? How do you know? If you are fairly sure of the answer, then still include additional sites. If you do not have an estimate, ask potential sites to survey their clinic population for 3 months documenting potentially eligible patients.

If you did not perform a pilot trial or preliminary survey that would have provided an estimate of patient availability, other determinants need to be assessed. For example, how many patients with the designated diagnosis are on the rosters of a typical clinic? Do not forget to consider Lasagna's Law (divide the number of patients you think are available by ten).

* * *

Problem: In a large multicenter trial of 50 centers, ten sites enrolled their patients from community hospitals, ten enrolled their patients from tertiary care hospitals, ten enrolled their patients from group practices, ten enrolled their patients from a mixture of practices, and ten enrolled their patients from overseas. Does each category have to be evaluated separately?

Answer: The purpose of the individual evaluation of sites is to show that the data obtained in each group are comparable and are able to be pooled. Imbalance in demographic data should be assessed among sites as well as between randomization groups.

* * *

Problem: I can't seem to find medicine-naive patients for my trial. All the patients have taken one of the medicines that makes them ineligible for the trial. What should I do?

Answer: Assuming that the population that you seek exists, there are several approaches. First, advertise for them. Second, send a letter to colleagues for referrals. Third, if your trial potentially has major importance, send a press release to the newspapers in your area. Fourth, go to medical meetings in your area and make a pitch to your colleagues. If this is a sponsored trial, hire a contractor to find patients (e.g., telephone recruiting). If the population no longer (or never) existed, then alter the inclusion criteria.

* * *

Problem: I've advertised for volunteers for a Phase I pharmacokinetic trial and only homeless people have shown up. Is it appropriate to enroll them?

Answer: There is nothing inherently wrong with including homeless volunteers in a clinical trial. The major issues include whether they are also alcoholics, drug abusers, or have other occult medical problems. If so, then that would be a major problem and should be included. The other problem is whether they will be cooperative and reliable in the trial. Will they show up at the clinic each time they are scheduled? If you believe that the people you are talking to are adequate in these regards and meet the inclusion criteria, then there is no particular reason not to enroll them. If you strongly prefer other types of patients, then modify your inclusion criteria and also modify your advertisements and in which newspapers they are presented.

* * *

Problem: I've advertised for volunteers for a Phase I trial and am mainly getting alcoholics or drug abusers. What is the problem?

Answer: The major issue is two-fold. First, where are you advertising? Is it in a big city newspaper or in a local community paper? Is it in a college paper? Second, what are you saying in your ad? Does it sound like you're providing food and shelter for a period of time to whomever wants to apply? Can you say that college students are preferred? This may give some of those volunteers who are answering the ad the idea that they need not apply. The inclusion criteria probably clearly require excellent health so this can be made clear in the advertising and during the initial screen. Make the initial telephone screen more precise to cut down the number of volunteers you do not wish to come to the clinic for screening.

* * *

Problem: I thought that I could enroll enough patients for my own clinical trial, but its been much more difficult than I anticipated. What are my options?

Answer: You could try all of the techniques listed in Chapter 8 to enhance enrollment. Rather than give up, consider inviting some colleagues to join you and expand the scope of the trial to multiple investigators (at the same or multiple sites). On the other hand, remember that closing down a trial that cannot enroll enough patients without spending an enormous amount of money (and effort) may be the best solution. Admitting that the trial was infeasible or too ambitious generally takes courage, but may be the best path to follow for both your sake and your patients.

* * *

Problem: I started my own clinical trial with a great deal of enthusiasm, but I now find that recruitment is tedious and boring. I'm ready to give up the entire clinical trial. Any suggestions?

Answer: Can you delegate the recruitment to others? This could include your current staff, new staff hired for that purpose (and possibly other purposes), or the staff of coinvestigators' you contact to join your trial. Other ideas are to find something in your trial that is of interest that you can focus on, or add something (e.g., a test) that is of interest. Explore other ideas discussed in Chapter 8 to improve motivation, or to simplify the protocol requirements and admission criteria.

* * *

Problem: I initiated a trial of acute care treatment options that requires patient enrollment in the emergency room. Between logistical problems and not being called, only four patients have been randomized instead of the 20 patients anticipated based on a pretrial survey. Should I give up and cancel the trial?

Answer: Before terminating the trial, reconsider your recruitment strategy. Are the emergency room staff (and ambulance staff if appropriate) aware of the trial? Do they know who to call and at what stage of the preliminary patient evaluation? Are you or your colleagues readily available at *all* times to respond to calls? How rapidly did you respond to the "firebell" for referrals that were not randomized? How many false alarms (inappropriate referrals) have you had and how did you handle them with the emergency room staff? Recruitment problems often relate to issues of communications and education. Should you bring boxes of snacks and sweets for the staff?

* * *

Problem: A new medicine widely touted as a significant advance in treatment is being tested in patients who are in the late stages of their disease. After sending informational letters to my colleagues, all the referrals have been for patients who are not remotely eligible for the trial. How can I reexplain the trial and inclusion criteria without offending my colleagues?

Answer: First, be sure to thank each colleague for having made a referral. Second, try one of several simple recruitment methods to clarify the inclusion criteria, particularly if your initial letter was not overly specific. Try sending posters that describe the essence of the trial and suggest that they be posted in the chart area for "ready reference about the trial." If utilized by your colleagues, a poster might be a clear stimulus to restrict referral to relatively appropriate patients. You are fortunate to have a stream of calls from your colleagues; it may just need some fine-tuning.

References

Ackerman, T. F. (1989): Compensation of human volunteers. In: *Development of new medicines: Ethical questions.* Champey, Y., Levine, R. J., and Lietman, P. S. (Eds.). pp. 51–62. Royal Society of Medicine Services Limited, London.

Agras, W. S., and Bradford, R. H. (1982): Recruitment for clinical trials: The Lipid Research Clinics Coronary Primary Prevention Trial experience: Its implications for future trials. *Circulation,* 66(Suppl. 4):IV-1–IV-78.

Agras, W. S., and Marshall, G. (1979): Recruitment for the Coronary Primary Prevention Trial. *Clin. Pharmacol. Ther.,* 25:688–690.

Agras, W. S., Marshall, G. D., and Kraemer, H. C. (1982): Planning recruitment. *Circulation,* 66(Suppl. 4):IV-54–IV-58.

Albanes, D., Virtamo, J., Rautalahti, M., Pikkarainen, J., Taylor, P. R., et al. (1986): Pilot study: The US–Finland lung cancer prevention trial. *J. Nutrition, Growth and Cancer,* 3:207–214.

American Medical Association Council on Scientific Affairs. (1991): Viability of cancer clinical research: Patient accrual, coverage, and reimbursement. *J. Natl. Cancer Inst.,* 83:254–259.

American Psychological Association. (1982): *Ethical principles in the conduct of research with human participants.* American Psychological Association, Washington, DC.

Annas, G. J., and Glantz, L. H. (1986): Rules for research in nursing homes. *N. Engl. J. Med.,* 315:1157–1158.

Anonymous. (1988): Recruiting patients for clinical trials. *J. Natl. Cancer Inst.,* 80:619–620.

Arnold, A., Johnstone, B., Stoskopf, B., Skingley, P., Browman, G., et al. (1989): Recruitment for an efficacy study in chemoprevention—the Concerned Smoker Study. *Prev. Med.,* 18:700–710.

Arthritis and Rheumatism Council Multicentre Radiosynoviorthesis Trial Group. (1984): Intra-articular radioactive yttrium and triamcinolone hexacetonide: An inconclusive trial. *Ann. Rheum. Dis.,* 43:620–623.

Aspirin Myocardial Infarction Study Research Group. (1980): A randomized, controlled trial of aspirin in persons recovered from myocardial infarction. *JAMA,* 243:661–669.

Baines, C. J. (1984): Impediments to recruitment in the Canadian National Breast Screening Study: Response and resolution. *Controlled Clin. Trials,* 5:129–140.

Barlow, P. B., Nelson, E. C., Howland, J., Meier, F. A., Brooks, A. H., et al. (1984): Locating community residents with chronic airway obstruction. A comparison of four strategies. *Am. Rev. Respir. Dis.,* 129:361–365.

Barofsky, I., and Sugarbaker, P. H. (1979): Determinants of patient nonparticipation in randomized clinical trials for the treatment of sarcomas. *Cancer Clin. Trials,* 2:237–246.

Bearman, J. E., Loewenson, R. B., and Gullen, W. H. (1974): *Muench's postulates, laws and corollaries or biometrician's views on clinical studies.* Biometrics note no. 4, National Eye Institute, Bethesda, MD, pp. 1–5.

Beck, R. W. (1988): The Optic Neuritis Treatment Trial. *Arch. Ophthalmol.,* 106:1051–1053.

Benedict, G. W. (1979): LRC Coronary Prevention Trial: Baltimore. *Clin. Pharmacol. Ther.,* 25:685–687.

Benfari, R. C., Eaker, E., McIntyre, K., and Paul, O. (1981): Risk factor screening and intervention. A psychological/behavioral cost or a benefit? *Controlled Clin. Trials,* 2:3–14.

Berry, H., Fernandes, L., Bloom, B., Molloy, M., Mace, B. E. W., et al. (1980): Expectation and patient preference—does it matter? *J. R. Soc. Med.,* 73:34–38.

Blankenhorn, D. H., Johnson, R. L., Nessim, S. A., Azen, S. P., Sanmarco, M. E., et al. (1987): The Cholesterol Lowering Atherosclerosis Study (CLAS): Design, methods, and baseline results. *Controlled Clin. Trials,* 8:354–387.

Borden, E. K., and Lee, J. G. (1982): A methodologic study of post-marketing drug evaluation using a pharmacy-based approach. *J. Chron. Dis.,* 35:803–816.

Borhani, N. O., Tonascia, J., Schlundt, D. G., Prineas, R. J., and Jefferys, J. L. (1989): Recruitment in the Hypertension Prevention Trial. *Controlled Clin. Trials,* 10(Suppl. 3):30S–39S.

Bradford, R. H. (1987): Participant recruitment to the Lipid Research Clinics Coronary Primary Prevention Trial. *Controlled Clin. Trials,* 8(Suppl. 4):31S–40S.

The Brain Resuscitation Clinical Trial II Study Group. (1991): A randomized clinical trial of calcium entry blocker administration to comatose survivors of cardiac arrest: Design, methods, and patient characteristics. *Controlled Clin. Trials,* 12:525–545.

Brauzer, B., and Goldstein, B. J. (1973): Symptomatic volunteers: Another dimension for clinical trials. *J. Clin. Pharmacol.,* 13:89–98.

Breckenridge, J. S., Zeiss, A. M., Breckenridge, J. N., Gallagher, D., and Thompson, L. W. (1985):

Solicitation of elderly depressives for treatment outcome research: A comparison of referral sources. *J. Consult. Clin. Psychol.*, 53:552–554.

Buchwald, H., Matts, J. P., Hansen, B. J., Long, J. M., Fitch, L. L., et al. (1987): Program on Surgical Control of the Hyperlipidemias (POSCH): Recruitment experience. *Controlled Clin. Trials*, 8(Suppl. 4):94S–104S.

Burns, P. A., Nochajski, T., Desotelle, P. C., and Pranikoff, K. (1990): Recruitment experiences in a stress incontinence clinical trial. *Neurourology and Urodynamics*, 9:53–62.

Byington, R. P., and the Beta-Blocker Heart Attack Trial Research Group. (1984): Beta-Blocker Heart Attack Trial: Design, methods, and baseline results. *Controlled Clin. Trials*, 5:382–437.

Calimlim, J. F., Wardell, W. M., Davis, H. T., Lasagna, L., and Gillies, A. J. (1977): Analgesic efficacy of an orally administered combination of pentazocine and aspirin. *Clin. Pharmacol. Ther.*, 21:34–43.

Calimlim, J. F., and Weintraub, M. (1981): Selection of patients participating in a clinical trial. In: *Statistics in the Pharmaceutical Industry.* Buncher, C. R., and Tsay, J. Y. (Eds.). pp. 107–138. Marcel Dekker, New York.

The Cardiac Arrhythmia Pilot Study (CAPS) Investigators. (1988): Recruitment and baseline description of patients in the Cardiac Arrhythmia Pilot Study. *Am. J. Cardiol.*, 61:704–713.

CASS Principal Investigators and Their Associates. (1983): Coronary Artery Surgery Study (CASS): A randomized trial of coronary artery bypass surgery: Survival data. *Circulation*, 68:939–950.

CASS Principal Investigators and Their Associates. (1984): Coronary Artery Surgery Study (CASS): A randomized trial of coronary artery bypass surgery: Comparability of entry characteristics and survival in randomized patients and nonrandomized patients meeting randomization criteria. *J. Am. Coll. Cardiol.*, 3:114–128.

Cassileth, B. R., Lusk, E. J., Miller, D. S., and Hurwitz, S. (1982): Attitudes toward clinical trials among patients and the public. *JAMA*, 248:968–970.

Chalmers, T. C. (1982): A potpourri of RCT topics. *Controlled Clin. Trials*, 3:285–298.

Chalmers, T. C., Celano, P., Sacks, H. S., and Smith, H. Jr. (1983): Bias in treatment assignment in controlled clinical trials. *N. Engl. J. Med.*, 309:1358–1361.

Charlson, M. E., and Horwitz, R. I. (1984): Applying results of randomized trials to clinical practice: Impact of losses before randomisation. *BMJ (London)*, 289:1281–1284.

Chlebowski, R. T., Blackburn, G. L., Nixon, D. W., Jochimsen, P., Scanlon, E. F., et al. (1989): Unpublished data summaries and the design and conduct of clinical trials. The Nutrition Adjuvant Study experience and commentary. *Controlled Clin. Trials*, 10:368–377.

Collet, J. P., Floret, D., Cochat, P., Gillet, J., Cogan-Collet, J., et al. (1991): Réunions collectives pour le recrutement des patients dans un essai thérapeutique en pédiatrie. *Therapie*, 46:139–142.

Collins, J. F., Bingham, S. F., Weiss, D. G., Williford, W. O., and Kuhn, R. M. (1980): Some adaptive strategies for inadequate sample acquisition in Veterans Administration Cooperative Clinical Trials. *Controlled Clin. Trials*, 1:227–248.

Collins, J. F., Williford, W. O., Weiss, D. G., Bingham, S. F., and Klett, C. J. (1984): Planning patient recruitment: Fantasy and reality. *Stat. Med.*, 3:435–443.

Covi, L., Lipman, R. S., McNair, D. M., and Czerlinsky, T. (1979): Symptomatic volunteers in multicenter drug trials. *Prog. Neuropsychopharmacol. Biol. Psychiatry*, 3:521–533.

Cramer, J. A., Collins, J. F., and Mattson, R. H. (1988): Can categorization of patient background problems be used to determine early termination in a clinical trial? *Controlled Clin. Trials*, 9:47–63.

Croft, J. B., Webber, L. S., Parker, F. C., and Berenson, G. S. (1984): Recruitment and participation of children in a long-term study of cardiovascular disease: The Bogalusa heart study, 1973–1982. *Am. J. Epidemiol.*, 120:436–448.

Croke, G. (1979): Recruitment for the National Cooperative Gallstone Study. *Clin. Pharmacol. Ther.*, 25:691–694.

Daugherty, S. A. (1983): Description of the enumerated and screened population. *Hypertension*, 5:IV-1–IV-43.

Detre, K., Hultgren, H., and Takaro, T. (1977): Veterans Administration Cooperative Study of surgery for coronary arterial occlusive disease: III. Methods and baseline characteristics, including experience with medical treatment. *Am. J. Cardiol.*, 40:212–225.

DeVries, B. M., Hughes, G. S. Jr., and Francom, S. F. (1989): Recruitment of volunteers for phase I and phase II drug development studies. *Drug Info. J.*, 23:699–703.

Deykin, D. (1991): Lessons learned from large-scale clinical trials. In: *Transactions of the American Clinical and Climatological Association*, 103rd annual meeting, October 1990, pp. 96–105.

Dicker, B. G., and Kent, D. L. (1990): Physician consent and researchers' access to patients. *Epidemiology*, 1:160–163.

Dunbar, J., and McKeown, M. B. (1982): Organization and management of recruitment. *Circulation*, 66(Suppl. 4):IV-49–IV-53.

Ederer, F. (1975): Practical problems in collaborative clinical trials. *Am. J. Epidemiol.*, 102:111–118.

Edlund, M. J., Craig, T. J., and Richardson, M. A. (1985): Informed consent as a form of volunteer bias. *Am. J. Psychiatry*, 142:624–627.

Facklam, D. P., Gardner, J. S., Neidert, G. L., and Westland, M. M. (1990): An epidemiologic post-marketing surveillance study of prescription acne medications. *Am. J. Public Health,* 80:50–53.

Fine, S. L. (1980): Macular Photocoagulation Study. *Arch. Ophthalmol.,* 98:832.

Fine, S. L. (1984): Clinical trials and the practice of ophthalmology. *Arch. Ophthalmol.,* 102:1282–1285.

Foley, J. F., and Moertel, C. G. (1991): Improving accrual into cancer clinical trials. *J. Cancer Education,* 6:165–173.

Ford, C. E., Langford, H. G., and Palmer, M. J. (1987): Recruitment in the Hypertension Detection and Follow-up Program. *Controlled Clin. Trials,* 8(Suppl. 4):54S–67S.

Ford, G. T., Wallace, E. L. (1975): Effects of donor recruitment methods on population responses. *Transfusion,* 15:159–164.

French, K., Porter, A. M. D., Robinson, S. E., McCallum, F. M., Howie, J. G. R., et al. (1982): At-tendance at a breast screening clinic: A problem of administration or attitudes. *BMJ (London),* 285:617–620.

Friedman, M. A. (1987): Patient accrual to clinical trials. *Cancer Treat. Rep.,* 71:557–558.

Ganz, P. A. (1990): Clinical trials: Concerns of the patient and the public. *Cancer,* 65(May 15 Suppl.):2394–2399.

Gaston, M., Smith, J., Gallagher, D., Flournoy-Gill, Z., West, S., et al. (1987): Recruitment in the Co-operative Study of Sickle Cell Disease (CSSCD). *Controlled Clin. Trials,* 8(Suppl. 4):131S–140S.

Gelber, R. D., and Goldhirsch, A. (1988): Can a clinical trial be the treatment of choice for patients with cancer? *J. Natl. Cancer Inst.,* 80:886–887.

Goldstein, S., Byington, R., and the BHAT Research Group. (1987): The Beta Blocker Heart Attack Trial: Recruitment experience. *Controlled Clin. Trials,* 8(Suppl. 4):79S–85S.

Gómez-Marín, O., Prineas, R. J., and Sinaiko, A. R. (1991): The sodium-potassium blood pressure trial in children: Design, recruitment, and randomization: The Children and Adolescent Blood Pressure Program. *Controlled Clin. Trials,* 12:408–423.

Greenlick, M. R., Bailey, J. W., Wild, J., and Grover, J. (1979): Characteristics of men most likely to respond to an invitation to be screened. *Am. J. Public Health,* 69:1011–1015.

Grufferman, S., Delzell, E., and Delong, E. R. (1984): An approach to conducting epidemiologic research within cooperative clinical trials groups. *J. Clin. Oncol.,* 2:670–675.

Hamilton, M. (1965): Computer programmes for the medical man: A solution. *BMJ (London),* 2:1048–1050.

Hellman, S. (1979): Editorial: Randomized clinical trials and the doctor–patient relationship: An ethical dilemma. *Cancer Clin. Trials,* 2:189–193.

Herson, J. (1980): Patient registration in a cooperative oncology group. *Controlled Clin. Trials,* 1:101–110.

Higby, D. J. (1990): Letter to Editor: Finder's fees for research subjects. *N. Engl. J. Med.,* 323:1710.

Hobbs, P., Kay, C., Friedman, E. H. I., St. Leger, A. S., Lambert, C., et al. (1990): Response by women aged 65–79 to invitation for screening for breast cancer by mammography: A pilot study. *BMJ (London),* 301:1314–1316.

Hsia, D. (1990): Letter to Editor: Finder's fees for research subjects. *N. Engl. J. Med.,* 323:1710–1711.

Hughes, G. H., Cutter, G., Donahue, R., Friedman, G. D., Hulley, S., et al. (1987): Recruitment in the Coronary Artery Disease Risk Development in Young Adults (CARDIA) Study. *Controlled Clin. Trials,* 8(Suppl. 4):68S–73S.

Hunninghake, D. B., Darby, C. A., and Probstfield, J. L. (1987): Recruitment experience in clinical trials: Literature summary and annotated bibliography. *Controlled Clin. Trials,* 8(Suppl. 4):6S–30S.

Hunninghake, D. B., Peterson, F., LaDouceur, M., Knoke, J., and Leon, A. (1982): Recruitment from clinical studies. *Circulation,* 66(Suppl. 4):IV-15–IV-19.

Hunter, C. P., Frelick, R. W., Feldman, A. R., Bavier, A. R., Dunlap, W. H., et al. (1987): Selection factors in clinical trials: Results from the Community Clinical Oncology Program Physician's Patient Log. *Cancer Treat. Rep.,* 71:559–565.

Hypertension Detection and Follow-up Program Cooperative Group (1977): Blood pressure studies in 14 communities: A two-stage screen for hypertension. *JAMA,* 237:2385–2391.

Jack, W. J. L., Chetty, U., and Rodger, A. (1990): Recruitment to a prospective breast conservation trial: Why are so few patients randomised? *BMJ (London),* 301:83–85.

Johnson, N., and Lilford, R. J. (1990): Computerized automation of clinical trials. *Baillieres Clin. Obstet. Gynaecol.,* 4:771–786.

Jonas, S. (1986): A proposed method for using a reimbursement moratorium to encourage recruitment for a randomized study of carotid endarterectomy. *Stroke,* 17:1335–1336.

Kass-Annese, B., Kennedy, K. I., Forrest, K., Danzer, H., Reading, A., et al. (1989): A study of the vaginal contraceptive sponge used with and without the fertility awareness method. *Contraception,* 40:701–714.

Katrušenko, A. G., and Šestov, D. B. (1981): Organizational methods used in an epidemiological study in Leningrad. *Bull. World Health Organ.,* 59:281–284.

Kaufmann, C. L. (1983): Informed consent and patient decision making: Two decades of research. *Soc. Sci. Med.*, 17:1657–1664.

Kaye, J. M., Lawton, P., and Kaye, D. (1990): Attitudes of elderly people about clinical research on aging. *The Gerontologist*, 30:100–106.

Kemp, N., Skinner, E., and Toms, J. (1984): Randomized clinical trials of cancer treatment—a public opinion survey. *J. Clin. Oncol.*, 10:155–161.

Kirkpatrick, M. A. F. (1991): Factors that motivate healthy adults to participate in phase I drug trials. *Drug Info. J.*, 25:109–113.

Kirscht, J. P., Haefner, D. P., and Eveland, J. D. (1975): Public response to various written appeals to participate in health screening. *Public Health Rep.*, 90:539–543.

Knatterud, G. L., and Forman, S. A. (1987): Patient recruitment experience in the Thrombolysis in Myocardial Infarction Trial. *Controlled Clin. Trials*, 8(Suppl. 4):86S–93S.

Koenig, H. G., Goli, V., Shelp, F., Kudler, H. S., Cohen, H. J., et al. (1989): Antidepressant use in elderly medical inpatients: Lessons from an attempted clinical trial. *J. Gen. Intern. Med.*, 4:498–505.

Krischer, J. P., Hurley, C., Pillalamarri, M., Pant, S., Bleichfeld, C., et al. (1991): An automated patient registration and treatment randomization system for multicenter clinical trials. *Controlled Clin. Trials*, 12:367–377.

Krupnick, J., Shea, T., and Elkin, I. (1986): Generalizability of treatment studies utilizing solicited patients. *J. Consult. Clin. Psychol.*, 54:68–78.

Langley, G. R., Sutherland, H. J., Wong, S., Minkin, S., and Llewellyn-Thomas, H. A., et al. (1987): Why are (or are not) patients given the option to enter clinical trials? *Controlled Clin. Trials*, 8:49–59.

LaRue, L. J., Alter, M., Traven, N. D., Sterman, A. B., Sobel, E., et al. (1988): Acute stroke therapy trials: Problems in patient accrual. *Stroke*, 19:950–954.

Lasagna, L. (1979): Problems in publication of clinical trial methodology. *Clin. Pharmacol. Ther.*, 25:751–753.

Leader, M. A., and Neuwirth, E. (1978): Clinical research and the noninstitutional elderly: A model for subject recruitment. *J. Am. Geriatr. Soc.*, 26:27–31.

Lee, J. Y., and Breaux, S. R. (1983): Accrual of radiotherapy patients to clinical trials. *Cancer*, 52:1014–1016.

Lee, J. Y., Marks, J. E., and Simpson, J. R. (1980): Recruitment of patients to cooperative group clinical trials. *Cancer Clin. Trials*, 3:381–384.

Levenkron, J. C., and Farquhar, J. W. (1982): Recruitment using mass media strategies. *Circulation*, 66(Suppl. 4):IV-32–IV-36.

Levine, R. J. (1986): *Ethics and regulation of clinical research*, second edition. Urban & Schwarzenberg, Baltimore.

Lind, S. E. (1990): Finder's fees for research subjects. *N. Engl. J. Med.*, 323:192–195.

The Lipid Research Clinics Program (1983): Participant recruitment to the Coronary Primary Prevention Trials. *J. Chron. Dis.*, 36:451–465.

Lipsitz, L. A., Pluchino, F. C., and Wright, S. M. (1987): Biomedical research in the nursing home: Methodological issues and subject recruitment results. *J. Am. Geriatr. Soc.*, 35:629–634.

Little, J. A. (1982): Recruitment from medical referrals and clinical laboratories. *Circulation*, 66(Suppl. 4):IV-36–IV-40.

Llewellyn-Thomas, H. A., McGreal, M. J., Thiel, E. C., Fine, S., and Erlichman, C. (1991): Patients' willingness to enter clinical trials: Measuring the association with perceived benefit and preference for decision participation. *Soc. Sci. Med.*, 32:35–42.

Lucas, M. G., Mitchell, A., and Lee, E. C. G. (1984): Failure to enter patients to randomised study of surgery for breast cancer. *Lancet*, 2:921–922.

Lumley, J., Lester, A., Renou, P., and Wood, C. (1985): A failed RCT to determine the best method of delivery for very low birth weight infants. *Controlled Clin. Trials*, 6:120–127.

Macintyre, I. M. (1991): Tribulations for clinical trials: Poor recruitment is hampering research. *BMJ (London)*, 302:1099–1100.

Mackillop, W. J., and Johnston, P. A. (1986): Ethical problems in clinical research: The need for empirical studies of the clinical trials process. *J. Chron. Dis.*, 39:177–188.

Macrae, F. A., Mackay, I. R., and Fraser, R. E. (1989): Participation of healthy volunteers in research projects. *Med. J. Aust.*, 150:325–328.

Macular Photocoagulation Study. (1984a): Age-related macular degeneration. *Am. J. Ophthalmol.*, 98:376–377.

Macular Photocoagulation Study Group. (1984b): Changing the protocol: A case report from the macular photocoagulation study. *Controlled Clin. Trials*, 5:203–216.

Marshall, G. D. (1982): Overview of recruitment to the Coronary Primary Prevention Trial. *Circulation*, 66(Suppl. 4):IV-5–IV-9.

Martin, J. F., Henderson, W. G., Zacharski, L. R., Rickles, F. R., Forman, W. B., et al. (1984): Accrual of patients into a multihospital cancer clinical trial and its implications on planning future studies. *Am. J. Clin. Oncol.*, 7:173–182.

Mattson, M. E., Curb, J. D., McArdle, R., and the AMIS and BHAT Research Groups (1985): Participation in a clinical trial: The patients' point of view. *Controlled Clin. Trials,* 6:156–167.

Mattson, R. H., Cramer, J. A., Collins, J. F., et al. (1985): Comparison of carbamazepine, phenobarbital, phenytoin, and primidone in partial and secondarily generalized tonic-clonic seizures. *New England J. of Med.,* 313:145–151.

Mattson, R. H., Cramer, J. A., Collins, J. F., McCutchen, C. B., Mamdani, M. B., et al. (1992): Valproate for treatment of partial and secondarily generalized tonic-clonic seizures in adults: A comparison with carbamazepine for efficacy and adverse effects. *N. Engl. J. Med.,* In Press.

McCusker, J., Wax, A., and Bennett, J. M. (1982): Cancer patient accessions into clinical trials: A pilot investigation into some patient and physician determinants of entry. *Am. J. Clin. Oncol.,* 5:227–236.

McDearmon, M., and Bradford, R. H. (1982): Recruitment by the use of mass mailings. *Circulation,* 66(Suppl. 4):IV-27–IV-31.

McKeown, M. B. (1982): Occupational screenings: Recruitment of government employees. *Circulation,* 66(Suppl. 4):IV-43–IV-46.

McTiernan, A., Weiss, N. S., and Daling, J. R. (1986): Bias resulting from using the card-back system to contact patients in an epidemiologic study. *Am. J. Public Health,* 76:71–73.

Melish, J. S. (1982): Recruitment by community screenings. *Circulation,* 66(Suppl. 4):IV-20–IV-23.

The MIAMI Trial Research Group. (1985): Patient population. *Am. J. Cardiol.,* 56:10G–14G.

MILIS Study Group. (1986): Hyaluronidase therapy for acute myocardial infarction: Results of a randomized, blinded, multicenter trial. *Am. J. Cardiol.,* 57:1236–1243.

Mitchell, H., Hirst, S., Cockburn, J., Reading, D. J., Staples, M. P., et al. (1991): Cervical cancer screening: A comparison of recruitment strategies among older women. *Med. J. Aust.,* 155:79–82.

Mitchell, J. E., Pyle, R., Eckert, E., Pomeroy, C., and Hatsukami, D. (1988): Patients versus symptomatic volunteers in bulimia nervosa research. *International Journal of Eating Disorders,* 7:837–843.

Morgan, J. P., Wardell, W. M., Weintraub, M., Mazzullo, J. M., and Lasagna, L. (1974): Clinical trials and tribulations. *Arch. Intern. Med.,* 134:380–383.

Moussa, M. A. A. (1984): Planning a clinical trial with allowance for cost and patient recruitment rate. *Computer Programs in Biomedicine,* 18:173–180.

Mullin, S. M., Warwick, S., Akers, M., Beecher, P., Helminger, K., et al.. (1984): An acute intervention trial: The research nurse coordinator's role. *Controlled Clin. Trials,* 5:141–156.

Neaton, J. D., Grimm, R. H. Jr., and Cutler, J. A. (1987): Recruitment of participants for the Multiple Risk Factor Intervention Trial (MRFIT). *Controlled Clin. Trials,* 8(Suppl. 4):41S–53S.

Newcomb, P. A., Love, R. R., Phillips, J. L., and Buckmaster, B. J. (1990): Using a population-based cancer registry for recruitment in a pilot cancer control study. *Prev. Med.,* 19:61–65.

O'Fallon, W. M., Rings, L., Gonzalez, R., Burnett, J., Golda, C., et al. (1987): Natural history study of congenital heart defects. *Controlled Clin. Trials,* 8(Suppl. 4):115S–120S.

Ogilvie, J. T., Mishkel, N. R., Mishkel, M. A., Welch, V. E., Insull, W. Jr., et al. (1982): Occupational screenings: Recruitment from private industry. *Circulation,* 66(Suppl. 4):IV-40–IV-43.

O'Hara, N. M., Brink, S., Harvey, C., Harrist, R., Green, B., et al. (1991): Recruitment strategies for school health promotion research. *Health Educ. Res.,* 6:363–371.

Orden, S. R., Dyer, A. R., and Liu, K. (1990): Recruiting young adults in an urban setting: The Chicago CARDIA experience. *Am. J. Prev. Med.,* 6:176–182.

Parkinson Study Group. (1989): DATATOP: A multicenter controlled clinical trial in early Parkinson's disease. *Arch. Neurol.,* 46:1052–1060.

Paskett, E. D., White, E., Carter, W. B., and Chu, J. (1990): Improving follow-up after an abnormal pap smear: A randomized controlled trial. *Prev. Med.,* 19:630–641.

Penman, D. T., Holland, J. C., Bahna, G. F., Morrow, G., Schmale, A. H., et al. (1984): Informed consent for investigational chemotherapy: Patients' and physicians' perceptions. *J. Clin. Oncol.,* 2:849–855.

Petrovitch, H., Byington, R., Bailey, G., Borhani, P., Carmody, S., et al. (1991): Systolic Hypertension in the Elderly Program (SHEP): Part 2: Screening and recruitment. *Hypertension,* 17(Suppl. 3):II-16–II-23.

Pocock, S. J. (1978): Size of cancer clinical trials and stopping rules. *Br. J. Cancer,* 38:757–766.

Probstfield, J. L., Wittes, J. T., and Hunninghake, D. B. (1987): Recruitment in NHLBI population-based studies and randomized clinical trials: Data analysis and survey results. *Controlled Clin. Trials,* 8:141S–149S.

Prout, T. E. (1979): Patient recruitment: Problems and solutions. *Clin. Pharmacol. Ther.,* 25(5 part 2, Suppl.):679–680.

Prout, T. E. (1981): Patient recruitment techniques in clinical trials. *Controlled Clin. Trials,* 1:313–318.

Quick, A. M., Khaw, P. T., and Elkington, A. R. (1989): Problems encountered in recruiting patients to an ophthalmic drug trial. *Br. J. Ophthalmol.,* 73:432–434.

Rowlands, M. W. D. (1987): Recruitment to inpatient trials of antidepressants. *Lancet,* 1:451–452.

Royce, W. S., and Arkowitz, H. (1977): Clarification of some issues concerning subject recruitment procedures in therapy analog studies. *Behavior Therapy,* 8:64–69.

Rude, R. E., Poole, W. K., Muller, J. E., Turi, Z., Rutherford, J., et al. (1983): Electrocardiographic and clinical criteria for recognition of acute myocardial infarction based on analysis of 3,697 patients. *Am. J. Cardiol.*, 52:936–942.

Sanders, T. A. B., Woolfe, R., and Rantzen, E. (1990): Controlled evaluation of slimming diets: Use of television for recruitment. *Lancet*, 336:918–920.

Saurbrey, N., Jensen, J., Rasmussen, P. E., Gjørup, T., Guldager, H., and Riis, P. (1984): Danish patients' attitudes to scientific-ethical questions. *Acta. Med. Scand.*, 215:99–104.

Schafer, A. (1982): The ethics of the randomized clinical trial. *N. Engl. J. Med.*, 307:719–724.

Schoenberger, J. A. (1979): Recruitment in the Coronary Drug Project and the Aspirin Myocardial Infarction Study. *Clin. Pharmacol. Ther.*, 25:681–684.

Schoenberger, J. A. (1987): Recruitment experience in the Aspirin Myocardial Infarction Study. *Controlled Clin. Trials*, 8(Suppl. 4):74S–78S.

Schröder, R. (1989): Flunarizine i.v. after cardiac arrest (Fluna-study): Study design and organisational aspects of a double blind, placebo-controlled randomized study. *Resuscitation*, 17(Suppl.):S121–S127.

Schrott, H. G., and Merideth, N. (1982): Recruitment by screening entire communities: The Iowa Lipid Research Clinic experience. *Circulation*, 66(Suppl. 4):IV-23–IV-26.

Sclar, D. A., Chin, A., Skaer, T. L., Okamoto, M. P., Nakahiro, R. K., et al. (1991): Effect of health education in promoting prescription refill compliance among patients with hypertension. *Clin. Ther.*, 13:489–495.

Shimm, D. S., and Spece, R. G. Jr. (1991): Industry reimbursement for entering patients into clinical trials: Legal and ethical issues. *Ann. Intern. Med.*, 115:148–151.

Shtasel, D. L., Gur, R. E., Mozley, P. D., Richards, J., Taleff, M. M., et al. (1991): Volunteers for biomedical research: Recruitment and screening of normal controls. *Arch. Gen. Psychiatry*, 48:1022–1025.

Silagy, C. A., Campion, K., McNeil, J. J., Worsam, B., Donnan, G. A., et al. (1991): Comparison of recruitment strategies for a large-scale clinical trial in the elderly. *J. Clin. Epidemiol.*, 44:1105–1114.

Smith, W. M., Vogt, T. M., Ireland, C. C., and Black, D. (1985): Resources in geriatric drug research. *Drug Info. J.*, 19:421–427.

Spilker, B. (1991): *Guide to clinical trials*. Raven Press, New York.

Stahl, S. M., Lawrie, T., Neill, P., and Kelley, C. (1977): Motivational interventions in community hypertension screening. *Am. J. Public Health*, 67:345–352.

Stern, M. P. (1982): Recruitment of participants from blood banks. *Circulation*, 66(Suppl. 4):IV-10–IV-15.

Strull, W. M., Lo, B., and Charles, G. (1984): Do patients want to participate in medical decision making? *JAMA*, 252:2990–2994.

Svensson, C. K. (1989): Representation of American blacks in clinical trials of new drugs. *JAMA*, 261:263–265.

Swinehart, J. M. (1991): Patient recruitment and enrollment into clinical trials: A discussion of specific methods and disease states. *J. Clin. Res. Pharmacoepidemiol.*, 5:35–47.

Sylvester, R. J., Pinedo, H. M., DePauw, M., Staquet, M. J., Buyse, M. E., et al. (1981): Quality of institutional participation in multicenter clinical trials. *N. Engl. J. Med.*, 305:852–855.

Taplin, D., Porcelain, S. L., Meinking, T. L., Athey, R. L., Chen, J. A., et al. (1991): Community control of scabies: A model based on use of permethrin cream. *Lancet*, 337:1016–1018.

Taylor, K. M., Margolese, R. G., and Soskolne, C. L. (1984): Physicians' reasons for not entering eligible patients in a randomized clinical trial of surgery for breast cancer. *N. Engl. J. Med.*, 310:1363–1367.

Tielsch, J. M., Sommer, A., Katz, J., Royall, R. M., Quigley, H. A., et al. (1991): Racial variations in the prevalence of primary open-angle glaucoma: The Baltimore Eye Survey. *JAMA*, 266:369–374.

Tiller, J. W. G., and Biddle, N. (1991): Obtaining outpatient referrals for clinical research. *Aust. N.Z. J. Psychiatry*, 25:132–133.

Toronto Leukemia Study Group. (1986): Results of chemotherapy for unselected patients with acute myeloblastic leukaemia: Effect of exclusions on interpretation of results. *Lancet*, 1:786–788.

Vestal, R. E. (1985): Methodological considerations for geriatric drug testing (phase 1 and 2 trials). *Drug Info. J.*, 19:435–445.

Vogt, T. M., Ireland, C. C., Black, D., Camel, G., and Hughes, G. (1986): Recruitment of elderly volunteers for a multicenter clinical trial: The SHEP pilot study. *Controlled Clin. Trials*, 7:118–133.

Waite, J., Grundy, E., and Arie, T. (1986): A controlled trial of antidepressant medication in elderly inpatients. *Int. Clin. Psychopharmacol.*, 1:113–126.

Waksberg, J. (1978): Sampling methods for random digit dialing. *J. Am. Stat. A.*, 73:40–46.

Weintraub, J., Leske, G. S., Ripa, L. W., and Levinson, A. (1980): Recruitment of a clinical field trial population: Reasons for nonparticipation. *J. Public Health Dent.*, 40:141–145.

Wilber, J. A., Millward, D., Baldwin, A., Capron, B., Silverman, D., et al. (1972): Atlanta community high blood pressure program methods of community hypertension screening. *Circ. Res.*, 30,31(Suppl. 2):101–109.

Wilhelmsen, L., Ljungberg, S., Wedel, H., and Werkö, L. (1976): A comparison between participants and non-participants in a primary preventive trial. *J. Chronic Dis.*, 29:331–339.

Williams, G. W., Snedecor, S. M., DeMets, D. L., and the NOTT Research Group. (1987): Recruitment experience in the Nocturnal Oxygen Therapy Trial. *Controlled Clin. Trials,* 8(Suppl. 4):121S–130S.

Williams, R. R., and Hunt, S. C. (1987): Recruitment of members of high-risk Utah pedigrees. *Controlled Clin. Trials,* 8:105S–114S.

Williford, W. O., Bingham, S. F., Weiss, D. G., Collins, J. F., Rains, K. T., and Krol, W. F. (1987): The "constant intake rate" assumption in interim recruitment goal methodology for multicenter clinical trials. *J. Chron. Dis.,* 40:297–307.

Wittes, R. E., and Friedman, M. A. (1988): Accrual to clinical trials. *J. Natl. Cancer Inst.,* 80:884–885.

Wood, T. A. (1989): The cost to patients of participating in clinical trials. *JAMA,* 261:1150–1151.

World Health Organization European Collaborative Group. (1980): Multifactorial trial in the prevention of coronary heart disease: 1. Recruitment and initial findings. *Eur. Heart J.,* 1:73–80.

Yu, L. C., Rohner, T. J., Kaltreider, D. L., Hu, TW., Igou, J. F., and Dennis, P. J. (1990): Profile of urinary incontinent elderly in long-term care institutions. *J. Am. Geriatr. Soc.,* 38:433–439.

Yusuf, S., Held, P., Teo, K. K., and Toretsky, E. R. (1990): Selection of patients for randomized controlled trials: Implications of wide or narrow eligibility criteria. *Stat. Med.,* 9:73–83.

Zifferblatt, S. M. (1976): Recruitment in large-scale clinical trials. In: *Proceedings of the National Heart and Lung Institute Working Conference on Health Behavior,* Weiss, S. M. (Ed.). pp. 187–195. DHEW publication no. 76-868.

Zimmer, A. W., Calkins, E., Hadley, E., Ostfeld, A. M., Kaye, J. M., and Kaye, D. (1985): Conducting clinical research in geriatric populations. *Ann. Intern. Med.,* 103:276–283.

Subject Index

Author Index